Caring for the
Older Adult

Caring for the Older Adult

A HEALTH PROMOTION PERSPECTIVE

Patricia A. O'Neill, RN, MSN, CCRN
Nursing Instructor
De Anza College
Cupertino, California

W.B. SAUNDERS COMPANY
A Harcourt Health Sciences Company
Philadelphia London New York St Louis Sydney Toronto

W.B. SAUNDERS COMPANY
A Harcourt Health Sciences Company

The Curtis Center
Independence Square West
Philadelphia, Pennsylvania 19106

Library of Congress Cataloging-in-Publication Data

O'Neill, Patricia.
Caring for the older adult: a health promotion perspective/
Patricia A. O'Neill.—1st ed.

p. cm.

Includes index.

ISBN 0–7216–8334–7

1. Aged—Health and hygiene. 2. Aged—Medical care.
   3. Health promotion. 4. Preventive health services for the aged.
   I. Title.

RA564.8.O54 2002   613′.0438—dc21   2001041119

NOTICE

Nursing is an ever-changing field. Standard safety precautions must be followed, but as new research and clinical experience broaden our knowledge, changes in treatment and drug therapy may become necessary or appropriate. Readers are advised to check the most current product information provided by the manufacturer of each drug to be administered to verify the recommended dose, the method and duration of administration, and the contraindications. It is the responsibility of the treating licensed prescriber, relying on experience and knowledge of the patient, to determine dosages and the best treatment for each individual patient. Neither the publisher nor the editor assumes any liability for any injury and/or damage to persons or property arising from this publication.

THE PUBLISHER

Vice President and Publishing Director, Nursing: Sally Schrefer
Senior Acquisitions Editor: Terri Wood
Senior Developmental Editor: Robin Levin Richman
Project Manager: Agnes Hunt Byrne
Production Manager: Peter Faber
Illustration Specialist: Lisa Lambert
Book Designer: Marie Gardocky Clifton

CARING FOR THE OLDER ADULT: A Health Promotion Perspective   ISBN 0–7216–8334–7

Printed in the United States of America.

Last digit is the print number: 9   8   7   6   5   4   3   2   1

To Tom and Audree O'Neill,
the most wonderful parents anyone could hope for

To Cerys Patricia Williams,
may you live a long and happy life

and

To Colin,
my husband, my inspiration, my soulmate

Contributors

Signe S. Hill, MA, BSN, RN
  Formerly Instructor, Practical Nurse Program
  Northeast Wisconsin Technical College
  Green Bay, Wisconsin
Promoting Psychosocial Health and Wellness; Leadership Role
of the LPN/LVN

Helen Stephens Howlett, MS, BSN, RN
  Formerly Instructor, Practical Nurse Program
  Northeast Wisconsin Technical College
  Green Bay, Wisconsin
Promoting Psychosocial Health and Wellness; Leadership Role
of the LPN/LVN

Mary Ann Matteson, PhD, RN, CNS, FAAN
  Professor Emerita
  The University of Texas Health Science Center at
  San Antonio School of Nursing
  San Antonio, Texas
Protecting the Vulnerable Older Adult; End-of-Life Care

Reviewers

Brenda E. Booth, MSEd, RN, C
Riverside School of Practical Nursing
Newport News, Virginia

Reitha Cabaniss, MSN, RN
Bevill State Community College
Walker College Campus
Jasper, Alabama

Marilyn Fisher, ADN, RN
Northwest Technical Institute
Springdale, Arkansas

Lillian Goodman, MEd, MA, RN
Los Angeles Unified School District
UCLA Education Extension
Los Angeles, California

Karen Kathryn Haagensen, RN, C
Howard College at San Angelo
San Angelo, Texas

Nancy B. Henry, MSN, RN
Delaware Technical and Community College
Georgetown, Delaware

Phyllis Sue Ramey Howard, BSN, RN
Ashland Technical College
Ashland, Kentucky

Donna Leach Kane, BS, RN
Louisiana Technical College
South Louisiana Campus
Houma, Louisiana

Janice Marie Kilgallon, MSN, RN, C, CNS
Passaic County Technical Institute
Wayne, New Jersey

Patricia Laing-Arie, BSEd, RN
Meridian Technology Center
Stillwater, Oklahoma

Valerie Leek, MS, RN, CS
Cumberland County Technical Education Center
Bridgeton, New Jersey
Cumberland County College
Vineland, New Jersey

Mary Jane Lofton, MA, BS, RN
Belmont Technical College
St. Clairsville, Ohio

Patricia McCormick, MA, RN
Central Lakes College
Brainerd, Minnesota

Janet Tompkins McMahon, MSN, RN
Pennsylvania College of Technology
Williamsport, Pennsylvania

Theresa Mendoza Mostasisa, PhN, MS, BSN, RN
City College of San Francisco
San Francisco, California

Sharon Powell-Laney, MSN, RN, CCRN
Indiana County Area Vocational Technical School
Indiana, Pennsylvania

Barbara Scattergood, BSN, RN
Upper Bucks Vocational Technical School
Perkasie, Pennsylvania

Julie A. Slack, MS, RN, ICCE
Dixie State College
St. George, Utah

Donna Welty Stoner, BSN, RN
Amarillo College
Amarillo, Texas

Delores N. Thompson, MSN, RN
Amarillo College
Amarillo, Texas

Mary Collins Wright, BA, RN
Vermont Technical College
Colchester, Vermont

Preface

Licensed practical nurses/vocational nurses are integral providers of nursing care for the older adult in acute, subacute, and long-term care settings, often assuming leadership roles. *Caring for the Older Adult: A Health Promotion Perspective* serves as a guide to basic bedside care of the gerontological client from a health promotion perspective and teaches students beginning management skills. The lively, engaging writing style presents basic information written specifically for the LPN/LVN student.

ORGANIZATION

Unit I: The Nursing Role in Care of the Older Adult

The concept of health promotion is introduced and interwoven throughout the text. *Healthy People 2010 Objectives* are first presented in Unit I, then given special emphasis in Unit II. Chapter 1 presents introductory information about gerontological nursing including demographics, theories of aging, and the role of the interdisciplinary team. Cultural views of aging and complementary and integrative therapies (including herbal remedies) are explored in Chapter 2. Chapter 3 addresses maintaining safe care environments for the older adult in the acute, subacute, long-term, and home-care settings. Pharmacology, including detailed information on alterations in pharmacokinetics and pharmacodynamics with age, and medication safety strategies are examined. Step-by-step assessment of the older adult is discussed in detail and the concept of atypical presentation of illness is explained. The risk for falls is discussed, along with interventions for reduction of this risk. Chapter 4 addresses self-care management of chronic illness, with an emphasis on healthy lifestyle habits.

Unit II: Promotion of Physical Health for the Older Adult

The core of the book, this unit addresses certain physical requirements for the healthy older adult, such as oxygenation (Chapter 9). Chapters are organized consistently beginning with a Case Study (where appropriate), then Age-Related Changes, Assessment, and Disorders Common to the Older Adult in the area of focus. The nursing process follows, with Nursing Diagnoses, Collaborating on the Plan of Care, Implementing Interventions for Health Promotion, and Gathering Data for Evaluation. The strength of the organization is that while each disorder in the chapter is discussed separately, care planning is addressed for chapter disorders together, thus encouraging the student to think conceptually. Of course, similarities and differences in appropriate nursing interventions among and between the various disorders are emphasized. Health promotion is used as the basis for discussing nursing interventions, which are discussed in the following order:

- promote health education
- promote lifestyle modification
- promote mobility
- promote nutrition
- promote rest and sleep

Unit III: Promotion of Psychosocial Health for the Older Adult

Chapter 12, "Promoting Psychosocial Health and Wellness," discusses emotional well-being, characteristics of centenarians, and the importance of family. Threats to psychosocial wellness and the nursing role in promoting wellness are examined, and a variety of nursing interventions are discussed.

Unit IV: Special Challenges in Care of the Older Adult

Nursing care to protect vulnerable older adults is discussed and ethical principles are defined and applied to case studies in Chapter 13. Restraint use is explored in detail, including types of restraints, hazards associated with use, and alternatives to restraint. Assessment and intervention for abuse are also discussed. Chapter 14 examines end-of-life care, including quality-of-life issues, pain and symptom management, advance directives, palliative care, and hospice. The process of dying, including its impact on client and family, is addressed.

Unit V: Management Skills in Care of the Older Adult

Chapter 15 explores leadership and management styles for the LPN/LVN. The concepts of delegation, assignment, and the expanded role of the LPN/LVN are examined in detail. Physical and psychosocial management activities are discussed and differentiated.

SPECIAL FEATURES

Chapter Opening Features

Each chapter contains numerous features designed to enhance learning. Each chapter begins with the following:

- **Objectives** and a **Chapter Outline** are clearly stated and give structure to and goals for the chapter content.
- **Key Terms** are defined in the Glossary at the end of the book.
- **Case Study** (selected chapters) is a brief client case history.

A wide variety of tables and other boxed material are distributed throughout most chapters.

Tips

Uniquely informative, "Tips" are brief, eye-catching, easily identified boxed features.

 Health Promotion Tip. Current health promotion and healthy lifestyle topics, for example, prevention of cataract development (see p. 187).

 Nutrition Tip. Information on good nutrition specific to the needs of the older adult, for example, antioxidants found in foods containing beta-carotene (see p. 140).

 Medication Safety Tip. Critical information on the safe administration and use of medications by older adults, including warnings about drug interactions and possible allergic reactions to medications, for example, medications that increase fall risk (see p. 48).

Signs and Symptoms Tip. Specific atypical signs and symptoms of disorders are discussed, for example, the symptom of confusion might be a sign of treatable disorders such as pneumonia or urinary tract infections (see p. 199).

Chapter Ending Features

Each chapter concludes with the following:

- **Summary** in a bulleted-list format
- **Study Questions** that include **Multiple-Choice Review** and **Critical Thinking** problems designed to stimulate further discussion. Answers to the Multiple-Choice Review questions are found on the inside back cover of the book.
- **Resources** list both Internet sites and organizations related to the chapter content.
- **Selected References** provide a current bibliography for students interested in further information about the chapter topic.

Appendices and Glossary

Appendix A provides a compilation of numerous assessment tools that will make this a truly practical textbook for student use. They include the Mini-Mental State Examination, Minimum Data Set, Stroke Risk Screening, Braden Scale for Predicting Pressure Sore Risk, and Determine Your Nutritional Health. Appendices B and C are Sample Advance Directives and Laboratory Value Alterations with Aging. A Glossary of all the Key Terms is provided.

ANCILLARIES

Supplemental materials include an **Instructor's Manual** with a test bank of multiple-choice, NCLEX-style questions with answers and rationales provided. The Instructor's Manual is free to adopters of the text.

PATRICIA A. O'NEILL

Acknowledgments

This book would never have taken form if not for the dedicated efforts of an enthusiastic, young editor named Terri Wood. Terri recruited me for this project and provided guidance and support, but more importantly, she inspired and motivated me to work more than I ever thought possible. One early statement made by Terri, which turned out to be prophetic, was to liken the writing of a book to having a baby: it begins with dreaming about the name and how it will look; later phases seem to last forever; and the finale consists of the "push" to production. Somewhere in the middle of writing this book I *did* have a baby, and I can attest to the similarities described. Thank you, Terri, for motivating me to finish the book and bringing in outstanding contributors to help do the job.

I would also like to thank Robin Richman, Senior Developmental Editor, and Cathy Ott, Senior Editorial Assistant, for their diligence, patience, and unending support throughout the process, and Helen Howlett, Signe Hill, and Mary Ann Matteson for their excellent contributions.

I would like to thank my former nursing instructors, Rita Cheek, Jack Weinberg, and Willie Rose of Montana State University for giving me the foundation and confidence to pursue graduate work, and Ginger Carreri for her excellent guidance at the University of California, San Francisco. I would also like to thank my LVN nursing students, De Anza College class of 2001, who inspire me to be a better nurse. I would like to acknowledge the nurses in my family: my mom, Audree, and my sisters, Mary and Sandy. You would have turned 50 today, Sandy, and I still miss you every single day of my life. I would also like to thank the former residents and staff of the Crest Nursing Home in Butte, Montana, for taking a chance 20 years ago by hiring a young girl to be a nursing assistant and making her fall in love with caring for older adults.

Thank you, Colin, for your unending love, support, and encouragement. Thank you Colin, Rena, Mom, Dad, and Mum, for your help and extra diaper duty. Cerys, my little Pooh Bear sleeping on my lap while I type this, Mommy can go play now!

PATRICIA A. O'NEILL
29 APRIL 2001

Contents

APPENDICES

Answers to the Multiple-Choice Review Questions are on the inside back cover.

I

The Nursing Role in Care of the Older Adult

Introduction to Health Promotion for the Older Adult

After completing this chapter, you will be able to:

- Examine your own attitudes toward aging.
- State the two broad goals of *Healthy People 2010*.
- Trace the development of gerontological nursing as a specialty.
- Identify three important federal laws that affect the nursing care of the older adult.
- Discuss the demographics of older adults.
- Refute misconceptions and stereotypes of aging.
- Discuss the major theories of aging.
- Describe the role of the interdisciplinary team in care of the older adult.

CHAPTER OUTLINE

Biological Theories of Aging
Psychosocial Theories of Aging
Relevance to Nursing Practice

CARE OF THE OLDER ADULT
THROUGH AN INTERDISCIPLINARY
TEAM APPROACH

KEY TERMS

Acute care

Ageism

Centenarians

Diagnosis-related groups

Gerontological nursing

Health promotion

Illness-wellness continuum

Interdisciplinary team

Long-term care

Medicare

Prospective payment

Subacute care

Wellness

People are living longer than ever before. Thanks, in part, to eradication of diseases, healthy living habits, and technological advances, most people can expect to live another 18 years beyond their 65th birthday (Strumpf, 2000) (Fig. 1–1).

Gerontological nursing has been around as long as there have been older people in need of care, although it has officially been recognized as a specialty only since 1966. There has been a recent explosive growth in the study of older people, as Baby Boomers approach their golden years. Think about it: how many television commercials have you seen advertising products for hair loss and bladder control, vitamin supplements, and nutritional products designed for older people? You have only to look around to see the focus of our society.

Fortunately, society is becoming more sensitive to the needs of older adults. Buildings are better designed for easy access, reading materials are available in large print, numerous books are available on cassette; people can even get groceries delivered to their homes. Of course, much work remains to be done in this area, and nurses are in a key position to ensure that society continues to support health promotion for older adults.

As a student you may be thinking, Why do I need to study gerontology? Almost every area of nursing, whether **acute care, subacute care, long-term care,** or home care, specializes in caring for older adults. Most available nursing positions involve care of the older adult. The

information included in this book will serve you well in your nursing career and will provide a valuable basis for further learning.

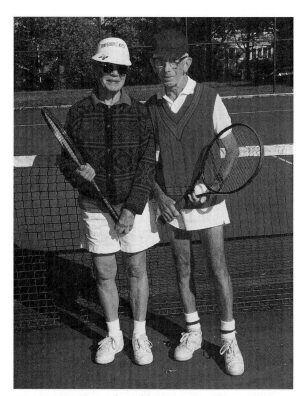

Figure 1–1. Examples of high-level wellness: The man is 85 years old; the woman is 78. (From Leahy, J. M., & Kizilay, E. [1998]. *Foundations of Nursing Practice.* Philadelphia: W. B. Saunders, p. 84.)

WHY HEALTH PROMOTION?

This book looks at the older adult through the focus of **health promotion**. Aging is not a disease, but rather, a unique life stage with its own rewards and issues. Health promotion is as important for the older adult as it is for all adults. By engaging in healthy habits, such as exercise, proper nutrition, and disease risk factor modification, one can hope to slow down the aging process and enhance the quality of the remaining years of life.

In 1979, the Surgeon General published a report, *Healthy People*, which led to a national health promotion and disease prevention initiative. *Healthy People 2000* followed in the 1990s, and was monitored by the U.S. Department of Health and Human Services. The current initiative, *Healthy People 2010*, is underway; it offers two broad health goals for all age groups to be met by the year 2010:

- Increase quality and years of healthy life
- Eliminate health disparities

There are 28 focus areas in *Healthy People 2010* along with 467 specific objectives. A sampling of some of the objectives can be found in Box 1–1.

Healthy People 2010 has served as the basis for the development of state and community plans with the goal of health promotion. Most states have built on the national objectives, tailoring them to their specific needs. Health-promoting behaviors can lead to valuable benefits such as prevention of falls, reduction in diseases such as heart disease and osteoporosis, and improvement in the length and quality of life. Throughout this book, health promotion information is easily identified by the symbol.

As a nurse, you will have a profound influence on the behaviors of the older adults you care for, probably a far greater influence than you can imagine. Toward this end, role modeling healthy behaviors is more effective than simply teaching them. In other words, it is not just what you say, but also how you behave that will be noticed by your patients. For example, it is difficult for older adults to listen to you lecture about the dangers of smoking if they smell tobacco on your breath. On a more positive note, your older adult client will take your nutritional advice more seriously if he or she observes you selecting healthy fruits and vegetables in the cafeteria. An important nursing intervention in the care of older adults is to encourage greater personal responsibility for one's own optimal **wellness**.

Older adults have a great deal to offer. Whatever the level of functioning of an older adult—that is, wherever he or she falls on the **illness-wellness continuum**—that individual has a unique potential that nurses have the opportunity, really the privilege, of helping to discover and develop. This is true health promotion for the older adult.

🦟 Box 1–1 Sample Objectives from *Healthy People 2010*

- Reduce the proportion of adults whose activity is limited owing to chronic lung and breathing problems.
- Reduce deaths from chronic obstructive pulmonary disease (COPD) among adults.
- Reduce the overall number of cases of osteoporosis.
- Reduce coronary heart disease deaths.

- Increase the proportion of adults who engage regularly (preferably daily) in moderate physical activity for at least 30 minutes per day.
- Reduce tobacco use by adults.
- Reduce visual impairment due to diabetic retinopathy.
- Increase the proportion of trips made by walking.

Source: U.S. Department of Health and Human Services. *Healthy People 2010: Understanding and Improving Health*, 2nd Edition. Washington, D.C.: U.S. Government Printing office, November 2000.

Box 1–2   Knowledge, Skills, and Attitudes of Effective Gerontological Nurses

Knowledge

- Normal changes of aging
- Diseases common to older adults
- Unusual disease symptoms with aging
- Interdisciplinary team concepts
- Altered pharmacology with aging

Skills

- Finely tuned assessment skills
- Communication with adults with sensory and cognitive impairment
- Good body mechanics

- Patience
- Listening skills
- Teaching skills
- The ability to work as an interdisciplinary team member
- Rehabilitative nursing techniques
- Ability to provide psychosocial support

Attitudes

- Positive attitude toward aging
- Belief in health promotion
- Comfort in working with diverse cultures

Adapted from Matteson, M. A., McConnell, E. S., & Linton, A. D. (1998). *Gerontological nursing: Concepts and practice.* Philadelphia: W. B. Saunders, pp. 43–44.

THE SPECIALTY OF GERONTOLOGICAL NURSING— PAST, PRESENT, AND FUTURE

What Is the Past?

Although gerontological nursing became an official specialty in 1966, the first American Nurses Association (ANA) Conference on Geriatric Nursing Practice took place 4 years earlier. There was rapid growth in the nursing home and hospital industries after **Medicare** was enacted in 1965. Numerous studies on aging took place in the 1960s and 1970s, and many nurses took advantage of federal funding to specialize in gerontological nursing. Some of these nurses became advanced practice nurses in gerontology, such as geriatric nurse practitioners (GNPs) and gerontological clinical nurse specialists (CNSs).

Where Is Gerontological Nursing Now?

Gerontological nurses today have many important responsibilities. These include providing direct care at the bedside, translating complex medical jargon to the client and family, providing emotional support during difficult times, assisting with daily activities, assessing older adults for age-related deficits and signs of illness, and providing patient teaching, as well as caring for older patients in many other ways. To be an effective gerontological nurse, you need to possess certain knowledge, skills, and attitudes (Box 1–2).

What Is the Future of Gerontological Nursing?

With the graying of America, gerontological nursing opportunities are abundant. As the numbers of older adults increase, opportunities for promoting the health of this segment of the population will continue to grow. There will continue to be nursing opportunities in a variety of settings, including hospital, subacute care, and long-term care, and there will be even greater opportunities in home care and other community service settings. These settings are discussed in Chapter 3.

The older adult of the 21st century is the Baby Boomer of today and is likely to be more mobile, more active, more educated, and more involved in health care decision making than the older person of the 20th century. As a result, nurses preparing to care for older adults are challenged to meet their increased expectations for gaining knowledge, receiving appropriate care, and making optimal health care choices for themselves.

LEGISLATION THAT AFFECTS THE PRACTICE OF GERONTOLOGICAL NURSING

Many laws have been passed that affect the nursing care of the older adult. The three laws highlighted in this section are (1) the Omnibus Budget Reconciliation Act (OBRA) of 1981, (2) the Tax Equity and Fiscal Responsibility Act (TEFRA) of 1983, and (3) OBRA 1987.

During the 1960s and 1970s, medical care was paid for on a cost-plus basis, in which decisions about medical care were made at the bedside without much regard to expense. The issue of cost for medical treatment was not a part of the decision-making process. Although this sounds ideal, the reality of the situation was that much waste, unnecessary expense, and sometimes duplication of services resulted.

OBRA 1981

Major changes in health care occurred in the 1980s, beginning with Omnibus Budget Reconciliation Act (OBRA) 1981. This law removed certain restrictions that had been in place regarding home health visits, such as the limited number of visits allowed and the rule that the patient must first have been hospitalized. As a result, the home health care industry grew rapidly, and nursing opportunities in the area of home health kept pace with that growth.

TEFRA

Another important law was passed in 1983: the Tax Equity and Fiscal Responsibility Act (TEFRA).

This law changed the way Medicare reimbursement is made. Before TEFRA, clients received whatever services the doctor deemed necessary. With passage of the new law, a **prospective payment** system was instituted, whereby reimbursement for medical treatment is made mostly on the basis of diagnosis (although complications, surgeries, and patient age are also considered). As a result, if hospitals are efficient in improving the client's health and discharging him or her quickly, the agency can make a profit. If the client experiences delays in treatment and is discharged later than scheduled, the agency loses money. This type of reimbursement is termed **diagnosis-related groups**, or DRGs. Implementation of DRGs since passage of the law has not only decreased client length of stay in the hospital, it has also enhanced the emphasis on wellness from a health care perspective.

OBRA 1987

The third law to be discussed is OBRA 1987, also known as the Nursing Home Reform legislation. This law defines requirements for the quality of care given to residents of nursing homes. It addresses many aspects of nursing home life, including nutrition, staffing, and required qualifications for personnel. Some of the regulations specified in this law can be found in Table 1–1.

Some of the positive outcomes of OBRA 1987 identified by residents and staff of long-term care facilities include empowerment of residents, focus on resident rights, reduction or elimination of physical restraint use, and improved staffing, although nursing research indicates that staffing

Table 1–1	
EXAMPLES FROM OBRA 1987 LAW	
Category	**Requirement**
Resident rights	The resident must be fully informed in advance and must participate in decisions about care and services or changes in care and services
Physical restraints	No restraints to be applied for discipline or convenience
Resident assessment	Comprehensive resident assessment to be performed and to serve as the foundation for planning and delivery of care
Licensed nursing services	There must be 24-hour licensed nursing services
Registered nurses	Registered nurse coverage 8 consecutive hours per day, 7 days per week
Nursing assistants	Nursing assistants must be trained and competency tested

Data from Marek, K. D., Rantz, M. J., Fagin, C. M., & Krejci, J. W. (1996). OBRA '87: Has it resulted in better quality of care? *Journal of Gerontological Nursing, 22*(10), 28–36; Marek, K. D., Rantz, M. J., Fagin, C. M., & Krejci, J. W. (1996). OBRA '87: Has it resulted in positive change in nursing homes? *Journal of Gerontological Nursing, 22*(12), 32–40.

remains only marginally optimal in some facilities. The Minimum Data Set (MDS) is an assessment tool that was developed as a result of this legislation. The MDS provides a system for assessment of each resident's functional, medical, mental, and psychosocial status; it is performed upon admission to a facility and at regular intervals thereafter. This comprehensive assessment has enabled health care professionals to improve care planning and provision of services for older adults (see Appendix A, Assessment Tools). Also as a result of OBRA 1987, the role of the licensed practical nurse/licensed vocational nurse (LPN/LVN) was expanded to include team leading and administration of intravenous therapy.

DEMOGRAPHICS OF OLDER ADULTS IN THE 21ST CENTURY

Who are the older members of our community? They are a very diverse group—ethnically, culturally, economically, functionally, and educationally. There is a saying in gerontological nursing: "If you've seen one older adult, you've seen one older adult."

Does old age begin at age 65? Although people generally consider 65 to be the beginning of the "golden years," one cannot place everyone over this age into one category. In fact, it is not uncommon for a client in the seventh decade of life to have youthful energy and vitality, just as a person in his or her 40s may be chronically ill and quite frail. *Chronological age is just one indicator of how old a person is.* Habits developed in younger years can help determine how an individual will behave in his or her later years—as the globe-trotting adventurer or the couch potato.

People between the ages of 65 and 75 are sometimes referred to as the *young old*; those between 75 and 85 the *middle old*; and those over age 85 the *oldest old*. Although members of the oldest age group are sometimes referred to as the *frail elderly*, that term is usually reserved for those who are in declining health or whose needs must be met by others. Older adults over age 85 are the fastest growing segment of the U.S. population. These remarkable people were born at the beginning of the 20th century, when life expectancy was only 49 years. Their life expectancy has doubled. They have outlived spouses, children, and friends. They were born before antibiotics were discovered, lived through two world wars, and have seen unthinkable technological advances.

Can you expect to double your life span today? Probably not; researchers say that the maximum life span remains at about 120 years. Although this maximum appears to be fixed, a greater percentage of people have been getting closer to this maximum age. Studying the older adults in your community will help you learn their secrets for long and healthy lives. **Centenarians**, the elite older adults who survive beyond age 100, will be discussed in Chapter 12.

The percentage of the U.S. population that is over age 65 is increasing (Fig. 1–2).

Most people over the age of 65 live in cities or suburbs rather than rural dwellings. Although some older adults are financially well off and most own their own homes, those residing in central cities, rural areas, and the South have higher than average rates of poverty (Profile of Older Americans, 1999). Differences in life expectancies, marital status, ratios of men to women after age 65, and ratios of men to women after age 85 are depicted in Table 1–2.

Most older adults are white, although the numbers of minority elders are increasing. Culture and ethnicity of the older adult will be discussed in Chapter 2.

MISCONCEPTIONS ABOUT AGING

Misconceptions about aging abound. Some of the more common ones are:

1. Most older adults live in nursing homes.
2. Older adults are senile.
3. Older people are preoccupied with dying.
4. Older adults are rigid, cantankerous, and set in their ways.
5. "You can't teach an old dog new tricks."

If you have read any one of these above statements and believe it to be true, you may be surprised when you learn the facts. Although some of these statements are widely believed, they certainly do not describe the majority of older people today. Many of these misconceptions reflect **ageism,** a negative attitude or bias toward older adults. Following is an examination of each misconception and clarification of the truth about each statement.

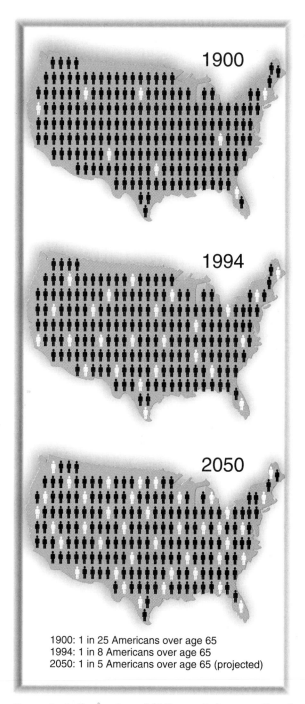

Figure 1–2. Proportion of U.S. population age 65 and older. (Data from the U.S. Bureau of the Census, 2000.)

Table 1–2 MALE-FEMALE DIFFERENCES AFTER AGE 65		
	♂	♀
Ratio of men to women at age 65	(2 men)	(3 women)
Ratio of men to women at age 85	(2 men)	(5 women)
Life expectancy (from birth)	72 years	79 years
Marital status	(couple)	(single woman)

Source: U.S. Census Bureau.

Misconception #1: Most Older Adults Live in Nursing Homes

Although a common misconception is that the older members of our society are locked away in nursing homes, the truth is that only about 4% of adults over age 65 reside in long-term care facilities (Profile of Older Americans, 1999). Those in nursing school may also unconsciously hold that opinion because many experiences of nursing students in working with older people occur in organized health care settings, such as hospitals and nursing homes. In addition, media attention is frequently focused on older adults in nursing home settings. The reality, however, is that most older adults live either at home independently (or with help), in an assisted living situation where help is available when needed, or with extended family, although it is true that this latter arrangement occurs less frequently in American culture than in some other cultures.

Misconception #2: Older Adults Are Senile

Senility is an outdated term that should never be used in any sentence about normal aging. In some disease processes, such as Alzheimer's disease, memory problems are a feature, but these should never be attributed to normal changes in the brain that happen as one gets older. Although the incidence of Alzheimer's disease increases after age 85, between the ages of 65 and 75 it is extremely low—between 2% and 4%. Some well-known scientists have conducted important research in their golden years. Linus Pauling was publishing in physics journals well into his 90s! Chapter 11 discusses strategies for promoting cognitive ability in the older adult.

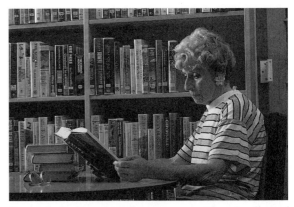

Figure 1–3. Ongoing learning provides intellectual stimulation to older adults. (From Leahy, J. M., & Kizilay, E. [1998]. *Foundations of Nursing Practice.* Philadelphia: W. B. Saunders, p. 358.)

Misconception #3: Older Adults Are Preoccupied with Dying

Although some older adults may think about their mortality from time to time—as do most people—it would not be fair to say that most of them are preoccupied with the thought. In the words of 105-year-old Josephine Smith: "I don't think about that; start thinking about it and you're out of luck."

Misconception #4: Older Adults Are Rigid, Cantankerous, and Set in Their Ways

Again, this is an unfair generalization. Research has shown that the people most likely to hold unrealistic generalizations about older adults are those people who have had limited exposure to members of that age group. In other words, these generalizations are simply based on ignorance. As for personality type, if you are an easy-going individual who can adapt to stress and change as a young adult, it is likely that you will be able to face challenges and stresses gracefully in your later years as well. When working with older adults, keep in mind that age does not change one's personality, and age does not automatically bring wisdom.

Misconception #5: "You Can't Teach an Old Dog New Tricks"

Memory and learning are complicated processes involving information storage and retrieval in the brain. As in other systems of the body, changes occur in the aging brain that affect the way information is learned and assimilated. However, some older adults are earning college degrees in their 70s (Fig. 1–3). Nurses can implement a few simple steps to help minimize the effects of aging on learning. Chapter 4 discusses strategies for teaching older adults.

THEORIES OF AGING

Why does aging occur? Theorists have set forth to try to explain aging. Of course, the hope is that if it can be determined with 100% certainty the reasons why aging occurs, then perhaps it can be slowed down to a snail's pace, or maybe even *reversed*. Various theories on aging have evolved over the years, and these basically fall into two categories: biological and psychosocial theories of aging. Following are brief discussions of some of the more popular theories in each category.

Biological Theories of Aging

The biological theories all state, in one way or another, that some sort of breakdown at the cellular

Table 1–3
BIOLOGICAL THEORIES OF AGING

Theory	Basic Premise	Comment
Biological programming theory	Genetic factors are a basis for aging	Supporters point to similar life expectancies some families as evidence
Cross-linkage theory	"Cross-linking agent" attaches to DNA	Abnormal parting in mitosis leads to cell death
Error theory	Cellular mutations occur during mitosis	Supporters of theory say radiation contributes
Free radical theory	Free radicals released from the oxygen molecule cause cell damage and aging	Antioxidant vitamins (A, C, E) are supposed to combat this
Immunity theory	Declining immune system leads to aging	Supporters of theory point to increased incidence of cancer and infection with aging as evidence
Wear and tear theory	Accumulated stress and damage, not chronological age, leads to aging	Not widely supported

Adapted from Matteson, M. A., McConnell, E. S., & Linton, A. D. (1998). *Gerontological nursing: Concepts and practice.* Philadelphia: W. B. Saunders.

level leads to aging and death of the cell, and therefore results in aging of the entire body. Each theory regards aging in a slightly different way. Biological theories of aging are summarized in Table 1–3.

Psychosocial Theories of Aging

Psychosocial theories of aging attempt to explore the behaviors, feelings, and mental processes of the aging individual. Three major psychosocial theories of aging have been proposed: the activity theory, the disengagement theory, and the continuity theory. Psychosocial theories are summarized in Table 1–4.

Relevance to Nursing Practice

Each theory on aging has followers, and no one theory is universally accepted. The important take-home message regarding theories is that it is important for nurses to have a basic understanding of what researchers have discovered so that they can better answer the questions of older clients.

Table 1–4
PSYCHOSOCIAL THEORIES OF AGING

Theory	Basic Premise	Comment
Activity theory	Staying socially more active leads to better adjustment to aging	Supporters of theory say activity leads to improved life satisfaction, higher morale, better mental health
Disengagement theory	With aging, people tend to withdraw from the social system and "step aside" for younger community members	Essentially the opposite of the Activity theory
Continuity theory	The ability to maintain continuity with previous life roles and activities helps one achieve healthy aging	Individualistic—supporters of theory believe that promotion of healthy aging means to "force" neither activity nor disengagement on an individual

Adapted from Matteson, M. A., McConnell, E. S., & Linton, A. D. (1998). *Gerontological nursing: Concepts and practice.* Philadelphia: W. B. Saunders.

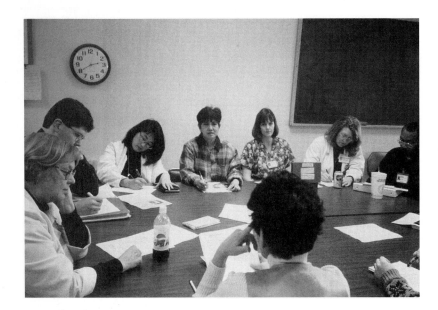

Figure 1–4. The interdisciplinary team meets regularly to discuss the plans of care for older adults in the long-term care setting.

CARE OF THE OLDER ADULT THROUGH AN INTERDISCIPLINARY TEAM APPROACH

Care of the older adult is generally accepted to be an **interdisciplinary team** project. In other words, the older adult does not "belong" to medicine, nursing, physical therapy, or any other discipline. Especially in long-term care settings, health care professionals work together as a team to meet the needs of the older adult.

Also, OBRA 1987 made it official that the various disciplines need to act as a team in caring for older adults in the long-term care setting. It states that the team must develop interdisciplinary care plans (ICPs) and must hold regular meetings to discuss these plans of care (Fig. 1–4). The interdisciplinary team can include the client and nurses (Gerontological Clinical Nurse Specialists, registered nurses [RNs], LPNs/LVNs, nursing assistants [NAs]), as well as a physician, social worker, pharmacist, dietitian, activities director, and rehabilitation specialists (from the areas of physical therapy, occupational therapy, and speech therapy); a podiatrist, psychiatrist, audiologist, and a dentist might also participate. Some states require that the client's family members or significant others be included in the interdisciplinary team meetings. The team meets on a regular basis and reviews the plan of care, with each team member offering his or her unique perspective. If nursing assistants are not part of the official meeting, it will be up to you, the LPN/LVN, to communicate closely with them. You must ensure that their viewpoint is represented because they are often the ones who work most closely with older adults as they provide much of the physical care in the long-term care setting. The involvement of all caregivers is crucial to the successful implementation of the interventions planned at the meeting.

Summary

- Gerontological nursing has been around as long as there have been older adults in need of care.
- Recently, caring for the older adult from a health promotion perspective has been advocated.
- Members of nearly every specialty in nursing care for older adults; so, knowledge of this group of clients is important in LPN/LVN nursing.
- Health promotion emphasizes the encouragement of healthy lifestyle to improve one's chances of living a long and healthy life.
- The U.S. government has set broad health goals for its residents in a document entitled *Healthy People 2010*.

- Important laws have been passed that affect provision of care to the older adult; these include OBRA 1981, TEFRA, and OBRA 1987. Each law affects the care of older adults differently, but all improve the quality of such care.
- Older adults are a very diverse group. Life expectancy has increased over the years, although the maximum human life span has not. Older adults keep increasing in numbers, and will make up a larger percentage of the population in the future, leading to many opportunities for practical/vocational nursing.
- Contrary to popular misconception, only 4% of people over age 65 reside in long-term care, senility is not a normal change of aging, and older adults are not all preoccupied with dying; nor are they all rigid, cantankerous, and unable to learn new things.
- Biological and psychosocial theories of aging attempt to explain aging of the body and psychosocial adaptations to aging.
- Care of the older adult is regarded as an interdisciplinary team responsibility.
- The LPN/LVN is a vital member of the team and will be in the future.

STUDY QUESTIONS
Multiple Choice Review

1. What is the average life expectancy today?
   1. 55 years
   2. 65 years
   3. 76 years
   4. 120 years
2. What is the probable maximum human life span?
   1. 65 years
   2. 75 years
   3. 120 years
   4. 150 years
3. What percentage of older adults lives in long-term care facilities?
   1. 4%
   2. 10%
   3. 50%
   4. 75%

4. Which of the following correctly states one of the two broad goals of *Healthy People 2010*?
   1. Increase quality and years of healthy life
   2. Stop Americans from smoking
   3. Increase the number of Americans able to be admitted to nursing homes
   4. Reduce death from falls and fall-related injuries
5. Which of the following laws led to nursing home reform?
   1. OBRA 1981 — Home Health
   2. TEFRA Medicare
   3. OBRA 1987
   4. *Healthy People 2010*

Critical Thinking

1. What are some possible reasons for passage of the various laws described in this chapter?
2. How is gerontological nursing likely to change in the future?
3. Describe how a long-term care unit might look when you are an older adult.
4. Which biological theory of aging would you like to learn more about? Explain.

Resources
Internet Resources
Centers for Disease Control and Prevention
http://www.cdc.gov
Healthy People 2010
http://web.health.gov/healthypeople/
Office of Disease Prevention and Health Promotion
http://www.odphp.osophs.dhhs.gov
U.S. Census Bureau
http://www.census.gov

Organizations
American Society on Aging
833 Market Street, Suite 511, San Francisco, CA 94103-1824
(415) 974-9600
Gerontological Society of America
1275 K Street, NW, Suite 350, Washington, DC 20005-4006
(202) 554-4444
National Gerontological Nurses Association (NGNA)
7250 Parkway Drive, Hanover, MD 21076
Office of Disease Prevention and Health Promotion
Room 738 G, Hubert Humphrey Building
200 Independence Avenue, SW, Washington, DC 20201
(202) 205-8583

Selected References

Centers for Disease Control and Prevention Survey: An Overview of Nursing Homes and Their Current Residents—Data from the 1995 National Nursing Home Survey. CDC Web Site: Available at http://www.cdc.gov/nchs www/nchshome.htm. Accessed August 12, 1998.

Habel, M. (1998). The oldest old: A new gerontological nursing challenge. *Nurseweek, 11*(14), 20–21.

Healthy People 2010. Available at http://www.web.health.gov/healthypeople/prevagenda/whatishp.htm. Accessed September 13, 2000.

Kaufmann, M. A. (1997). Wellness for people 65 years and better. *Journal of Gerontological Nursing, 23*(6), 7–8.

Marek, K. D., Rantz, M. J., Fagin, C. M., & Krejci, J. W. (1996). OBRA '87: Has it resulted in better quality of care? *Journal of Gerontological Nursing, 22*(10), 28–36.

Marek, K. D., Rantz, M. J., Fagin, C. M., & Krejci, J. W. (1996). OBRA '87: Has it resulted in positive change in nursing homes? *Journal of Gerontological Nursing, 22*(12), 32–40.

Matteson, M. A., McConnell, E. S., & Linton, A. D. (1998). *Gerontological nursing: Concepts and practice*. Philadelphia: W. B. Saunders.

Profile of Older Americans: 1999. Administration on Aging. Available at http://www.aoa.dhhs.gov/aoa/stats/profile/default.htm Accessed September 14, 2000.

Sixty-Five Plus in the United States: U.S. Census Bureau Statistical Brief. Available at http://www.census.gov/ socdemo/ www/agebrief.html. Accessed September 14, 2000.

Stone, J. K., Wyman, J. F., & Salisbury, S. A. (1999). *Clinical gerontological nursing: A guide to advanced practice*. Philadelphia: W. B. Saunders.

Strumpf, N. E. (2000). Improving care for the frail elderly: The challenge for nursing. *Journal of Gerontological Nursing, 26*(7), 36–44.

Waldner, E. (1998, August 5). Seton Coastside resident recalls a century. *Half Moon Bay Review*, p. 3A.

Promoting Health in a Culturally Diverse Older Adult Population

OBJECTIVES

After completing this chapter, you will be able to:

- Compare the terms *culture* and *ethnicity*.
- Recognize common beliefs about health and aging from various cultures.
- Identify the effect your culture has on your beliefs and values.
- Describe the importance of culture on delivery of nursing care.
- Examine the culture of health care.
- State nursing interventions that can assist you when caring for an older adult from another culture.
- Discuss the significance of herbal medicines.

CHAPTER OUTLINE

KEY TERMS

Beliefs

Cultural diversity

Culturally sensitive care

Culture

Eastern medicine

Ethnic group

Ethnicity

Herbal therapies

Religion

Traditional healers

Transcultural nursing

Values

Western medicine

CASE STUDY*

Mr. F. was a client in an Intensive Care Unit (ICU) who was on a ventilator and in a coma. He was pronounced brain-dead by his physician on Friday; he had been in the ICU 1 week. Although in most cases the topic of withdrawal of life support would be discussed with the family at this time, the physician wrote orders to "continue full support over the weekend."

The nursing staff immediately assumed that the family was having difficulty coping with the reality of the terrible situation. They immediately developed a care plan to assist the family's coping efforts. The nurses were also confused by the family's focus on seemingly unimportant details, such as keeping two pillows under the client's head to keep his mouth closed. In addition, the nurses were concerned about the expense of keeping a brain-dead client on a ventilator over the weekend; in one nurse's words, "it was not my idea of death with dignity."

What was going on? Could the nurses have done anything differently?

As the story unfolded, the care planning efforts of the nurses were completely misguided. The important piece of information not being considered was the culture of the family: the family was Jewish. The client was pronounced dead very close to the start of the Jewish Sabbath, which lasts from sundown Friday to sundown Saturday. According to Jewish custom, a body cannot be moved on the Sabbath. It is also very important in Jewish culture that the mouth of the patient remain closed.

What could the nurses have done differently? They could have assessed the family's **culture.** Had the nurses learned the true meaning behind the actions being taken, more **culturally sensitive care** could have been given.

CULTURALLY SENSITIVE NURSING CARE

The United States is a very diverse and exciting place to live. Most people living in the United States come from families transplanted from some other land—only the American Indians, Aleuts, and Eskimos are considered native to this land, as they migrated here thousands of years before the arrival of the Europeans.

It is important to consider culture when planning and providing nursing care because it can

have a profound effect on clients' health behaviors. Without consideration of a client's culture, it is easy to assume that everyone shares the same **beliefs, values,** and preferences. Even simple things, such as the preference for ice in one's water pitcher or water at room temperature, can have cultural roots. If you ignore culture, your client teaching will probably be ignored, if it conflicts with cultural practices. For example, if your dietary instructions are culturally unacceptable and the client does not bring this to your attention, it is very likely that all dietary teaching will be ignored.

Nutrition Tip

Always consider the client's culture when providing dietary teaching.

Health care professionals must try to avoid such situations by learning about other cultures (Fig. 2–1).

As a nurse, you must first be aware of your own culture and how it affects your beliefs and values. Then you must consider the client and what his or her cultural beliefs and values *might* be. You cannot assume that just because a person belongs to a certain cultural or **ethnic group,** they necessarily subscribe to a certain set of beliefs or practices; that would be stereotyping. But it is helpful in learning about your client to have some notion of traditional beliefs and values from his or her cultural group and to consider the influence they *might* have on the client's view of

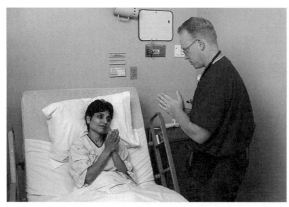

Figure 2–1. Nurse giving traditional greeting to a Hindu. (From deWit, S. [2001]. *Fundamental concepts and skills for nursing.* Philadelphia: W. B. Saunders. p. 176.)

health care and health care practices. Only as you get to know the client will you gain insight as to how much influence his or her culture has on health care choices.

What Is Culture?

Culture is a system of values, beliefs, and practices that guide a person's behavior. Culture is learned or shared; it is a way of thinking, feeling, and acting. It is passed from one generation to the next. **Religion** is often an important part of one's cultural identity. **Ethnicity** is a person's identification with a certain ethnic group. This is based on shared traditions, national origin, physical characteristics, and other markers such as language, religion, food, and dress. Definitions related to **transcultural nursing** care can be found in Box 2–1.

In recent decades, more cultural groups have declared the United States their home. The population of the United States continues to increase, as does the ethnic and **cultural diversity** in all age groups (Fig. 2–2).

As cultural diversity increases, you will work with older adults whose beliefs and attitudes about health and health care practices are different from your own—not better or worse, just different. It is important to learn about the beliefs associated with other cultures and to understand some of the major differences from one culture to another.

Just as the number of older adults in the population of the United States is increasing, so is racial and ethnic diversity increasing. For example, at present 4% of older adults in the United States are Hispanic; this number is expected to increase to 16% by the year 2050. Nurses will be caring not only for greater numbers of older adults but also for greater numbers of *culturally diverse* older adults. Having an understanding of the diverse cultures of American society is essential for the nurse who strives to give comprehensive nursing care.

CULTURAL AND SPIRITUAL VIEWS OF HEALTH AND AGING

Culture affects how an older adult perceives and defines the meaning of illness. One's beliefs about the meaning of health and illness influence what he or she is likely to do when illness strikes. If your cultural belief is that evil spirits cause illness, western medicine will be of value only if it is expected to interfere with the spirits, or if it is administered by someone with power against such spirits. If illness is perceived as a form of revenge for bad deeds, then prayer or asking for

---

Box 2–1 Transcultural Nursing Definitions

Transcultural nursing: Integration of the concept of culture into all aspects of nursing care

Acculturation: The process of learning a different culture to adapt to a new or changing environment

Assimilation: The process of completely giving up or replacing one's values, beliefs, and practices with those of another culture

Subculture: A group that shares some of the characteristics of the larger group of which it is a part but that is seen as a distinguishable subgroup

Race: a biological classification of the human species that differs from other divisions based on common hereditary traits

Ethnocentrism: the view that your own culture is superior to that of others

Data from *Saunders manual of nursing care.* (1997) Philadelphia: W. B. Saunders.

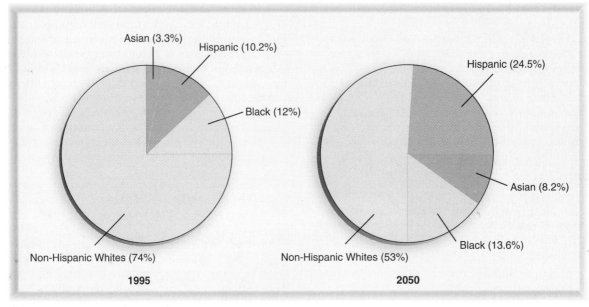

Figure 2–2. Projected changes in U.S. population (all age groups). (Data from the National Center for Policy Analysis, Washington, D.C., 1997.)

forgiveness may be an important part of the healing process.

Health Promotion Tip

It is important to understand a client's cultural beliefs about health and illness to assist with health promotion for that individual.

Aging is also viewed differently by people of different cultures. Attitudes toward aging can affect health care practices, health promotion activities, and numerous other aspects of everyday living. If your cultural belief states that aging means an inevitable decline in your physical abilities, you may be less likely to participate in health-promoting activities such as exercise. On the other hand, if your culture promotes the belief that older adults are an important source of knowledge for the community, you may place a higher value on learning to keep your mind sharp.

As a licensed vocational nurse (LVN), you will be caring for older adults from many cultural backgrounds. The information in this section is presented by geographic region of origin,

beginning with people native to this land, the American Indians. Remember, of course, that numerous factors influence how closely your client identifies with his or her cultural group, including the generation of immigration and individual life experiences. For example, the experience of being a Japanese American is different for a young client whose grandparents immigrated to this country than it is for an older Japanese American who experienced being placed in an internment camp during World War II.

American Indians

American Indians view health as a process that involves restoring balance and harmony to self, loved ones, Indian nations, the environment, and the universe. Caring values and spiritual values are extremely important in the healing process. Health means living in harmony with nature and having the ability to survive under extremely difficult circumstances.

Traditional treatment of illness includes the use of herbs, plants, and **traditional healers** (medicine man or woman), since the traditional American Indian believes the cause of illness to be of a spiritual nature. American Indians may consult traditional healers before seeking western medical care.

The Indian Health Service has provided most of the health care services available to American Indian populations since 1954. In recent years, however, tribes have been allowed to manage their own health care programs. The Indian Health Service consists of inpatient facilities, outpatient clinics, and public health nursing services. Community health representatives are tribal members who identify health problems within the community, encourage people to use medical facilities, and transport people to the clinic as needed.

Diabetes, alcohol abuse, and domestic violence are increasing among American Indians. Traditional American Indians believe that the spread of such health problems is related to decreased observation of many native traditions.

American Indians respect the older members of their community as teachers and leaders. The self-esteem of an older American Indian is based in large part on his or her ability to help guide younger tribal members and to be regarded as a source of wisdom.

African Americans

Most African Americans are descendants of people who were imported from the West Coast of Africa to this country as slaves during the 17th century. Voluntary immigration of blacks to the United States occurred in later years; these blacks came from African countries, the West Indies, the Dominican Republic, Haiti, and Jamaica. African Americans reside in every part of the United States and are represented in every socioeconomic group; however, one third live in poverty. African Americans have survived despite the deplorable conditions imposed upon them by the people of this country, both during and after slavery.

Traditional African American views of health involve harmony with nature; illness is a state of disharmony. Many African Americans believe in the power of some people to help and heal others. Traditional African American views of health perceive the mind, body, and spirit as interconnected. The African American community cares for both its old and young members. Older adults are held in high esteem as they are filled with knowledge and wisdom.

Life expectancy is shorter for older African Americans than for older whites, although the gap is narrowing (Table 2–1). Health care services are expensive and often inaccessible to older African American women who are poor and have multiple health problems, such as coronary artery disease, elevated blood cholesterol levels, and diabetes mellitus (Burggraf, 2000, pp. 184–185). Studies have also shown that, compared with other groups, African Americans tend to delay seeking treatment when experiencing a heart attack (Lee, H., 1997).

African American older adults depend mostly on their families to provide care for chronic ailments; fewer African American older adults can be found in long-term care facilities than white older adults. This may reflect the higher value placed by African Americans on family care as opposed to institutional care, but it may also reflect the difficulty that minority older adults have in accessing health care services. On the other hand, no significant differences have been found between African Americans and other cultures in terms of use of community-based health care services, such as home health aides and visiting nurses.

Hispanic Americans

Hispanic is a term used to refer to people from many countries: Puerto Rico, Cuba, Mexico, South America, Central America, and Spain. Hispanic people include individuals from every race (blacks, whites, and those of American Indian and Asian descent). Hispanic Americans are the fastest growing minority in the United States. Between the years 1990 and 2030, the older adult Hispanic population is expected to increase by 555%.

Table 2–1	
LIFE EXPECTANCY FOR OLDER WHITES AND BLACKS IN THE UNITED STATES	
Group	Life Expectancy
White men	73.8 years
White women	79.6 years
Black men	66.1 years
Black women	74.2 years

Source: Sheryl Gay Stolberg, "U.S. Life Expectancy Hits New High," New York Times, Sept. 12, 1997.

Many Hispanic people regard good health as God's reward for living a good life, treating the body with respect, and praying. Illness can be a punishment from God. Religious medals and amulets may be worn to help prevent illness; relics may be kept in the home. Many Hispanics believe in the theory of hot and cold in describing illness. Illnesses, foods, and medicines are classified as either hot or cold. When an individual experiences illness, the treatment and foods taken must be of the opposite type. For example, after a woman gives birth, a hot experience, she cannot eat pork because it is considered a hot food. Instead, she needs a cold food, such as whole milk or bananas.

Nutrition Tip

The licensed practical nurse/licensed vocational nurse (LPN/LVN) should ask the Hispanic client about his or her perception of the illness and of what foods or treatments might be most effective.

Many older Hispanic Americans live below the poverty line, are uninsured, and suffer from severe illnesses such as diabetes, stomach and cervical cancer, and obesity. The Hispanic older adult may utilize alternative health care practices such as folk healing or home remedies.

Older adults are highly regarded in the Hispanic culture, and they are usually cared for in the home. Older Hispanic adults depend mostly on their families to provide care for chronic ailments, and they may feel isolated or even betrayed when placed in a long-term care facility. Traditional gender roles are valued by the Hispanic older adult, and respect and courtesy are expected. The older Hispanic male may have a difficult time accepting changes or any physical decline associated with aging or disability, because these may result in loss of traditional gender roles.

Asian Americans

Asian Americans discussed in this section include older adults with ancestors from China, Japan, Korea, and the Philippines.

Chinese Americans

Traditional Chinese beliefs are that *yin* (female negative energy) and *yang* (male positive energy) must be in harmony for health to prevail. Herbs, acupuncture, and acupressure may be used in addition to or instead of western medical treatments. Sometimes **western medicine** is used for acute illness and **eastern medicine** during chronic illnesses.

Living to an old age is viewed as a blessing in Chinese culture. Members of the Chinese community view older members with esteem and often seek their advice. The family unit considers it a responsibility to care for its older members.

Japanese Americans

Like the Chinese, Japanese may prefer eastern medicine and traditional health practices to western medical approaches. The Japanese culture values self-sufficiency and self-control. Respect and tact are expected. It is viewed as an insult to give a command to a Japanese older adult.

Japanese view their older members with great respect. They expect to care for older family members, and few place older adults in a nursing home. In recent years, however, more Japanese Americans have been forced into the difficult decision of nursing home placement for a loved one. Japanese nursing homes in some cities try to preserve Japanese traditions.

Korean Americans

Traditional Koreans may employ Chinese medicine, western medicine, folk medicine, and spirituality. In traditional Korean culture, there is more emphasis on interdependence than independence; the strong view is "we care for one another."

Most older adults, with or without physical disabilities, reside in the home environment. The usual caregiver in these situations is the daughter-in-law, the wife, or the daughter. Gradually, Koreans are becoming more westernized: independence is becoming more valued than the traditional value of interdependence. However, nursing home care is still not culturally accepted.

Growing old is viewed in a positive way in the Korean culture. The older Korean adult is understood to have acquired wisdom from lifelong experiences and is regarded as an historian. Korean society gives to older adults respect, reverence, and honor for their wisdom and gray hair. Many older Koreans have experienced lifelong struggles, such as gaining independence from the Japanese, fighting in the Korean War, and experiencing hunger and famine. The older Korean wishes to maintain dignity during illness and dying. Many Koreans embrace a social code based on Confucianism, that is, the obligation to care for sick and elderly parents. Caring for one's parents is often viewed as a source of pride.

Filipino Americans

Traditional Filipinos believe that individuals should unquestioningly accept what life brings: destiny is God's will. Religious faith may provide a sense of security, especially in times of stress. Some Filipino older adults carry religious medals and rosaries or pin a piece of cloth imprinted with the image of a religious figure close to their bodies. A member of the Filipino community may view illness, disease, or accidents as outside one's personal control and related to factors such as overwork or exposure to heat or cold. A Filipino American may try to avoid conflict by giving in to health care advice, even when he or she does not agree with it. Traditional Filipino health care practices include faith healing and the use of herbs.

In the Philippines, the older adult assumes a dominant role within the family structure. The culture places a high value on wisdom acquired through life experience. If an older adult immigrates to the United States through sponsorship by a son or daughter, this places the older adult in a situation of role reversal. Being addressed by one's first name instead of surname by a stranger is a sign of disrespect to the Filipino older adult.

European Americans

Most Western European countries embrace the principle of solidarity in their view of health care: the common belief is that people should care for one another. The more pervasive view in the United States is from an individualistic perspective. While in the United States we view health care as a shared responsibility on a family or extended-family basis, most European countries view it as a shared responsibility on a national level. Europeans who have recently immigrated to the United States may be surprised at the individualistic view we hold.

All countries face the challenge of increasing health care costs. Many European countries are offering expanded services to accommodate people with health care needs, such as 24-hour care at home and payment for relatives who care for older adults at home. Some of these countries are also reducing the number of long-term care beds and are taking on the financial burden of repairing or upgrading homes (Fig. 2–3).

Most European Americans subscribe to the germ theory of infection. Some European Americans believe in other causes of illness, such as stress, drafts, and environmental change, or in the evil eye and punishment from God. Many Scandinavians deeply value freedom of choice, autonomy, and the ability to live as unrestricted a life as possible. Many Europeans are shocked to discover any use of restraint devices in American health care facilities.

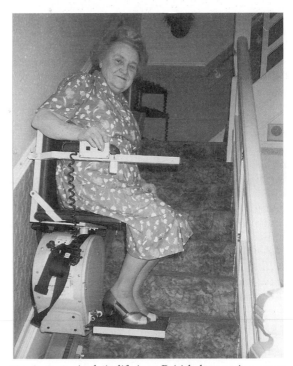

Figure 2–3. A chair lift in a British home gives more freedom of mobility to this older adult.

In the country of origin, it was typical to live in multigenerational households. It is not uncommon for an adult emigrating from Europe today to have grown up with his or her grandparents, and perhaps an uncle or aunt, living in the family home.

Some believe that the European American view of older adults has declined since the Industrial Revolution. Before the Industrial Revolution, family members depended on one another and the older members were a great source of knowledge. Following the Industrial Revolution, the great emphasis shifted to physical strength; an older adult who was weaker than younger members became undervalued (Eliopoulos, 1997, p. 4).

Now we are in an information age, in which many view intellectual strength as superior to physical strength. Therefore, older adults are beginning to regain the respect they deserve. There is also strength in numbers: the post–World War II Baby Boomers are aging and becoming members of the "Senior Boom." Older adults are organizing their collective power, and elected officials are paying attention to their needs and requests.

Jewish Americans

Although Jewish Americans come from a variety of countries, it has been estimated that half of the world's Jewish population lives in America.

Jewish tradition recognizes two components of health: the body and the spirit. Prayer is used to ask God for healing. According to the Torah, visiting the sick imitates God, decreases isolation, and promotes community. Western medical care is encouraged, although consultation with a rabbi may be desired when life-sustaining measures or transplantation is considered. A Jewish client in your care may decline medical procedures on the Sabbath or other holy days. Jewish clients who follow kosher dietary practices must avoid mixing meat with dairy products, and eating shellfish and pork are forbidden.

> ### 🍴 Nutrition Tip _____
>
> Your older Jewish client may observe dietary restrictions such as not mixing meat and dairy products and abstaining from pork or pork-based products (such as insulin) and shellfish.

The older adult in the Jewish community is highly regarded. Older adults often serve as community leaders. In the United States, Jewish communities are developing a network of community and institutional services for the older adult that preserve Jewish traditions.

HEALTH CARE CULTURE

Thus far we have examined the influence that culture may have on your beliefs and practices, as well as on those of your client. A third culture is superimposed on both of these—that of health care. Health care providers wear different clothes than their clients and speak a common medical language. Some of the rituals may appear strange to some clients: awakening the client to hold a circular, metal listening device to the chest; bathing the client in bed; examining and measuring body fluids; and imposing endless lists of rules to which clients must adhere. Often, one is not allowed to bring food into the health care setting from the outside culture. Simple activities that one normally does independently, such as walking about in the room, are often supervised. Our health care culture can be very frightening to some clients.

In addition, the visitor to health care culture is placed in a dependent role. He or she is stripped of clothing, instructed to wear pajamas, and assumes a supine position in bed; while the health care provider wears a culturally sanctioned uniform and takes the standing position. The visitor is culturally illiterate regarding health care language; the health care provider speaks in a foreign language, using words such as "prn" and "stat."

Sometimes health care providers become so used to medical terminology that they forget that the client is not accustomed to or familiar with the language. For example, imagine that you are an 80-year-old man, who has been admitted to the hospital for enlargement of the prostate. You are slightly confused from lack of sleep and because of the pain medications you have been given. At 2:00 in the morning, a nurse enters the room and says, "I'm going to take your vitals." You shriek in horror and proceed to defend yourself. (Later, the progress notes state, "client combative.")

NURSING IMPLICATIONS OF CULTURE

Specific implications for nurses of the cultural diversity of clients include the following:

- Many cultures, such as Hispanic and Filipino, have a "present time" orientation. Client teaching may be most effective if focus is placed on short-term goals.
- Older adults from many cultures experience poverty. Before labeling a client as noncompliant, consider the possibility that medical therapy and treatments ordered may be too expensive. The older adult may have a strong sense of pride and be reluctant to disclose this as a factor.
- Language barriers may exist between health care workers and older adult clients from various cultures. Many older adults are recent immigrants to the United States and may be fluent only in their native language. Strategies for enhancing communication include keeping the message simple, using diagrams and pictures with explanations, and rephrasing the message if it is not understood. Often a person will smile and nod even if he or she does not understand what you are saying. Validate your communication with questions, or ask the older adult to state back to you the information just presented.
- Many cultures possess a strong sense of family and view family as essential for the healing process. It is important to allow the older adult in your care to benefit from the strength of the large family visit, unless it is medically contraindicated. Family members can help translate when there is a language barrier, may wish to spend the night at the older adult's side, and can reduce the anxiety of an unfamiliar environment for their loved one; some may wish to participate in the personal care of the older adult.
- Be careful not to overgeneralize. Although information in this chapter may be helpful to you as you try to understand an older adult client from another culture, it is wrong to assume that the client will possess every (or any) of the characteristics described. You must get to know the beliefs, values, and views of your older adult client as an individual.

COMPLEMENTARY AND INTEGRATIVE THERAPIES

Complementary and integrative therapies are becoming popular ways for individuals to try to promote physical and psychological wellness. The term *complementary* refers to therapies used in addition to traditional western medical treatment, whereas *integrative* implies a blending or integration of systems to address the needs of the whole client. Table 2–2 lists examples of complementary and integrative therapies.

Table 2–2
COMPLEMENTARY AND INTEGRATIVE THERAPIES

Chinese therapies
- Acupuncture
- Acupressure
- Chinese herbal medicine

Natural healing
- Aquatherapy
- Aromatherapy
- Homeopathy
- Color therapy

Nutrition and diet
- Diet therapies
- Naturopathic medicine

Body work and movement therapies
- Yoga
- Rolfing
- Reiki
- Massage
- Qigong
- T'ai chi
- Reflexogy
- Shiatsu
- Therapeutic touch
- Healing touch
- Dance therapy
- Chiropractic treatment
- Cranial osteopathy

Plant therapy
- Flower essence therapy
- Herbal medicine

Mind/body medicine
- Meditation
- Music therapy
- Visualization and imagery
- Hypnotherapy
- Biofeedback
- Light therapy

Ayurvedic medicine

From Zerwekh, J., & Claborn, J. C. (2000). *Nursing today: Transitions and trends* (3rd Ed.). Philadelphia. W. B. Saunders, p. 306.

Herbal therapies are included in this category of complementary medicine. They are becoming a popular way for many clients to self-treat various health-related problems without having to seek traditional medical advice. Many cultures, however, consider herbal remedies "traditional" medicine and our western medical practices to be foreign.

To many health care providers, herbal therapies represent an unknown and mysterious part of clients' health care practices. Often health care providers ignore or are unaware of the influence that herbal therapies can have on a client's health, both positive and negative. Health care providers may view herbal therapies somewhat like "black magic," or perhaps may overlook herbs as a benign influence.

Health care providers need to become better educated about herbal therapies and learn how these agents interact with western medical treatments. Many herbs work in a similar way to medicines that are available only by prescription. If a client consumes a medication and an herb that act on the same cell receptors, overdosage can occur. Herbs can also reduce the effectiveness of certain medications. For example, cases have been reported of St. John's Wort interacting with cyclosporin, leading to rejection of heart transplants.

Medication Safety Tip

If a client takes a prescription medication in addition to an herbal remedy

- it can greatly increase the potency of the prescription medication, or
- it can counteract the prescription medication

Use patterns of herbal remedies are different between the United States and other countries. In Europe, for example, herbal therapy is considered to be traditional medicine and is used for chronic diseases and minor illnesses that do not require drug therapy. In the United States, however, a different pattern of usage is noted. Americans tend to use prescription medications more readily for minor illnesses and to seek out herbal therapies for serious or life-threatening illnesses; in other words, they often seek out herbal medicines out of desperation. This can lead to serious consequences because the client with this pattern of usage is likely to already be taking prescription medications.

Because the Food and Drug Administration has no jurisdiction over herbal therapies, hidden dangers may be associated with their use. The potency of herbs can vary from batch to batch if the herb is not from a standardized preparation. To combat this problem, American standards have been published for nine of the most popular herbs; those that meet the standard can add the letters NF (national formulary) to their label. A second very serious problem is that of purity. Certain shipments of ginseng have been found to contain a high level of fungicide (Gorman, 1998). Pregnant and lactating women should avoid the use of many herbs.

Another more serious problem is that herbal therapies are classified as food supplements and are sold in health food stores, although many of them act in similar ways to prescription medications and should carry similar warnings on their labels. Approximately 60% of Americans who use herbal therapies do not tell their health care providers that they are taking herbs. Health care providers need to recognize the potential for medication interactions and adverse drug effects associated with these therapies so that clients can be better educated about the potential benefits and dangers of such agents. Table 2–3 contains information on some of the more popular herbal therapies, along with special considerations and nursing implications.

Summary

- Culture can have a profound effect on our clients' health behaviors. You must recognize your own culture and be aware of how it affects your beliefs and values, then consider the client's cultural beliefs and values.
- Culture includes values, beliefs, and practices. Older adults in the United States are increasing in both number and cultural diversity.
- Culture affects how an older adult defines illness and influences what measures are taken when illness strikes.
- Aging is viewed differently by different cultures. Attitudes toward aging can affect one's health care practices, health promotion activities, and other aspects of everyday living.

Table 2–3
COMMON HERBAL THERAPIES

Name	Popular Uses	Mechanism of Action	Precautions
St. John's Wort	• Mild depression • Wounds (used topically) • Viral infections	Similar to MAO inhibitors	• Not to be used with prescription antidepressant medications • Client should avoid foods high in tyramines (aged cheese, fava beans, Chianti wine, etc.) • Increases sensitivity to sunlight
Valerian	• Insomnia • Mild anxiety (often paired with St. John's Wort)	May inhibit enzyme-induced breakdown of gamma-aminobutyric acid (GABA), leading to sedation	• Not to be used with prescription antianxiety drugs • Foul smell
Gingko Biloba	• Circulation problems (intermittent claudication) • Memory impairment	Reduces platelet aggregation; antioxidant	• Side effects can include GI upset, headache • If entire plant used (traditional Chinese medicine), can have cross-allergy to poison ivy • Can interact with blood-thinning medications
Ginger	• Nausea • Anti-inflammatory • Antioxidant	Weak antiemetic agent	• Can be taken as plant, pill, or tea • May enhance the effects of anticoagulants
Kava-Kava	• Anxiety and tension	Thought to bind gamma-aminobutyric acid (GABA) receptors, blocking norepinephrine uptake. May block monoamine oxidase B	• Not to be paired with prescription barbiturates or antidepressants • Side effects include allergic reactions, yellowing of the skin • Not to be used in pregnancy
Echinacea	• Colds and flu • Vaginal yeast infections (taken *orally*)	Thought to stimulate the immune system	• People with allergies to daisies will be allergic • Not to be used for longer than 8 weeks • Not to be used in people with autoimmune disorders (e.g., lupus)
Evening Primrose Oil (EPO)	• Eczema • PMS • Cyclic breast pain	Prostaglandin modifier	• Expensive
Saw Palmetto	• Benign prostatic hyperplasia	Similar action as finasteride (Proscar) (alpha reductase inhibitor)	• Not to be used in prostate cancer • Not to be handled by woman who is or may be pregnant • Mild GI disturbances, decreased libido, headache
Vitex ("Chaste Flower")	• PMS • Hot flashes • Menstrual irregularities	Increases production of progesterone during luteal phase; modulates production of prolactin	• Not to be used in pregnancy or with hormone replacement therapy

| Table 2–3 | | | |
| (continued) | | | |

Name	Popular Uses	Mechanism of Action	Precautions
Bilberry	• Noninfectious diarrhea	Slows GI motility Reduces platelet aggregation	• Not to be used in infectious diarrhea • Adverse reactions, toxic effects unknown
Asian Ginseng	• Fatigue	Unknown	• Not to be used in client with uncontrolled hypertension • Not to be used with high-dose caffeine • May cause GI upset, menstrual abnormalities, breast tenderness • Interacts with MAO inhibitors • Not the same as Siberian Ginseng
Feverfew	• Migraine headaches		• Avoid use of other migraine medications • Avoid in pregnancy and lactation • Avoid if allergic to daisies
Cranberry	• Urinary tract infections	Prevents adherence of *Escherichia coli* to bladder wall	• Should not be substituted for antibiotic therapy
Chamomile	• Inflammatory bowel disease • Gingivitis, thrush (as a mouthwash) • Poison ivy (as compresses)	Reduces inflammation	• Not to be used in clients with allergy to ragweed
Milk Thistle	• Liver disease	Helps hepatocytes to regenerate	• Can have a transient laxative effect
Garlic	• High cholesterol • Intermittent claudication	Lowers cholesterol, reduces platelet aggregation, reduces cholesterol biosynthesis, lowers blood pressure	• Drug-drug interaction with anticoagulants

Data from Anding, R. (1998, May). Herbal essence: The good, the bad, and the deadly. National Teaching Institute and Critical Care Exposition. Symposium conducted at the meeting of the American Association of Critical Care Nurses, Los Angeles, CA; McEnany, G. (2000). Herbal psychotropics. Part 3: Focus on Kava, Valerian, and Melatonin. *Journal of American Psychiatric Nurses Association, 6*(4), 126–130; and O'Neil, C. K., Avila, J. R., & Fetrow, C. W. (1999). Herbal medicines: Getting beyond the hype. *Nursing 99, 29*(4), 58–61.

• The American Indian view of health involves living in harmony with nature. Traditional treatment of illness includes the use of herbs, plants, and traditional healers. American Indians respect older adults as teachers and leaders.

• Traditional African American views of health involve harmony with nature, with mind, body, and spirit interconnected. Older adults are held in high esteem as they are filled with knowledge and wisdom.

• Hispanic people view good health as God's reward for living a good life, treating the body with respect, and praying. Many Hispanic individuals believe in a theory of hot and cold in describing illness; this theory requires that treatment provided must be opposite in temperature to the illness. Older adults are highly regarded and are usually cared for in the home.

- Traditional Chinese people believe that yin and yang must be in harmony for health to prevail. Herbs, acupuncture, and acupressure may be used in addition to or instead of western medical treatments. Living to an old age is viewed as a blessing.
- Japanese may prefer eastern medicine and traditional health practices to western medicine. The Japanese culture values self-sufficiency and self-control. Japanese view their older members with great respect.
- Traditional Koreans may employ Chinese medicine, western medicine, folk medicine, and spirituality. The older Korean adult is understood to have acquired wisdom and is regarded as an historian.
- Filipino health care practices may include faith healing and herbs. The older adult assumes a dominant role within the family structure.
- Western European countries embrace the principle of solidarity and view health as a shared responsibility on a national level.
- The European American view of older adults may have declined during the Industrial Revolution when greater emphasis was placed on physical strength. In today's information age, many view intellectual strength as superior to physical strength; older adults are regaining respect.
- The Jewish tradition recognizes two components of health: the body and the spirit. A Jewish client may decline medical procedures on the Sabbath and may observe dietary restrictions. The older adult is highly regarded.
- Health care also has a culture of its own, including language, foods, and rituals. The patient, who is a visitor to health care culture, is placed in a dependent role, stripped of clothing and power.
- Complementary and integrative therapies are becoming very popular. In the United States, herbal therapies are classified as food supplements, although many of them act in similar ways to prescription medications. Health care providers must recognize the potential for medication interactions and adverse drug effects.

STUDY QUESTIONS

Multiple-Choice Review

1. Which cultural group is considered "native" to the United States?
   1. Western Europeans
   2. American Indians
   3. Hispanics
   4. Whites
2. Which of the following is a true statement regarding culture?
   1. Culture is learned or shared.
   2. Culture is the same as ethnicity.
   3. Not all people have a culture.
   4. Culture determines exactly what a person will do when faced with illness.
3. Which of the following best describes African American older adults?
   1. They are usually cared for in long-term care facilities.
   2. They are held in high esteem by younger members of the black community.
   3. They tend to survive longer than white older adults do.
   4. They always consult faith healers before medical doctors when faced with a health problem.
4. Characteristics of health care culture include:
   1. Dress
   2. Language
   3. Customs
   4. All of the above
5. Herbal therapies
   1. Often work in similar ways to drug therapies
   2. Work by "placebo effect"
   3. Are becoming less popular in all cultures
   4. Are always dangerous

Critical Thinking

1. If, in the year 2050, whites make up less than half of the people under age 18 yet are still the majority of those over age 65, what might the sentiment of the somewhat poorer Hispanics be toward paying benefits for the relatively well-off, aging, white Baby Boomers?

2. What should you tell your older adult client who asks your advice on herbal medicines?

3. What alterations could the health care system make to create a "hospital culture" that is friendlier to outsiders?

4. Compare your own culture with the information on other cultures presented in this chapter. In what ways are your cultural practices similar to those described? In what ways are you different?

Resources

Internet Resources

Minority Aging Research Institute:
http://www.unt.edu/depts/mari/index.html

Ethnic Heritage Council: http://www.cultural.org/ehc/

Southwest School of Botanical Medicine (herbal medicine):
http://chili.rt66.com/hrbmoore/HOMEPAGE/
HomePage.html

Organizations

National Asian-Pacific Center on Aging, Melbourne Tower, 1511 Third Avenue, Suite 914, Seattle, WA 98101; telephone (206) 624-1221

National Association for Hispanic Elderly, 3325 Wilshire Boulevard, Suite 800, Los Angeles, CA 90010; telephone (213) 487-1922

National Association on Spanish Speaking Elderly, 2025 I Street NW, Suite 219, Washington, DC, 20006

National Caucus and Center on Black Aged, 1424 K Street NW, Suite 500, Washington, DC 20005; telephone (202) 637-8400

National Indian Council on Aging, 6400 Uptown Boulevard NE, Suite 510W, Albuquerque, NM 87110; telephone (505) 242-9505

Selected References

Administration on Aging (1999). Profile of Older Americans: 1999. Available at *http://www.aoa.dhhs.gov/aoa/stats/profile/ default.htm* Accessed 9/14/00.

Anding, R. (1998, May). *Herbal essence: The good, the bad, and the deadly.* National Teaching Institute and Critical Care Exposition. Symposium conducted at the meeting of the American Association of Critical Care Nurses, Los Angeles, CA.

Arsenault, S. F. (1997). Assessing the family: The importance of culture. *Critical Care Nurse, 17*(4), 96.

Beck, C., & Chumbler, N. (1997). Planning for the future of long-term care: Consumers, providers, and purchasers. *Journal of Gerontological Nursing, 23*(8), 6–12.

Burggraf, V. (2000). The older woman: Ethnicity and health. *Geriatric Nursing, 21*(4), 183–187.

Devine, N. (1999). Dangerous combinations: Understanding the risks of mixing herbal products and drugs. *Nurseweek, 13*(8), 26.

Eliopoulos, C. (1997). *Gerontological nursing.* Philadelphia: Lippincott.

Evans, L. K. (1997). Trends in aging care in Scotland and Scandinavia. *Journal of Gerontological Nursing, 23*(9), 32–36.

Gorman, C. (1998). Is it good medicine? *Time, 152*(21), 69.

Greenwald, J. (1998). Herbal healing. *Time, 152*(21), 59–67.

Jan, R., & Smith, C. A. (1998). Staying healthy in immigrant Pakistani families living in the United States. *Image: Journal of Nursing Scholarship, 30*(2), 157–159.

Lee, H. (1997). Typical and atypical clinical signs and symptoms of myocardial infarction and delayed seeking of professional care among blacks. *American Journal of Critical Care, 6*(1), 7–13.

Lee, H., Kim, S., & Kwang-Su, Y. (1997). Learning from other lands: Caring for elderly demented Koreans. *Journal of Gerontological Nursing, 23*(9), 21–30.

Marek, K. D., Rantz, M. J., Fagin, C. M., & Krejci, J. W. (1996). OBRA '87: Has it resulted in positive change in nursing homes? *Journal of Gerontological Nursing, 22*(12), 32–40.

McEnany, G. (2000). Herbal psychotropics. Part 3: Focus on kava, valerian, and melatonin. *Journal of American Psychiatric Nurses Association, 6*(4), 126–130.

Murashima, S., Zerwekh, J. V., Yamada, M., & Tagami, Y. (1998). Around-the-clock nursing care for the elderly in Japan. *Image: Journal of Nursing Scholarship, 30*(1), 37–41.

National Center for Policy Analysis Idea House. *Social Policy: Census Bureau Projections Suggest Ethnic Shift.* Available at http://www.public-policy.org/~ncpa/pd/social/sociala.html

National Center for Policy Analysis Idea House. *Social Policy: Life Expectancy Increasing.* Available at http://www.public-policy.org/~ncpa/pd/social/socsep97d.html

Oldendick, R., Coker, A., Weiland, D., Raymond, J. I., Probst, J. C., Schell, B. J. & Stoskopf, C. H. (2000). Population-based survey of complementary and alternative medicine usage, patient satisfaction, and physician involvement. *Southern Medical Journal, 93*(4), 375–381.

O'Neil, C. K., Avila, J. R., & Fetrow, C. W. (1999). Herbal medicines: Getting beyond the hype. *Nursing 99, 29*(4), 58–61.

Reuters Medical News (2000). St. John's Wort may interact with cyclosporin to cause heart transplant rejection. Available at http://www.medscape.com/reuters/prof/2000/02/02.16/cl02160c.html Accessed 2/17/00.

Saunders Manual of Nursing Care. (1997). Philadelphia: W. B. Saunders.

Schiavenato, M. (1997). The Hispanic elderly: Implications for nursing care. *Journal of Gerontological Nursing, 23*(6), 10–15.

Spector, R. E. (1996). *Cultural diversity in health and illness.* Stamford, CT: Appleton & Lange.

Talsma, A., & Abraham, I. L. (1997). Nursing and health care for an aging society: The case of the Netherlands. *Journal of Gerontological Nursing, 23*(9), 37–44.

Tom-Orme, L. (1998). Waters running deep. *Reflections, 24*(2), 22–23.

U.S. Census Bureau Statistical Brief. *Sixty-Five Plus in the United States.* Available at http://www.census.govftp/pub/socdemo/www/agebrief. html

Wong, F. K. Y. (1998). The integration of traditional Chinese health practices in nursing. *Reflections, 24*(2), 20–21.

Zerwekh, J., & Claborn, J. A. (2000). *Nursing today: Transitions and trends.* Philadelphia: W. B. Saunders.

Promoting a Safe Care Environment

CARING FOR THE OLDER ADULT
    UNDERGOING A SURGICAL
    PROCEDURE
    Preoperative Phase
    Intraoperative Phase
    Postoperative Phase

PREVENTING FALLS IN THE OLDER
    ADULT
    Assessment of Risk for Falls
    Prevention of Falls

KEY TERMS

Absorption	Hyperthermia
Activities of daily living	Hypothermia
Adverse drug reactions	Metabolism
Assisted living	Noncompliance
Atypical presentation	Pharmacodynamics
Clinical pathways	Pharmacokinetics
Distribution	Polypharmacy
Drug toxicity	Protein binding
Excretion	Rehabilitative techniques
Half-life	Skilled nursing facilities
Home care	Typical presentation

CARE OF THE OLDER ADULT IN VARIOUS SETTINGS

Older adults receive nursing care in numerous settings, including acute care, subacute care, long-term care, and home care. In each of these settings, the older adult requires specific medical and nursing interventions that are important for his or her recovery. It is important that you view every older adult client as a unique individual and not merely, for example, "the pneumonia in room 202." In each of the following settings, you must provide appropriate care for the older adult, while ensuring a safe care environment.

Acute Care Environment

The acute care, or hospital, environment can be a stressful place for the older adult. Often the situation that led up to hospitalization was an accident or injury, or an illness that became too difficult to manage at home. Sometimes you will encounter an older adult who is experiencing his or her first hospital stay. You might find such a person to appear bewildered and frightened. Other times, your client will have been hospitalized numerous times owing to chronic illnesses, and will be somewhat used to the hospital routine and expectations. Thus, different older adults have different nursing care needs.

Pretend for a moment that you are a 70-year-old woman with diabetes mellitus on your first hospital stay. You were rushed to the hospital late last night with a diagnosis of pneumonia. You are exhausted because you had to wait in the emergency department until 2:00 AM before a bed could be assigned to you. Once in bed, you slept fitfully for a few hours, but nurses kept coming into and out of your room, asking if you were all right, over and over again. Why were they so worried? They pricked your finger every 4 hours but they never explained why. After each prick, the nurse gave you another injection of insulin. You have never taken so much insulin before. Every 4 hours the nurse came in and put her cold stethoscope on your back and told you to take several deep breaths, but it hurt to take deep breaths. You have a tube jabbing into your right wrist, and your wrist is stiffening up from your arthritis. Your back hurts because the mattress is thin; you have a bad back, and no bed is as comfortable as your bed at home anyway. You were awakened by a phlebotomist taking blood with a steel needle—some kind of heart test. How can they tell anything about your heart from your blood? Nobody explains things. This morning you needed a portable chest x-ray. The technician and the nurse helped position you onto a hard, cold plate behind your back, then asked you to take *another* deep breath. Later in the morning, you were wheeled to another department for some more tests. You froze as the chilly hospital air breezed through your thin hospital gown. You felt groggy from the medications being pumped into your veins. Later in the day, you had a visitor before you even had a chance to comb your hair and apply lipstick. Based on the look on the visitor's face, you must look terrible. You're scared because nobody has told you exactly what is going on.

Such a scenario is not as unusual as you might think. From the older adult's perspective, the hospital can be a very frightening, impersonal place that is insensitive to his or her needs.

Proper nursing and medical care of an older adult may include numerous types of interventions. Different disciplines may be involved, such as respiratory therapy, physical therapy, and occupational therapy. The older adult may have intravenous lines, including central venous lines, and may require frequent laboratory work and assessments.

The hospital routine is busy; interventions and treatments occur on a round-the-clock basis. This can be detrimental to the older adult in numerous ways: quality sleep can be difficult to achieve; the mix of medications or electrolyte imbalances can leave the older adult confused; and staff members can seem too busy to take the extra time needed to assist an older person who needs help with **activities of daily living** (ADL). The hospital setting can provide limited space and privacy, unusual noises and odors, and sensory overload. In the acute care setting, the primary objective is to get the medical condition resolved. Sometimes other priorities, such as letting the older adult perform his own ADL, seem less important. Ask yourself,

though, Have you really done your older adult client a service if, upon discharge, the pneumonia is "fixed," but the older adult is no longer able to ambulate? In other words, the nurse must keep in mind the big picture and incorporate **rehabilitative techniques** into the acute care environment. It is just as important to ambulate the older adult as it is to give the antibiotic on time.

Health Promotion Tip

Health promotion in the acute care setting:

- Interview the older adult (or speak with usual caregiver, if applicable) to find out his or her usual self-care abilities.
- Encourage the older adult to perform all ADL possible, taking extra time if needed.
- Inquire about usual dietary preferences and communicate these to the kitchen to facilitate optimal nutrition.
- On every shift, encourage physical activity that is tailored to the medical disorder and the physician orders.

In developing a care plan for older adults, it is important that you consider *their* priorities and preferences, as well as your own. Findings from a recent pilot study of older adults suggest that humanistic caring was one of the most important required components of good nursing care, surpassed only by technical competence (Marini, 1999). Another study was done that compared older adults' perceptions about the importance of specific nursing activities with nurses' perceptions of the same activities (Hudson & Sexton, 1996). A list of 50 activities was given to recently hospitalized older adults and practicing medical-surgical nurses. People participating in the study were asked to rank each activity in order of importance, from 1 to 50. Activities included items such as "see that the bedpan or urinal is provided when needed," "relieve my anxiety by explaining reasons for my symptoms," "assist me with meals," and "see that the unit is clean and tidy," along with 46 others. The results of the study are very illuminating. On some items both groups more or less agreed on the relative importance of the activity; for example, both groups rated pain management as high and recreation as low. However, in terms of other activities, there were striking differences, which can be explained in two ways. First, the older adult may not understand the importance or the extent of the nurse's responsibility with items ranked higher by nurses and lower by older adults. Second, when certain items are ranked very high by the older adults but much lower by the nurses, perhaps the nurses underestimate the importance of these interventions in the eyes of the older adult. Maybe the significance in calming a frightened older adult is underestimated. Likewise, even though housekeeping isn't necessarily the job of the nursing staff, an untidy nursing unit reflects poorly on nurses, whether they realize it or not. See Figure 3–1 for differences in rankings between nurses and older adults.

Chronically ill older adults who are discharged home have a high rate of hospital readmission when they do not have adequate support at home. Nurses need to encourage family members of hospitalized older adults to seek and use social support services that are offered.

Subacute Unit

Since the late 1980s, subacute care units, which provide a cost-effective alterntive to acute care, have sprung up all over the country. The subacute unit can be viewed as a bridge between acute care and long-term care. Most subacute units are located in freestanding **skilled nursing facilities;**

TOP 10 ISSUES AS RANKED BY ELDERS

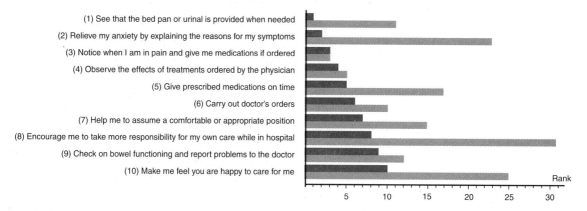

TOP 10 ISSUES AS RANKED BY NURSES

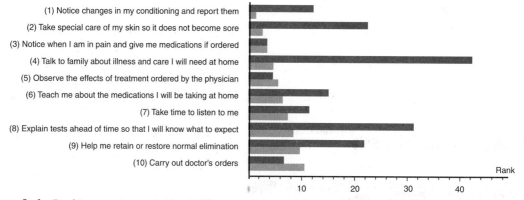

Figure 3–1. Ranking nursing activities. Differences between the results as ranked by nurses and by older adults. (From Hudson, K. A., & Sexton, D. L. [1996]. Perceptions about nursing care: Comparing elders' and nurses' priorities. *Journal of Gerontological Nursing, 22*[12], 41–46.)

others are former hospital units that have been reclassified to provide subacute care. Subacute units offer a stronger rehabilitative focus and a shorter length of stay than long-term care. The level of care provided in subacute units is nearly of the same intensity as that in an acute care hospital. In fact, the typical older adult found in a subacute unit today is comparable to the typical medical-surgical client of the 1980s.

How is this happening? It is a combination of our increased life span and changes in hospital reimbursement procedures. Modern medicine is saving lives that, prior to technological advances, were unable to be saved. This has led to a ripple effect: those people who would not have survived before these technological advances are now occupying beds in the intensive care unit (ICU). People who used to occupy the ICU beds can be found on the medical-surgical floor. Those who used to occupy beds on the medical-surgical floor are now discharged out of the hospital—but often their problems are too complex for care in the home, hence, the evolution of the subacute unit.

Since the inception of diagnosis-related groups (DRGs) (see Chapter 1), a client's hospital time may be limited because of limitations in reimbursement. These strict DRG reimbursement rules for acute care do not, however, apply to subacute care that is provided in a skilled nursing facility setting. Cost savings are an important reason for the growth of subacute care: average cost savings per day are estimated to be 40% to 60% when subacute care costs are compared with those in the hospital setting.

Older adults with numerous disorders can be found on subacute units. Clients can receive many different therapies, including intravenous medication administration via peripheral or central venous catheters, complex dressing changes, even mechanical ventilation. The four most common client care needs in subacute care are physical rehabilitation, stroke rehabilitation, wound care, and recovery from hip fracture. The nurse employed in a subacute unit must have a variety of assessment, rehabilitative, medical-surgical, and leadership skills. One must have the assessment and technical skills of a medical-surgical nurse, along with the knowledge of the Omnibus Reconciliation Acts (OBRAs) and the interdisciplinary team skills of a long-term care nurse.

Health Promotion Tip

Health promotion in the subacute setting:

- Set specific goals with older adult clients to increase their level of self-care; add this to the care plan
- Encourage older adults to perform all ADL.
- Communicate dietary preferences to the kitchen.
- With older adult clients, set progressive physical activity goals that are tailored to the medical disorder and the physician orders.

Long-Term Care Environment

Care of the older adult in a long-term care environment is required when the older adult needs help meeting everyday needs. Long-term care facilities are also known as nursing homes or extended-care facilities. Because the long-term care facility becomes a home for the older adult, on either a long-term or a short-term basis, the older adult is referred to as a *resident* rather than a *client*.

The enactment of OBRA in 1987 led to the requirement that long-term care facilities must use greater numbers of licensed nursing staff. This created greater opportunities for employment for the licensed practical nurse/licensed vocational nurse (LPN/LVN). Other aspects of the OBRA law helped expand the role of the practical/vocational nurse to include areas such as intravenous therapy and leadership/management responsibilities. The leadership role of the LPN/LVN is discussed in Chapter 15.

Generally, two categories of residents are found in a long-term care facility. The first category is the short-term, sometimes called short-stay, resident. Typically, this type of resident has been transferred from an acute care facility to which they had been admitted for an acute illness or the worsening of a chronic illness. The resident is admitted to long-term care principally for rehabilitation and is expected to be discharged within 6 months. There are many similarities between this type of resident and the resident of a subacute unit. The second category is the long-term resident. This is the traditional resident who lives in the facility until he or she dies or is transferred to an acute care facility. This resident may have numerous nursing care needs and may be cognitively impaired. Most residents in the typical long-term care facility are of the traditional category described, although the current trend is to admit more short-term residents. As a result, the overall nursing care needs of long-term care residents have become more complex in recent years.

Health Promotion Tip

Health promotion in the long-term care setting:

- Review data obtained from the Minimum Data Set (MDS) assessment form, specifically information regarding activity level and nutrition.
- Set specific goals with the older adult regarding activity and nutrition, and document these in the Interdisciplinary Care Plan.
- Identify environmental modifications and assistive devices needed to maximize independence for the older adult.
- Identify and eliminate hazards in the environment.
- Encourage preventive measures (such as pneumovax immunization) to avoid the development of complications.

Table 3–1 provides information on the characteristics of nursing home residents.

In recent years, there has been a drop in the proportion of older adults entering long-term care facilities; this is mostly a result of both other care alternatives, such as **assisted living** and **home care**, and our improved health status. There are fewer but larger nursing homes today. Providing care for an older adult in the home is

Table 3–1	
CHARACTERISTICS OF NURSING HOME RESIDENTS	
Older adults residing in U.S. nursing homes	1.4 million
Average age on admission (yrs)	82
Percentage needing help with bathing or showering	96
Most frequent admission diagnosis	Disease of the circulatory system

Source: Americans Less Likely to Use Nursing Home Care Today. Press release Jan. 23, 1997. US Department of Health and Human Services. Available at http://www.cdc.gov/nchswww/releases/97news/97/news/nurshome.htm Accessed 8/16/98.

less expensive than care offered in a long-term care facility, unless the older adult has a high degree of physical impairment (Lee, 2000).

Home Care Environment

Although, as in the previous section, the term "long-term care" is often used interchangeably with "nursing home," the truth is that many older adults receive long-term care at home. The older adult receiving care at home receives a great deal of this care from family members, such as adult children or a spouse, as well as from organized sources such as visiting nurses. The typical older adult receiving home care services is female, is older than 75 years of age, and requires assistance only when bathing or showering; however, home care clients can receive complex medical therapies such as mechanical ventilation and kidney dialysis.

Care of the older adult at home may involve a great deal of participation from loved ones. Older women may be caring for older family members (such as a spouse), as well as children, grandchildren, and great-grandchildren in multigenerational households. Without the support of the family unit in care of the older adult, admissions into long-term care facilities would undoubtedly increase, perhaps tripling. In addition, caring for the older adult at home costs about half the cost of care in a long-term care setting.

The typical caregiver at home is a female over the age of 65 who does not use formal health care services. Nurses need to recognize this important core of care for older members of the community, advocate for services to help these families continue to provide this vital function, and educate those who are not using community services about the existence and specifics of such programs. Important services to help family members care for older adults at home are outlined in Box 3–1.

The numbers of both long-term care residents and home care clients are expected to increase over the next 20 years. However, the need for home care services is expected to increase two to three times over the need for long-term care (Fig. 3–2).

In Chapter 1, we discussed legislation affecting care of the older adult. Recall that OBRA 1981, which removed certain restrictions for home care

Box 3–1 — **Services for Those Caring for Older Adults at Home**

- *Respite Care*: Scheduled stays for the older adult needing care at a long-term care facility (e.g., 1 week every 4 months) to give "time off" to caregiver and older adult with needs
- *Day Care*: A setting that provides structured activities during the day, similar to day care for children
- *Home Health Assistance*: Assistance with ADLs (provided by a Home Health Aide) or with nursing care (provided by a Home Health Nurse)
- *Nutrition Programs*: Congregate meals (at Senior Center) or home delivery of one hot meal per day (Meals on Wheels) for a nominal fee
- *Senior Centers*: Government-funded centers that provide recreational activities, lunch, health screening, classes, and transportation to and from the site if needed
- *Transportation services*: Dial-a-ride service for transporting clients to grocery shopping or medical appointments

recipients, led to rapid growth in the home care industry. As shown in Figure 3–2, this growth is expected to continue. Until recently, home care has always had a cost-reimbursement system in place, much as hospitals did before the enactment of TEFRA (see Chapter 1). A new system of care reimbursement has been enacted, called the interim payment system, that sets strict limits on payment rates. The challenge for home care agencies under the new system is to save money while not sacrificing client care. Agencies use various strategies such as educating staff about the system, using clinical pathways, and implementing team conferences and case managers to help coordinate and ensure safe client care. The implication of this new system for the LPN/LVN is that some agencies are using more LPN/LVNs as a high-quality, lower cost care alternative than registered nurses (RNs) for stable home clients.

Because of the recent shift in all areas of health care reimbursement to prospective payment, it is more important than ever for nurses to encourage maintenance of health and prevention of illness, in other words, to practice health promotion. Nurses in the home setting are in a key position to teach health promotion strategies.

 Health Promotion Tip

Health promotion in the home setting:

- Identify educational needs and provide older adult with appropriate resources.
- Set specific goals with older adult regarding activity and nutrition.
- Identify environmental modifications needed in the home to maximize independence for the older adult.
- Discuss preventive care strategies (such as immunizations and health screenings) related to the older adult's health history.
- Encourage participation in programs related to fitness, smoking cessation, and stress management, as appropriate.

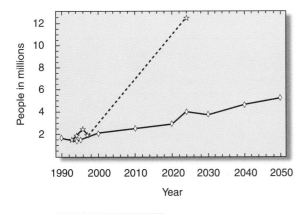

Figure 3–2. Projected long-term care and home care needs. (Data from Centers for Disease Control, National Center for Health Statistics, Atlanta, 1997.)

PROMOTING SAFE MEDICATION USE IN THE OLDER ADULT

Most people over age 65 have at least one chronic illness; therefore, the typical older adult takes some form of prescription medication

Table 3–2
COMMON MEDICATIONS USED BY OLDER ADULTS

Classification	Common Example
Antacids	aluminum carbonate with magnesium (Maalox)
Antiarrhythmics	digoxin (Lanoxin)
Anticoagulants	warfarin (Coumadin)
Antidiabetics	glipizide (Glucotrol)
Antiglaucoma agents	timolol (Timoptic)
Antihyperlidipemics	lovastatin (Mevacor)
Antihypertensives	captopril (Capoten)
Beta-adrenergic blockers	metoprolol (Lopressor)
Bronchodilators	ipratropium bromide (Atrovent)
Calcium channel blockers	nifedipine (Procardia)
Diuretics	furosemide (Lasix)
H2 antagonists	famotidine (Pepcid)
Laxatives	magnesium hydroxide (milk of magnesia)
Nitrates	isosorbide (Isordil)
Nonsteroidal anti-inflammatory drugs (NSAIDs)	ibuprofen (Motrin)
Sedative-hypnotics	zolpidem (Ambien)

regularly. With aging, the body responds differently to medications. Metabolism slows down and drugs are processed more slowly than in younger adults. Nurses must understand how medications affect older adults differently in order to promote safe medication use by this population. Common medications used by older adults can be found in Table 3–2.

Before discussing medication management with the older adult, it is important that you examine both the **pharmacokinetics** and the **pharmacodynamics** of the drugs. Pharmacokinetics refers to how the drug is used by the body. It involves four phases: absorption, distribution, metabolism, and excretion. Pharmacodynamics refers to the effect the medication has on the body, including drug actions and drug effects (Box 3–2).

Aging is associated with changes in pharmacokinetics and pharmacodynamics; these are briefly discussed in the following paragraphs, along with pertinent nursing implications.

Age-Related Changes in Pharmacokinetics

Absorption

Absorption is the passage of the medication into the body's bloodstream. With aging, the stomach contents become more alkaline, leading to an increase in their pH value. This change may affect the effectiveness of oral medications, which require an acidic (low pH) environment for proper absorption. In addition, blood flow to the intestinal tract is slowed, as is motility. The effect of these

---

✎ Box 3–2   Pharmacodynamics

Drug Actions

- *Depression*: lessened activity or function of a body part
- *Stimulation*: increased activity or function of a body part
- *Irritation*: drugs that produce irritation at site of administration
- *Demulcence*: soothing at the site of administration

Drug Effects

- *Cumulation*: drugs that remain in the body to toxic levels
- *Addition or summation*: drugs that produce additive effects to one another to a limited degree
- *Synergism or potentiation*: drugs that produce additive effects to one another to a greater degree than addition or summation
- *Antagonism*: when one drug counteracts the effects of another drug

- *Tolerance*: when drug effects on the body are lessened owing to prolonged exposure to the drug
- *Adverse reaction*: unpleasant or harmful effect of a drug; not the intended effect
- *Anaphylaxis*: medical emergency caused by an extreme hypersensitivity to a drug
- *Idiosyncratic or paradoxical effect*: a response to a drug that is not what was intended; can be the opposite of the desired effect
- *Addiction*: physiologic and emotional dependence upon a substance

Sites of Action

- *Local*: drugs producing their actions and effects where they are applied
- *Systemic*: drugs that are absorbed into the bloodstream and have effects throughout the body

age-related changes is that drugs may be absorbed more slowly in the older adult than in the younger adult. Likewise, if a medication is given via injection, whether intramuscularly, subcutaneously, or intravenously, absorption can be slowed down in older adults owing to less efficient circulation.

Nursing Implications. As a result of these metabolic changes, it may take a surprisingly long time before the desired effects of a particular medication are seen in an older adult. It is important not to overreact and overmedicate the client. For example, if you give your older adult client acetaminophen because he or she is complaining of a headache, it might take 30 minutes or longer before the client feels any therapeutic effect. Likewise, it is important to administer medications on time. Imagine the consequences of giving your client's pain medication late, then knowing its therapeutic effect may be delayed.

Medication Safety Tip

REMEMBER: It is very important to administer medications to the older adult on time because of age-related changes in absorption.

Distribution

Distribution of a medication refers to how it spreads throughout the body via the circulatory system and how it arrives at its desired location. The amount of drug in the bloodstream that can have an effect on the body depends partly on the amount of protein in the bloodstream. This is because part of the drug travels freely in the blood and part of the drug is bound to protein in the blood, primarily albumin. Some medications, such as digoxin and warfarin, bind very tightly to protein; others are less protein-bound. **Protein binding** is important for three reasons:

1. The unbound or free part of the drug is the part that produces effects.
2. Many older adults have decreased albumin levels, which means there is less protein for the drug to bind with; therefore, the effects of the drug will be greater.
3. If the albumin level is decreased, then older adults can experience toxic effects from a drug even though the blood level is within the normal range.

Distribution can also be affected by blood flow and body composition. If an older adult's circulation is impaired, distribution of a drug to sites throughout the body will be slower. With aging, there is lower total body water and an increase in body fat. Some medications are lipophilic, or stored in fat tissues. With increased body fat, medications can have a sustained-release effect and remain in the body of an older adult longer than usual. Some drugs, such as antianxiety or antipsychotic medications, can even take weeks or months before they completely leave the body.

Nursing Implications. It is important to remember that the effects of a medication can last longer in an older adult. Monitor closely for **drug toxicity**: assess the client, not just the blood level. Be especially careful in administering prn (as needed) pain medications to an older adult; remember the saying regarding dosages, "Start low and go slow." Adverse reactions to a medication can be seen even after a drug has been discontinued.

Medication Safety Tip

The older adult who is malnourished or dehydrated can have greater drug concentrations in the bloodstream.

Metabolism

Metabolism, also called biotransformation, is the process by which the drug is detoxified, or turned into harmless substances. This process occurs primarily in the liver. Drug metabolism is measured by a term called **half-life,** the time it takes for the body to inactivate half of the medication. Because liver size and blood flow normally decrease with aging, the process can take longer in an older adult, leading to a longer drug half-life and longer lasting effects.

Nursing Implications. Drugs last longer in older adults. Because of age-related changes in metabolism, a little goes a long way.

Medication Safety Tip

Drug half-life can be even more prolonged in an older adult who has impaired liver function.

Excretion

Excretion is the process of eliminating the drug from the body, usually by way of the kidneys. This process can be slowed down by age-related reductions in kidney blood flow and function. For example, a dose of diazepam (Valium) may take 20 hours to be excreted in a young adult, but up to 90 hours in an older adult, and even longer if you consider the metabolites of the drug that are stored in fat tissue.

Nursing Implications. Many drugs are prescribed in lower dosages for older adults because of decreased excretion rates. Always check dosages carefully and question the physician if the dosage is greater than that recommended in your drug handbook.

Medication Safety Tip

Drug excretion can be further decreased when an older adult is on multiple medications.

Age-Related Changes in Pharmacodynamics

Medications can have unusual effects on the older adult, including the following:

- *Increased sensitivity:* The older adult can be more sensitive to a drug; for example, older adults are more sensitive to diazepam (Valium) and related drugs that affect the central nervous system.

Medication Safety Tip

Greater central nervous system effects of drugs can place the older adult at risk for falls and other injuries.

- *Decreased sensitivity:* The older adult can be less sensitive to certain drugs, such as a group of cardiac medications called beta-blockers.
- *Adverse drug reactions:* The older adult is more prone to adverse drug reactions. In addition, these are not always the typical adverse reactions associated with a drug; they can even arise after a drug has been discontinued.

Nursing Implications. It is very important that the nurse monitor the older adult's response to medication and document it carefully in the chart. Report all adverse reactions immediately.

POLYPHARMACY AND THE OLDER ADULT

Most older adults take between one and six prescription medications. The typical older woman takes more than five prescription medications and three over-the-counter (OTC) medications concurrently. **Polypharmacy** is a term that refers to this concept of taking several medications in the same time period. Although many authors have written about polypharmacy, not everyone agrees on exactly how many medications being consumed constitutes polypharmacy; some define it as anything more than *one* drug. Another definition of polypharmacy is simply taking more medications than are needed, regardless of the exact number. In other words, according to this definition, if an older adult takes only one medication, but that medication is unnecessary, then this would be considered polypharmacy. In addition, many older adults add to their complex regimen OTC and herbal products, which can interact with medications.

Dangers of Polypharmacy

When multiple medications are taken, although each medication is usually prescribed for a good reason, the combination of drugs can have unexpected effects in the older adult because of the additive or synergistic effects of medications (see Box 3–2). In addition, adverse drug reactions are more likely to occur when multiple medications are being taken.

Polypharmacy can also lead to unnecessary expense for the older adult because many health plans do not pay for the cost of medications. This expense can result in a medication being used intermittently rather than according to schedule. Other risks of polypharmacy include increased incidence of depression, decreased mental status, and decreased social activity. It has even been found to be a risk factor for placement in a long-term care facility.

Adverse Drug Reactions

An adverse drug reaction is any unintended or unpleasant side effect of a medication. Adverse drug reactions occur three times more frequently in older adults than in younger persons. Drug-related problems have been estimated to account for up to nearly one quarter of all hospital admissions by older adults and are frequently the cause of incorrect diagnosis. Although all medications undergo rigorous testing before becoming FDA approved in the United States, most drugs are not tested on older adults. The older adult may react differently to the medication than a younger person, and he or she may experience more extreme or even dangerous side effects.

Adverse drug reactions are more common in older adults, in part, because of the age-related changes in pharmacokinetics and pharmacodynamics discussed earlier. Because drugs are present in the body for a greater length of time, they have a greater opportunity to produce an adverse effect. Another reason for the increased incidence of adverse drug reactions among the elderly is the fact that many older adults are taking more than one medication. As the number of drugs being taken increases, so does the likelihood of adverse reactions. Risk factors for adverse drug reactions in the older adult are outlined in Box 3–3.

Signs and symptoms of adverse drug reactions are not always easy to detect in an older adult. Signs that can be mistaken for other disorders

Table 3–3
FACTORS LEADING TO UNDERUSE OR ERRATIC USE OF MEDICATIONS AMONG OLDER ADULTS

Factors	Rationale
Loss of manual strength Decreased dexterity	Older adult may be unable to open "childproof" containers
Visual changes from aging	Small typeface on prescription label may be misread
Memory deficits	Complex medication regimen may be difficult to remember; polypharmacy can cause confusion
Knowledge deficit	Older adult may be unaware of importance of taking medication according to exact schedule
Cultural values	Older adult may have cultural bias about medications not shared with caregivers
Financial concerns	Medications may be skipped or schedule altered owing to expense of the medications

include loss of balance, falls, incontinence, and change in bowel habits; symptoms can include confusion or nausea. Because these signs and symptoms are so common to many disorders, any of these can easily be mistaken for an illness—and lead to yet more drugs being prescribed.

MEDICATION USE AND ABUSE

It has been estimated that up to half of older adults misuse medications. However, not all medication abuse is intentional. Some factors that can lead to medication misuse include a regimen that includes a large number of medications, complex medication schedules, and knowledge deficit regarding medications. Factors that can lead to underuse or erratic use of medications are outlined in Table 3–3.

Noncompliance occurs when a client does not follow the recommendations of the health care team. This term may be used to describe a client who is not taking the medications recommended by the physician. Sometimes an older adult may not take the medications for a logical reason, such as wanting to avoid side effects, or because it is too expensive. The older adult may not always share this information with the physician. Problems may occur, however, when the older adult becomes hospitalized and is administered

---

Box 3–3	**Risk Factors for Adverse Drug Reactions**

- Presence of multiple diseases
- Poor health status
- Polypharmacy
- Previous history of adverse drug reaction
- Age-related changes in pharmacokinetics and pharmacodynamics
- Fragmented medical care
- Medication errors

Data from Matteson, M. A., McConnell, E. S., & Linton, A. D. (1998). *Gerontological nursing: Concepts and practice* (2nd Ed.). Philadelphia: W. B. Saunders.

what is thought to be his regular medication regimen. At this point, adverse drug reactions or signs of drug toxicity may occur. In such a circumstance, you must be especially vigilant in assessing for adverse drug reactions.

Medication overuse may occur if an older adult visits more than one physician and neglects (or forgets) to inform the doctors of medications already being taken. Overuse of medications can be deliberate, for example, if the older adult believes that more of the drug will provide a greater benefit. It can also be accidental, however, in a forgetful individual. Serious consequences can occur in older adults who overuse medications.

Sometimes an older adult may have a difficult time coping with the changes of aging or the death of loved ones and may turn to medications for escape. Drug abuse occurs any time an individual uses a drug for other than its intended purpose or exceeds the recommended dosage. Although it is virtually unheard of for an older adult to abuse street drugs such as opiates or stimulants, prescription medications are often abused. Older adults may hoard medications for later use, avoid taking scheduled medications if they do not have symptoms, and consume higher than recommended dosages when they do feel the need to self-medicate. Among the most commonly abused prescription medications are benzodiazepines (such as Valium) and products containing codeine.

Over-the-counter (OTC) medications commonly overused by older adults include laxatives, analgesics, sleep medications, and combination preparations containing alcohol, caffeine, and antihistamines. These can interact with other prescription and nonprescription medications being taken by the older adult. It is possible for clients to develop magnesium toxicity and coma from long-term consumption of large doses of milk of magnesia.

Medication overuse can result in physical and psychological dependence. Consequences can range from life-threatening complications, such as magnesium-induced coma, to less obvious effects, such as decreased physical activity and muscle atrophy. Even decreased physical activity is a significant concern because the individual will be at greater risk for the complications of immobility. Activity and rest will be further discussed in Chapter 5.

STRATEGIES TO ASSIST OLDER ADULTS WITH SAFE MEDICATION USE

As an LPN/LVN, you should assist the older adult to use medications safely. An important part of this effort is to educate your client on the purpose of each of the medications they are taking. Many older adults are prescribed more than one medication, which increases the chance that a mistake in self-administering medication may occur. Strategies that can promote the safe use of medications by the older adult are depicted in Figure 3–3.

As an LPN/LVN, you may encounter some older adults who are unwilling or uninterested in taking an active role in learning about medications. Older adults grew up during a time when it was not expected that an individual would take an active role in managing his or her health care, let alone question the doctor. Health promotion, however, implies that individuals take responsibility for their own health, which includes learning about medications and treatments that affect them. Encouraging this self-responsibility in your older adult clients ultimately helps them achieve a higher level of wellness.

RECOGNIZING COMMON DISORDERS IN OLDER ADULTS

An important part of caring for the older adult involves the ability to recognize and interpret the normal signs of aging and distinguish them from disorders that an older adult may experience. Assessment is the first and most important step of the nursing process. A thorough assessment provides the foundation on which nursing interventions can be planned.

It is important to discuss assessment specific to the older adult for the following reasons. First, certain normal changes of aging require a different approach in assessment of the older adult for accurate assessment data to be obtained. Second, patience and a longer time frame may be required to assess the older adult. Third, and most importantly, many illnesses have unusual signs and symptoms in an older adult. These signs and symptoms can be vague or even *absent*; therefore, determining what is wrong with the older adult can involve a fair

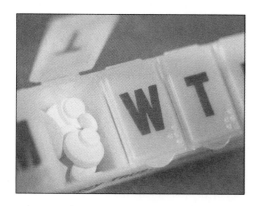

Pill Dispensing Box

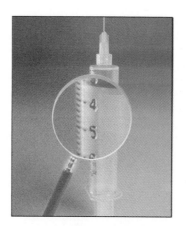

Magnifying Glass

MARCH						
Sun	Mon	Tues	Wed	Thurs	Fri	Sat
				1	2	3
4	5	6	7	8	9	10
11	12	13	14	15	16	17
18	19	20	21	22	23	24
25	26	27	28	29	30	31

Calendars

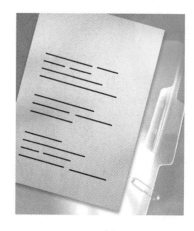

Medication List

Figure 3–3. Strategies to improve medication safety.

degree of detective work. These unusual signs and symptoms are called **atypical presentation**, or atypical illness presentation, or nonspecific disease presentation.

Although assessment and normal changes of aging specific to various body systems are discussed in detail in future chapters, the following is an overview of assessment of the older adult.

ASSESSMENT OF THE OLDER ADULT

An accurate initial assessment is crucial to care planning for the older adult in any setting.

Although the primary responsibility for the assessment lies with the RN, the LPN/LVN gathers much of the information needed for a complete and accurate assessment. Your skilled assessment will allow you and the RN to formulate the best plan of care for the older adult.

Allow adequate time for a thorough assessment. Take time to develop a comfortable rapport. Sometimes a novice examiner experiences tunnel vision in which he or she is so completely focused on a task (such as blood pressure measurement) that the big picture is overlooked. This often happens when the examiner is nervous, anxious, or overly tired, or is working too fast.

Assessment begins with observation. Before you even reach for your stethoscope, take a good look at the older adult. Observe posture, observe the client walking. Does he or she stand erect and tall? Is the client's gait smooth? Is movement symmetrical and fluid? Do you notice any tremors? When you ask questions, does the client seem to understand your questions and respond with pertinent answers in a timely manner? Does the client ask you to repeat information?

Physical Examination

The physical examination part of the assessment usually begins with the measurement of vital signs. Normal ranges of vital signs for the older adult can be found in Table 3–4. The normal temperature for an older adult can be lower than that of a young adult. Although it is considered normal for one's systolic blood pressure to increase somewhat with age, the normal range remains the same as that for young adults.

After the measurement of vital signs, follow a head-to-toe direction for the assessment. Begin with the head, observe the eyes, ears, and mouth of the older adult. Notice any discharge, erythema (redness), or edema. Inspect the mouth and teeth. If the older adult has dentures, ask him or her to take them out. Inspect the gums and lips for swelling, cracking, or ulcerations. Cracking or ulcerations can indicate nutritional deficiencies; swelling can be a sign of ill-fitting dentures. Inspect the dentures. Also inspect the scalp of the older adult for flaking, dryness, or lesions. Assess the neck; gently determine range of motion and the presence or absence of neck pain or tenderness. Hypertrophy, or overdevelopment, of neck muscles may indicate lung disease.

Assess the level of orientation of the older adult. It is important to determine if the client is oriented to person, place, and time. An assessment tool such as the Mini Mental State Examination (MMSE) (Appendix A) may be used. Neurologic assessment is discussed in greater detail in Chapter 11.

Next, examine the chest area and upper back. It is normal with age for the thorax to take on a more rounded, or barrel-chest, appearance. Auscultate the heart and lungs with your stethoscope. Lung sounds are best heard from the back of the client, although the right middle lobe must be auscultated from the anterior or lateral aspect of the chest. Although most assessment books advise that auscultation begin at the top of the lungs (apices) and move to the bottom (base), you may get better assessment data with the older adult by doing the opposite. Beginning at the bases allows the older adult to generate his or her best respiratory effort to your instructions to take a deep breath. After four or five deep breaths, the older adult is often beginning to fatigue, and subsequent deep breaths may be less deep than the first ones; if you begin at the apices, you may merely hear and chart diminished bases, when, in fact, there could be abnormal lung sounds present. Next, auscultate heart sounds anteriorly. Instruct your client that he or she may now breathe normally. You may find the apical pulse difficult to locate because of the barrel-shaped chest. Heart sounds may be easier to hear in the client's lower left chest area. After auscultation of heart sounds is completed, the older adult will be ready to again provide deep enough breaths to allow auscultation of breath sounds from the anterior chest.

Observe the arms, looking for edema or bruising. Bruising may be observed if the client is taking certain medications, such as aspirin or prednisone, but it can also be a sign of elder abuse. You may note decreased muscle tone. Test strength by asking the older adult to move his or her arm against your resistance. Assess range of motion of shoulders, elbow joints, and hands. Listen for any crepitation (cracking); observe for pain or tenderness.

Ask about usual bowel and bladder habits; perform a general inspection of the perineal area for edema, discharge, or erythema. Auscultate for the presence of bowel sounds in all four abdominal quadrants.

Assess the lower extremities, looking for bruising and edema, and evaluate muscle tone and peripheral pulses. Hair loss in the lower extremities

Table 3–4	
VITAL SIGN RANGES FOR THE OLDER ADULT	
Vital Sign	**Normal Range**
Temperature	96.4° to 99.1°F (oral)
Pulse	60 to 100 beats per minute
Respiration	10 to 20 respirations per minute
Blood pressure	110–140/60–90 mm Hg

can be a sign of vascular insufficiency. Check the feet for thickened toenails and dry or cracking skin. White, yellow, or thickened toenails can be signs of a fungal infection or decreased circulation. Poor hygiene in this area can be a clue that the older adult has diminished sense of smell or sight or has limited mobility and is unable to reach this area of the body easily.

The physical assessment is important in all settings of care for the older adult. The area of emphasis of the physical assessment varies according to the older adult's chief complaint, signs or symptoms experienced by the older adult, medical diagnoses, and new findings discovered by the examining nurse during the assessment.

Functional Assessment

It is important that the older client's level of functioning regarding performance of ADL be assessed. ADL include grooming, bathing, dressing, eating, elimination, and mobility. Each of these areas must be adequately assessed. Assessment quality is always enhanced by direct observation; therefore, it is good to ask the older adult to demonstrate certain activities, such as hair brushing, eating, or ambulating. Information regarding other ADL, such as those related to elimination, can best be gained by interviewing the client and following up later with nursing observations.

In the acute care setting, it is important that a complete assessment of ADL be performed and documented as part of the initial patient assessment; this enables the nurse to be aware of exactly what the older adult can and cannot do for him- or herself. With the older adult's ADL strengths and limitations in mind, the nurse can appropriately plan for discharge from the hospital; this process can include recruitment of additional help or resources that the older adult will need at home or in another facility. In subacute and long-term care, ADL must be accurately assessed and considered in development of the interdisciplinary care plan. Expected outcomes should address maintaining and improving the older adult's abilities in performing ADL. In home care it is important that the nurse assess ADL as well as the adequacy of their completion. For example, the nurse's assessment may reveal that the older adult had adequate range of motion and mobility to bathe, yet the client may give the appearance that

this is not being done. This discrepancy gives the nurse an opportunity to explore the reasons why. There may be numerous explanations, including memory loss, loss of sense of smell, or depression. In other words, the home care nurse must assess not only what the client can do, but also what he or she is doing.

Instrumental Activities of Daily Living

Instrumental activities of daily living (IADL) are those activities that are more complex than ordinary ADL. These include tasks such as shopping, cooking, managing finances, and so forth. Assessment of IADL is performed primarily by interviewing the client, along with verification of information by family members.

In acute, subacute, and long-term care, assessment of IADL is important primarily from the standpoint of planning for discharge. In home care, assessment of IADL is even more important, and results can be an indicator of how well an older adult is managing at home. When assessing a client's IADL, the nurse must also evaluate the adequacy of the older adult's support systems. For example, an older man may have great difficulty cleaning the home because of limited mobility, but he may still have a sharp mind for balancing the checkbook; with the help of his wife, he can manage well. However, any change in the family, such as onset of illness in the wife, can place the independence of the family at risk.

TYPICAL VERSUS ATYPICAL PRESENTATION OF ILLNESS

Most illnesses have an expected set of signs and symptoms that health care providers, as well as the general public, associate with them. For example, if you are caring for a client who is experiencing a heart attack, you might expect chest pain. If your client was admitted to the hospital with pneumonia, you may expect to observe shortness of breath. These are known as **typical presentations,** the usual signs and symptoms of illness or disease.

In some patients, however, the typical signs and symptoms of disease are not present. Have you heard of a client who has experienced a silent heart attack? This person had a myocardial

Table 3–5
ILLNESS PRESENTATIONS IN OLDER ADULTS

Disorder	"Typical" Presentation	"Atypical" Presentation
Pneumonia	Cough, shortness of breath, production of sputum	Absence of the usual symptoms; malaise, anorexia, confusion
Myocardial infarction	Severe, substernal chest pain; shortness of breath; nausea	Mild or no chest pain; confusion, weakness, dizziness
Urinary tract infection	Dysuria, frequency, hematuria	Absence of dysuria; confusion, incontinence, anorexia
Thyrotoxicosis (hyperthyroid emergency)	Rapid heart rate, restlessness, agitation, tremor	Lethargy, cardiac arrhythmias, fatigue, weight loss
Acute appendicitis	Right lower quadrant abdominal pain, fever, tachycardia	Diffuse abdominal pain, confusion, urinary urgency; absence of fever or tachycardia
Infection	Fever, tachycardia, elevated white blood cell count	Temperature normal or below normal, absence of tachycardia, slightly elevated white blood cell count
Depression	Sad mood, increased sleep time, fluctuations in weight	Confusion, apathy; absence of subjective feeling of depression

Adapted from Emmett, K. R. (1998). Nonspecific and atypical presentation of disease in the older patient. *Geriatrics, 53*(2), 50–60.

infarction but no chest pain. This is an example of an atypical presentation of illness. In caring for the older adult, one must be aware of these atypical presentations because most people who experience these unusual signs and symptoms, or the lack thereof, are older adults. Sometimes, a client with an atypical presentation of illness has no signs or symptoms whatsoever. In other cases, clients have signs or symptoms, but they are unrelated or are even the opposite of what is usually expected. Table 3–5 lists some of the more common atypical presentations of illnesses.

The reasons why older adults often have atypical symptoms are not known for certain, but possible reasons are listed in Box 3–4. The

important message for nurses is that understanding illness in the older adult requires careful assessment. Subtle clues are often the only hint that something may be seriously wrong with a client. Left unexplored, serious situations can develop seemingly without warning.

ALTERED THERMOREGULATION WITH AGING

Older adults have impaired thermoregulation. In other words, the ability of their bodies to heat up and cool down when needed is slowed with aging, owing to a less efficient circulatory system and age-related changes in the hypothalamus. It takes approximately twice as long for an older person to recover from extreme heat or cold compared with a younger adult. During summer and winter months, news stories often feature older adults who die during extremes in temperature.

Protection from Hypothermia and Hyperthermia

An important nursing responsibility is to take the knowledge of the older adult's impaired thermoregulatory abilities and apply it to provide a safe care environment for the older client. Although they are unusual, these disorders can be deadly for the older adult.

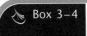

Box 3–4   Possible Causes of Atypical Illness Presentation in Older Adults

- Age-related physiologic changes
- Age-related loss of physiologic reserve
- Interactions of chronic conditions with acute illnesses
- Underreporting of symptoms

Adapted from Emmett, K. R. (1998). Nonspecific and atypical presentation of disease in the older patient. *Geriatrics, 53*(2), 50–60.

Table 3–6
CAUSES OF HYPOTHERMIA IN OLDER ADULTS

Category	Examples
Drugs	Alcohol, barbiturates, tranquilizers, antidepressants, salicylates, acetaminophen, general anesthesia
Disorders	Diabetes mellitus, cardiovascular disease, cerebrovascular disease, sepsis, pneumonia, confusion, falls, fractures
Physiologic changes of aging	Decreased heat production, loss of subcutaneous fat, impaired thermoregulation, decreased sensation
Social influences	Limited income, inadequate housing, social isolation, physical limitations

Adapted from: Matteson, M. A., McConnell, E. S., & Linton, A. D. (1998). *Gerontological nursing: Concepts and practice.* Philadelphia: W. B. Saunders.

Hypothermia

Hypothermia is defined as a body temperature below 95°F (35°C) rectally. Causes of hypothermia in older adults are outlined in Table 3–6.

Signs of hypothermia include the slowing down of many body functions, which can be seen as decreased heart and respiratory rates, diminished reflexes, and reduced mental functioning, eventually leading to coma. Skin color is a combination of pallor and cyanosis, resulting in a gray color. As body functions slow down, shivering ceases.

Hypothermia is a medical emergency, and the registered nurse and physician must be notified immediately. Treatment is directed toward slow rewarming, at a rate of about 0.5°F per hour. As the older adult is warmed, cells become more metabolically active, which leads to acidosis. The blood vessels also expand, causing hypovolemia and resulting in the need for intravenous fluid volume replacement.

Hyperthermia

Hyperthermia is defined as a body temperature above 105°F (40°C) rectally. Risk factors contributing to hyperthermia are outlined in Table 3–7.

Hyperthermia is characterized by excessive storage of body heat and an inability of the body to rid itself of this heat by the usual methods (convection, conduction, radiation, and evaporation). Hyperthermia is a medical emergency, and the registered nurse and physician must be notified immediately. Treatment is aimed at cooling the body. The older adult must be moved immediately to a cooler environment and excess clothing removed. Fluids must be given, usually intravenously, unless the client is conscious. Cool sponge baths with vigorous massage to counteract the peripheral vasoconstriction help cool the body. Circulatory shock and pulmonary edema are risks associated with cooling the older person; vital signs must be monitored at least every 10 minutes. Cooling measures are slowed down when the older adult reaches a temperature of 101°F, as the risk of hypothermia induction is enhanced.

Table 3–7
RISK FACTORS CONTRIBUTING TO HYPERTHERMIA IN OLDER ADULTS

Category	Examples	Comment
Drugs	Phenothiazines, anticholinergics, tranquilizers	Decreased sweat gland activity
Cardiovascular disease	Circulatory disorders	Decreased ability to move heat from core to periphery
Aging	Impaired thermoregulation, decreased thirst sensation	Older adult may not consume sufficient fluids
Altered mental status	Delirium (temporary) or dementia (permanent)	Older adult may not remember the importance of fluids
Social influences	Lack of money	May be unable to afford air conditioning in hot environments

Adapted from Matteson, M. A., McConnell, E. S., & Linton, A. D. (1998). *Gerontological nursing: Concepts and practice.* Philadelphia: W. B. Saunders.

CARING FOR THE OLDER ADULT UNDERGOING A SURGICAL PROCEDURE

Older adults are at greater risk of complications from surgical procedures than are younger adults. As in the general population, emergency surgery carries greater risk for older adults than does elective surgery. Nurses are in an excellent position to minimize the risk of surgery for an older adult.

Preoperative Phase

Care of the older adult during the preoperative phase is most important in helping to prevent postoperative complications. The older adult should be at his or her optimal level of functioning. For example, if an older adult is malnourished, an elective surgery will often be postponed until the client's nutritional status can be improved.

Nursing care begins with a thorough history and assessment. Document baseline data and assist with development of a plan of care to assist nurses involved in the intraoperative and postoperative phases. Include information about the older adult's present level of ADL and IADL performance, support systems, and living situation. In the health history, include information on past illnesses and chronic conditions. For example, an older adult with a history of cardiac or respiratory disorders may experience a slower recovery from surgical procedures. A client with a history of arthritis may notice stiffness after surgery. Nurses who care for the client will find your documentation of arthritis useful in anticipating potential discomfort in the client during the postoperative phase.

The nursing assessment should include the head-to-toe assessment described earlier in the chapter, along with information on nutritional status, level of fluid balance, and patient mobility. Thoroughly document the skin assessment preoperatively, as certain surgical procedures require that the client assume an uncomfortable position on the operating table for prolonged periods of time. Carefully document the client's level of physical mobility. Perform and document a mental assessment. A tool such as the MMSE may be employed.

During the preoperative phase, the client must be prepared. The older adult should be told and shown what to expect after surgery. Some surgeries, such as open-heart surgery, require that postoperative time be spent in an ICU, which will be filled with a bombardment of sensory experiences. In many hospitals, the nurse accompanies the client on a tour of the ICU and points out the unusual noises, lights, tubes, and wires, and possibly discusses restraints that the patient may expect. It is thought that this advance preparation results in a less stressful awakening to the environment than would occur without such preparation.

Teaching is another important aspect of the preoperative role of the nurse. Teach the older adult undergoing major surgery about the postoperative routine of turning, coughing, and deep breathing. Instruct him or her on how to use the incentive spirometer, including a return demonstration by the client. For the older adult undergoing joint surgery, explain expectations of mobility, and reassure him or her that postoperative pain will be managed.

Intraoperative Phase

When operating on an older adult, the anesthesiologist or nurse anesthetist may choose alternatives to general anesthesia, such as spinal or epidural anesthesia, to minimize the risks of complications. In the operating room, position older adults carefully with padding and support devices, as they often have fragile skin and decreased fat tissue. Monitor vital signs frequently, especially body temperature, as older adults are more prone to hypothermia. Box 3–5 lists interventions the operating room team may use to minimize the chances of hypothermia.

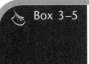

> **Box 3–5** **Intraoperative Interventions to Minimize Hypothermia in Older Adults**
>
> - Monitor temperature and other vital signs frequently
> - Warm intravenous fluids and blood administered
> - Warm gowns and blankets
> - Cover areas of the body not involved in the surgical procedure
> - Humidify oxygen to be administered

Postoperative Phase

The goal of care during the postoperative period is to encourage the older adult to resume his or her previous level of functioning as soon as possible. Recovery may be prolonged in an older adult. It may take as long as 4 to 6 months for the older client to fully recover from major surgery.

The LPN/LVN caring for an older adult in the postoperative phase must carefully monitor for complications. Perform a thorough head-to-toe assessment, compare it with the preoperative assessment, and review both with the registered nurse. It is important that a thorough report be received from the operating room nurse regarding the surgery and the client's response to the procedure. Important items to inquire about are outlined in Box 3–6.

Review carefully all postoperative orders for the older adult with the operating nurse and the registered nurse. If any unexpected events or complications during surgery are described to you during the report, you must inform the registered nurse immediately.

It is crucial that you give nothing by mouth to the client who has been given general anesthesia until he or she is fully awake. Check physician orders carefully and question the registered nurse regarding what type of diet should be resumed and when. If you are unsure about the appropriateness of the recommendations, be sure to question the registered nurse again and ask her to personally evaluate the client. Older adults are more prone to aspiration, so extreme caution is recommended when a diet is resumed.

| Box 3–6 | **Important Information to Obtain in Postoperative Report** |

- Type of surgical procedure performed
- Type of anesthesia used (general, local, spinal, etc.)
- Fluids administered (amounts and types)
- Blood products administered
- Fluid output (amounts and types)
- Most recent vital signs
- Total operating room time
- Any complications or unexpected events

Monitor vital signs closely during the postoperative phase. Most surgical units have a set monitoring routine, such as every 15 minutes for the first hour, every 30 minutes for the next 2 hours, then every hour for the next 4 hours. Keep a vital sign sheet at the bedside and follow this routine *exactly*. Report any abnormalities immediately to the registered nurse because abnormal vital signs are often the first clue of a complication.

Monitor the client for postoperative pain and administer medication when needed. Smaller dosages of medication at frequent time intervals are often more effective for the older adult because medications are metabolized more slowly in older than younger people.

Another important nursing intervention is to promote deep breathing and mobility. Once the client is awake, encourage deep-breathing exercises according to physician orders. For the older adult who has been given general anesthesia, this usually means using the incentive spirometer every 1 to 2 hours. The client may be reluctant to take a deep breath because it causes pain. Mobility orders are very important to carry out as well. If the orders state that the client is to be out of bed three times a day, that means *at least* once on your shift. The first few times out of bed are likely to be very difficult for your client, depending on what type of surgery he or she has had. Pain medication administered 20 to 30 minutes before the planned activity is helpful; also, the help of additional staff members may be required for the first few times, as your client will likely be weaker than before surgery.

You may feel uncomfortable as a new nurse enforcing these doctor's orders because you may feel that you're causing discomfort to the patient. After all, you wanted to become a nurse to help people's suffering, not to cause pain. It is so important that you understand this: it is *much* more cruel to not carry out these orders. Imagine the following scenario: you are a new nurse caring for an older gentleman who had abdominal surgery yesterday. It has been 12 hours since he was up in the chair, although his activity orders state, "chair three times a day." He looks so comfortable that you hate to disturb him; you heard from report how difficult it was to move him and that he had experienced pain. Although it is human nature to wish to leave the client undisturbed, you may actually be causing him *more* pain later if you fail to carry out the order: he could develop pneumonia or another complication, or he may have to endure a longer hospitalization, possibly intensive care, invasive procedures, and a larger hospital bill, to name a few possibilities. Sometimes as a nurse, you must take a deep breath, remember the larger picture, and know that you really *are* being kind, even though the client may not appreciate it at the moment. With your help and encouragement, the older adult will get on his or her way to resuming his or her previous, or a better, level of functioning and enjoying more years of life.

PREVENTING FALLS IN THE OLDER ADULT

Falls are a serious health threat to the older adult. One out of three older Americans falls each year. Falls can lead to injuries, fractures, or hospitalization; they are the sixth leading cause of accidental death among adults over age 65. Even when not life threatening, a fall can result in loss of independence for an older adult. Helping to prevent falls in the older adult is an integral part of maintaining a safe care environment for the older client.

Assessment of Risk for Falls

Nurses play a key role in preventing falls. The first and most important nursing responsibility in caring for an older adult at risk for falls and injury is to perform a thorough assessment of the risk for falls and document the results. Risk levels for falls are often multifactorial; the more risk factors an older adult has, the greater his or her

risk of falling. Many medications increase an older adult's risk of falling. Nursing researchers have identified numerous risk factors for falls, some of which can be found in Box 3–7.

> ### Medication Safety Tip
>
> Medications that increase an older adult's risk for falls include:
>
> - Alcohol
> - Antihypertensives
> - Barbiturates
> - Benzodiazepines
> - Cardiac medications
> - Diuretics
> - Eye medications (nonmyotic)
> - Narcotics
> - Oral hypoglycemics
> - Phenothiazines
> - Tricyclic antidepressants
>
> Adapted from Stone, J. T., Wyman, J. F., & Salisbury, S. A. (1999). *Clinical gerontological nursing: A guide to advanced practice.* Philadelphia: W. B. Saunders.

Prevention of Falls

After completing a thorough assessment of fall risk factors, the nurse must plan carefully for the older adult client to minimize the risks for falling and experiencing injury. It is important that this plan be individualized, based on the older adult's unique risk factors. Frequent checks of the client are essential, as he or she may be reluctant to use the call light. Box 3–8 outlines several

> ### Box 3–7 | Fall Risk Factors in the Older Adult
>
> - Cognitive impairment
> - Problems with mobility (decreased muscle strength, unsteady gait, loss of balance)
> - Acute or chronic illness
> - Sensory impairment
> - Environmental hazards: extension cords, loose rugs, poor lighting, slippery floors
> - Unfamiliar environment (e.g., hospitalization)
> - Medications
> - Normal changes of aging (visual, musculoskeletal, cardiovascular)
> - Dehydration

> ### Box 3–8 | Interventions to Decrease Fall Risk in the Older Adult
>
> - Strengthening exercises
> - Physical activity to improve strength, mobility, and flexibility
> - Environmental modifications: installation of grab bars and railings; elimination of throw rugs, clutter, extension cords, and other hazards
> - Clothing modifications: nonskid footwear, avoidance of long robes
> - Adequate staffing/supervision
> - Judicious use of medications that have sedating effects
> - Education regarding proper use of mobility aids

important nursing interventions that may be useful in preventing a fall for an older adult in your care.

Summary

- As an LPN/LVN, you will care for older adults in many settings.
- In the acute care setting, you must recognize normal changes of aging, allow the older adult to perform self-care activities, and consider nursing care from the client's perspective.
- In the subacute setting, you must possess strong assessment, technical, and interdisciplinary team skills.
- The role of the LPN/LVN in long-term care settings has expanded to include management responsibilities and administration of IV therapy.
- More LPN/LVNs are employed in home care since Medicare reimbursement has changed to an interim payment system.
- Older adults process medications more slowly. Pharmacokinetics consists of four phases: absorption, distribution, metabolism, and excretion. Pharmacodynamics refers to the effect that medication has on the body. With aging, there are changes in both pharmacokinetics and pharmacodynamics. The effects of medications last longer in the older adult.
- Administer medications to the older adult carefully, usually in smaller amounts, and watch for side effects over a longer time frame.
- Polypharmacy refers to an individual taking more drugs than needed, including OTC drugs and herbal remedies.
- Medication abuse can include underuse, erratic use, noncompliance, overuse, and contraindicated use. Numerous problems may result, as the medication will not work as expected or may produce dangerous side effects. Health promotion strategies for medication safety in the older adult include use of special pill containers, special reminders, and magnifying glasses.
- Assessment of the older adult is the first step of the nursing process. After measuring vital signs, perform your assessment in a head-to-toe direction. Document edema, lesions, bruising, or abnormalities in appearance; include ADLs and IADLs in the assessment.

- Typical illness presentation refers to the usual signs and symptoms experienced by a client with an illness. Older adults sometimes have atypical illness presentations, such as a heart attack with no chest pain, infections without fever, or elevated white blood cell count and pneumonia without sputum or cough.
- Older adults have impaired thermoregulation; their ability to heat and cool the body when needed is slowed with aging. In extreme situations, the older adult is at risk for hypothermia or hyperthermia.
- When caring for the older surgical client, you should perform a thorough preoperative assessment to document baseline functioning and to help you in planning care. Make intraoperative adjustments, including warming of fluids, changing position, and providing padding. Postoperative nursing priorities include assessing the patient, managing pain, and encouraging activity.
- The LPN/LVN has a crucial role in preventing falls for the older adult. Carefully assess an older adult's risk factors for experiencing a fall, and plan interventions specific to the risk factors.

STUDY QUESTIONS
Multiple-Choice Review

1. Which of the following settings serves as a bridge between acute care and long-term care?
   1. Hospital setting
   2. Subacute care setting
   3. Nursing home
   4. Home care setting
2. Which of the following settings has recently expanded the role of the licensed practical/vocational nurse owing to enactment of the OBRA law?
   1. Acute care
   2. Subacute care
   3. Long-term care
   4. Home care
3. Which of the following is a correctly stated normal change of aging that affects pharmacokinetics?
   1. The pH of the stomach is decreased
   2. Gastrointestinal motility is increased

3. Blood flow to the intestinal tract is increased
4. Gastrointestinal motility is slowed

4. One example of an "atypical presentation" of illness would be:
   1. Chest pain occurring with a heart attack
   2. Pain and dysuria occurring with a urinary tract infection
   3. Nervousness and anxiety occurring with hyperthyroidism
   4. Confusion as the only sign of pneumonia

5. Which of the following is the most appropriate time to discuss potential postoperative complications?
   1. Preoperatively
   2. Intraoperatively
   3. Postoperatively
   4. Perioperatively

Critical Thinking

1. How would you explain the routine of the acute care facility to a 70-year-old woman who has never been hospitalized?
2. If you could redesign an acute care hospital unit to better serve the older adult, what would it look like?
3. Bearing in mind the changes that have affected first acute care, then home care reimbursement, what do you predict might happen to subacute care in the 21st century?
4. Why is it important for nurses to understand how normal aging affects pharmacokinetics and pharmacodynamics?
5. Why does emergency surgery carry a greater risk to the older adult than elective surgery?

Resources

Internet Resources

American Association of Homes and Services for the Aged: http://www.aahsa.org/

National Council on Aging: http://www.ncoa.org/

AgeNet (Fall Risk Document): http://www.agenet.com/cut_falling_risks.html

Organizations

SRx Regional Program, 1182 Market Street, Suite 204, San Francisco, CA 94101. Available for purchase: medication fact sheets in English, Spanish, Chinese, and Vietnamese, personal medication record, client educational materials.

American Association of Retired Persons, 1909 K Street, Northwest, Washington, DC 20049. Booklet available: Dangerous Products, Dangerous Places.

National Safety Council, 444 North Michigan Avenue, Chicago, IL 60611. Telephone: 1-800-621-7619, ext. 6900. Pamphlets available: Preventing Falls: A Safety Program for Older Adults; Falling: The Unexpected Trip.

Selected References

Beck, C., & Chumbler, N. (1997). Planning for the future of long-term care: Consumers, providers, and purchasers. *Journal of Gerontological Nursing, 23*(8), 6–12.

Centers for Disease Control and Prevention Advance Data 274: An overview of home health and hospice care patients—1994 national home and hospice care survey. CDC Web Site url: *http://www.cdc.gov/nchswww/*products/pubs/pubd/ad/280-271/ad274.htm Accessed 8/16/98.

Centers for Disease Control and Prevention Advance Data 279: Characteristics of elderly home health care users—data from the 1994 national home and hospice care survey. CDC Web Site url: *http://www.cdc.gov/nchswww/*products/ pubs/pubd/ad/280-271/ad279.htm Accessed 8/12/98.

Centers for Disease Control and Prevention Fact Sheet: Unintentional Injury. CDC Web Site url: *http://www.cdc.gov/ncipc/duip/falls.htm* Accessed 8/12/98.

Centers for Disease Control and Prevention Survey: Characteristics of elderly nursing home residents—data from the 1995 national nursing home survey. CDC Web Site url: *http://www.cdc.gov/nchswww/*products/pubs/pubd/ad/290-281/ad289.htm Accessed 8/16/98.

Coccia, R. J., & Cameron, E. A. (1999). Caring for elderly individuals in nursing homes. *Journal of Gerontological Nursing, 25*(12), 38–40.

Cox, E. R., Gardner, M., & Brandman, J. (1998). Expanding opportunities for pharmacists in geriatric care. *Drug Benefit Trends, 10*(4), 33–48.

Crist, L. (1997). Outcomes system implementation for subacute care. *Nursing Case Management, 2*(1), 33–41.

De La Cruz, P. (1997). Subacute nursing: Different stages of development. *MedSurg Nursing, 6*(4), 219–221.

Eckler, J. A. L., & Fair, J. M. S. (1996). *Pharmacology Essentials.* Philadelphia: W. B. Saunders.

Emmett, K. R. (1998). Nonspecific and atypical presentation of disease in the older patient. *Geriatrics, 53*(2), 50–60.

Gueldner, S. H. (1997). Creating an elder sensitive acute care climate: A health care imperative. *Journal of Gerontological Nursing, 23*(4), 7–9.

Hodgson, B., & Kizior, R. (1999). *Saunders Nursing Drug Handbook 1999.* Philadelphia: W. B. Saunders.

Hudson, K. A., & Sexton, D. L. (1996). Perceptions about nursing care: Comparing elders' and nurses' priorities. *Journal of Gerontological Nursing, 22*(12), 41–46.

Kelley, S. J., Yorker, B. C., & Whitley, D. (1997). To grandmother's house we go . . . and stay: Children raised in intergenerational families. *Journal of Gerontological Nursing, 23*(9), 12–20.

Lee, R. D. (1998). Polypharmacy: A case report and new protocol for management. *Journal of the American Board of Family Practice, 11*(2), 140–144.

Lee, T. (2000). The relationship between severity of physical impairment and costs of care in an elderly population. *Geriatric Nursing, 21*(2), 102–106.

Marini, B. (1999). Institutionalized older adults' perceptions of nurse caring behaviors: A pilot study. *Journal of Gerontological Nursing, 25*(5), 11–16.

Matteson, M. A., McConnell, E. S., & Linton, A. D. (1998). *Gerontological nursing: Concepts and practice.* Philadelphia: W. B. Saunders.

Neigh, J. E., & Forster, T. M. (1998). Coping with the interim payment system: Practical notes from the front line. *Caring, 17*(2), 22–26.

Nursing home admission drops while population ages. (1997). *Nurseweek* 10(3), 19.

Rawsky, E. (1998). Review of the literature on falls among the elderly. *Image: The Journal of Nursing Scholarship, 30*(1), 47–52.

Robinson, K. M. (1997). The family's role in long-term care. *Journal of Gerontological Nursing, 23*(9), 7–10.

Schwartz, K. A. (2000). Predictors of early hospital readmissions of older adults who are functionally impaired. *Journal of Gerontological Nursing, 26*(6), 29–36.

Stone, J. T., Wyman, J. F., & Salisbury, S. A. (1999). *Clinical gerontological nursing: A guide to advanced practice.* Philadelphia: W. B. Saunders.

Chapter 4

Promoting Self-Care Management of Chronic Illness

OBJECTIVES

After completing this chapter, you will be able to:

- Describe healthy lifestyle habits.
- State two safety habits appropriate for an older adult.
- Differentiate between acute and chronic pain.
- Discuss cultural differences in one's response to pain.
- Identify pharmacologic and nonpharmacologic pain relief measures.
- Discuss strategies for adapting a teaching/learning session to the needs of the older adult.

KEY TERMS

Acute pain *- short, severe course of pain to sx*	Functional assessment
Age-associated memory impairment	Nonpharmacologic pain treatment
Chronic illness	Pharmacologic pain treatment
Chronic pain	Preventive health care *- Dx prevention + health maintenance*
Food Guide Pyramid	Safety habits

ENCOURAGING HEALTHY LIFESTYLE HABITS

As discussed in Chapter 1, the document *Healthy People 2010* included two broad health goals to be met by the year 2010:

1. Increase quality and years of healthy life
2. Eliminate health disparities

Healthy lifestyle habits are an important part of health promotion for everyone, young and old alike, and will help us as a society to meet these goals. People tend to form habits over an entire lifetime. Some habits are healthy, such as eating nutritious foods, exercising regularly, managing stress effectively, and maintaining an appropriate weight for one's body size. These habits can be called health-promoting activities. Other habits are not conducive to health and can be dangerous, such as not exercising, carrying excess weight, smoking, and consuming excessive amounts of alcohol. These habits do not promote optimal health. Of course it is difficult to be perfect, but nurses are in an optimal position to both encourage healthy habits and model them.

Can a Zebra Change Its Stripes?

Although many habits are formed over a long time, this does not mean that they cannot be changed. Change is usually not very easy, however, and the more radical the change, the more challenging the task.

Although change in one's lifestyle habits may be suggested repeatedly by others (the older adult's spouse, the physician, the nurse, a friend), usually the impetus for change occurs when the individual finally realizes that a change is needed. This realization can be brought on by a crisis in his or her physical health, such as a serious medical diagnosis. Other times, an individual may decide to change unhealthy lifestyle habits because of a crisis in someone else's life, for example, losing a loved one to lung cancer.

The Carrot or the Stick?

What is the best way to encourage healthy lifestyle habits? Although scolding might work to alter the behavior of a 2-year-old, this approach usually has the opposite effect on an adult. Most adults have some lifestyle habits that are less than healthy, and they know this. Stating to Mr. Jones, "That cigarette will kill you" is a bit dramatic, and Mr. Jones probably has been informed of this many times. On the other hand, when Mr. Jones verbalizes frustration that he does not seem to be able to give up his bad habit, you could both acknowledge how difficult quitting smoking must be, then offer to guide him to some resources that can help.

It is very important to maintain a nonjudgmental attitude. Sometimes this is difficult, as nurses are human. Sometimes a client may remind you of the frustrations you experience when dealing with a friend or family member who engages in similar unhealthy habits. You must separate yourself from whatever comparisons you are making and provide nonjudgmental nursing care, or ask to be reassigned to another client. Every client in need of nursing care deserves the best care available, whether or not we agree with his or her lifestyle choices.

Why Change?

There are numerous benefits to encouraging healthy lifestyle habits and discouraging unhealthy ones.

 Health Promotion Tip

Encouraging healthy lifestyle habits may:

- Enhance perception of quality of life
- Increase length of life
- Encourage independence
- Discourage disease progression
- Decrease personal expense of health care costs

Nutrition and the Prevention of Illness

Consuming a nutritious diet with the proper quantity of nutrients can decrease one's chances of acquiring a serious illness. For example, increasing fiber in the diet can reduce the chance of developing certain types of colon disorders, including cancer, and decreasing saturated fats in the diet can reduce the risk of heart disease. In addition, certain chronic illnesses require dietary modifications to help control symptoms of the disease; for example, foods such as chocolate and orange juice can worsen the symptoms of gastroesophogeal reflux disease (GERD) for some clients. Detailed information regarding nutritional modifications recommended for various disorders is presented throughout Unit II of this book. In addition, information on nutritional requirements associated with aging and related disorders is presented in Chapter 6.

The **Food Guide Pyramid** was issued by the U.S. Department of Agriculture in 1992 and is meant as a guide for promoting nutrition (Fig. 4–1).

Although the Food Guide Pyramid has been around since 1992, older adult clients are probably more familiar with the Basic Four Food Groups. It is important to remind the older adult of the recommended changes and to suggest ways of incorporating these into his or her daily life. Major differences between the Pyramid and the Basic Four include a greater emphasis on fruits, vegetables, and grains, and less emphasis on meat

and dairy products in the newer guidelines. The older adult may be resistant to the suggested increase in fruit and vegetable servings. Client education regarding the benefit of fruits and vegetables in the prevention of chronic disease may help your client establish healthier dietary habits.

Nutrition and Culture

Like many other aspects of health care behavior, an individual's culture has a profound effect on dietary habits. If you proceed with automatic dietary instructions without considering a client's culture, your advice will likely be ignored. It is important to collaborate with the older adult, learn what his or her cultural dietary preferences are, and work to establish a dietary plan that will provide the needed nutrients while adhering to the diet of his or her culture. It may be helpful to ask a dietitian to speak with the older adult and his or her family to formulate a balanced plan.

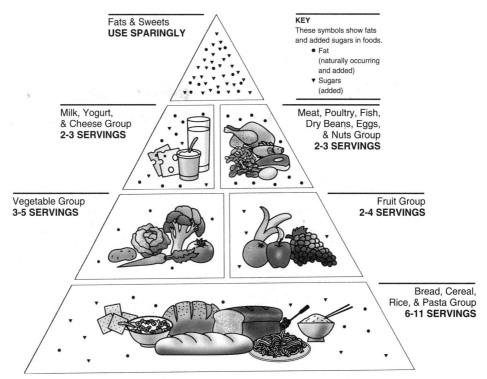

Figure 4–1. Food Guide Pyramid (©1999 Tufts University School of Nutrition Science and Policy, Medford, MA.)

Exercise

Activity is an important part of everyday living. Regular exercise is an important part of the plan of care for an older adult. Exercise has numerous benefits for the older adult.

 Health Promotion Tip _____

Benefits of regular exercise:

Decrease risk of injury from falls by

- Increasing strength
- Increasing muscle mass
- Improving balance and coordination
- Increasing bone density

Improve general well-being by

- Alleviating symptoms of depression
- Improving quality of sleep
- Lessening requirements for pain medication
- Reducing stress

Improve symptoms of various diseases such as

- Cardiovascular disease
- Arthritis
- Parkinson's disease
- Diabetes mellitus

_____

Adapted from Butler, R. N., Davis, L., Lewis, C. B., Nelson, M. E., & Strauss, E. (1998). Physical fitness: Benefits of exercise for the older patient. *Geriatrics, 53*(10), 46, 49–52, 61–62.

Most older adults can engage in almost any type of physical exercise. An aerobic activity combined with the use of large muscle groups (e.g., swimming, walking, or cycling) can be a very effective way to keep active. Older adults with arthritis or musculoskeletal disorders may find water activities to be more comfortable owing to their low-impact nature. Older women and men at risk for osteoporosis may wish to choose a weight-bearing form of activity, such as walking or jogging, to help maintain bone mass. An important nursing role is to assist the older adult in selecting an exercise program that best suits his or her needs and abilities (Box 4–1).

Some older adults have never made physical activity a part of their daily routine and may be reluctant to begin now. They may lack confidence in their physical abilities, or they may see a

 Box 4–1 | **Guidelines for an Exercise Program for Older Adults**

Note: Examination by the older adult's physician must be undertaken prior to beginning a new exercise program.

- Tailor the program to the older adult's strengths, weaknesses, and interests.
- Teach the older adult how and when to take his/her pulse; identify target heart rate range.
- Begin each session with gentle stretching and a "warm up" period of low-intensity activity.
- Encourage activities that move muscle groups through their entire range of motion.
- Gradually increase level of activity from less difficult to more difficult.
- End each session with a "cool down" period of low intensity.

_____

Adapted from Tyson, S. R. (1999). *Gerontological nursing care.* Philadelphia: W. B. Saunders, p. 181.

physical exercise program as too large of an obstacle to confront. Other older adults may be physically limited and may dismiss the idea of exercise. The nurse can be an important source of encouragement for these types of individuals. It is important to help the client start with small goals, while pointing out the physical and psychologic benefits of activity. Physical activities that can be performed from a chair include:

- Neck rolls
- Arm, leg, or foot circling
- Leg lifts
- Shoulder rolls
- Deep breathing
- Torso twist

Even a bed-bound client can benefit from exercises done in the bed, which can help guard against further deconditioning and promote tissue circulation. Exercises that can be performed in bed, in addition to those described previously, can be found in Box 4–2.

Preventive Health Care

Preventive health care remains an important way of minimizing physical decline, both for

> **Box 4–2** **Exercises for Bed-Bound Older Adults**
>
> - Knee to chest (supine or side-lying): Raise one knee to chest, wrap arms around, hold and breathe, straighten leg slowly
> - Pelvic tilts (on back, feet flat with knees bent): Tuck in abdomen, relax
> - Bridging (on back, feet flat on bed): Raise hips, lower slowly
> - Head raising (prone or supine)
> - Rolling from side to side
> - Arm raising through full range of motion (supine)
>
> Adapted from Matteson, M. A., McConnell, E. S., & Linton, A. D. (1997). *Gerontological nursing: Concepts and practice* (2nd Ed.). Philadelphia: W. B. Saunders, pp. 473–474.

healthy older adults and for older adults with chronic illness. Annual physical examination (or more often, if needed) by one's physician can help detect small health problems before they become larger and less manageable.

Regular assessment of vision and hearing is important to enable the older adult to compensate

> ### Health Promotion Tip
>
> Preventive health care for the older adult:
>
> - Annual physical examinations
> - Blood pressure screening every 1 to 2 years
> - Serum cholesterol every 5 years
> - Annual vaccination against influenza
> - Pneumovax immunization at least once
> - Tetanus-diphtheria immunization every 10 years
> - Mammogram every 1 to 2 years, or as directed by physician
> - Pap smear every 1 to 3 years, or as directed by physician
> - Regular eye and ear examinations
> - Dental examinations every 1 to 2 years (even if client wears dentures)
> - Annual fecal occult blood screening
> - Digital rectal examination (screening for prostate cancer) every year, or as directed by physician
> - Osteoporosis screening for high-risk individuals
>
> Adapted from Stone, J. T., Wyman, J. F., & Salisbury, S. A. (1999). *Clinical gerontological nursing: A guide to advanced practice.* Philadelphia: W. B. Saunders, p. 72.

for any age-related decline with appropriate devices such as glasses and hearing aids. Augmenting the hearing and vision of an older adult has safety benefits and helps him or her to avoid unnecessary injury.

Safety Habits

Good safety habits can help to prevent or minimize injury in the event of an accident. It is important for nurses working with older adults to encourage the practice of **safety habits**.

FUNCTIONAL ASSESSMENT

The older adult with a chronic illness may have difficulty performing certain activities because of symptoms associated with, or limitations imposed by, the chronic illness. For example, it might be a difficult chore for an older adult with shortness of breath to clean the house. It might be too challenging (and perhaps dangerous) for an older adult with limited mobility to get into and out of the bathtub every morning. A **functional assessment,** described in Chapter 3, involves observing the older adult's ability to perform activities of daily living (ADL) and instrumental activities of daily living (IADL). A functional assessment helps the health care professional to determine what activities the older adult is capable of performing, and which activities he or she will need assistance with. The nurse uses the information gained in a functional assessment to help the older adult devise a plan to maximize his or her independence. Resources for older adults who need assistance with ADL and IADL can be found in Box 4–3.

>
>
> **Box 4–3** **Resources for Older Adults Who Need Assistance with ADL and IADL**
>
> ADL
> - Home health nurses
> - Home health aides
> - Occupational therapy
>
> IADL
> - Grocery delivery services
> - Meals on Wheels
> - Senior centers
> - Volunteers (e.g., to help with taxes at tax time)

Seat belts are instrumental in minimizing injury caused by automobile accidents; however, because they have been mandatory in most states only since the mid-1980s, older adults have driven most of their adult lives without them. In addition, the older adult may be driving an older car that does not have the shoulder restraint/seat belt combination. It can be a challenge to change a lifelong habit.

 Health Promotion Tip

Safety tips for the older adult:

- Use safety belts while driving/riding in a car.
- Use helmets when riding a bicycle or motorcycle.
- Wear sunscreen when out in the sunshine.
- Avoid throw rugs in the home.
- Hold onto railing when walking up or down the stairs.
- Avoid extension cords in the home.
- Clean up spills promptly.
- Use optimal lighting in the environment.
- Decrease clutter in the home.
- Avoid smoking.
- Ask for help when necessary.
- Have frequent checks of water heater, furnace, and smoke detectors.

Motivation in Performing Self-Care Activities

Although it is important for the health care professional to determine what an older adult is capable of doing in the realm of self-care activities, it is more important to assess what the client actually does. In other words, even though the older adult is perfectly capable of caring for him- or herself, he or she may lack the motivation to do so for many reasons. This lack of motivation could lead to other areas of self-neglect and a downward spiral, ultimately resulting in a loss of independence. It is important to look at lack of motivation as a factor in self-care, and to consider decreased motivation as a nursing opportunity. Lack of motivation can be directly related to depression in the older adult.

It has been shown that older adults are more motivated to perform functional activities when they receive verbal encouragement and reinforcement, when they feel cared for and cared about,

and when unpleasant sensations such as pain and fear are decreased (Resnick, 1998).

 Health Promotion Tip

Interventions to strengthen motivation:

- Provide verbal encouragement.
- Encourage actual practice of the activity.
- Explore thoughts and feelings related to physical sensations (e.g., pain, fear).
- Demonstrate kindness and caring.
- Use humor.
- Provide positive reinforcement.
- Recognize individual needs and differences.
- Explore the meaning of spirituality and, if appropriate, encourage the older adult to participate in this.
- Teach the significant other to verbally encourage and reinforce desired behaviors.
- Develop goals with the older adult that are clear, specific, and challenging but attainable.

Adapted from Resnick, B. (1998). Motivating older adults to perform functional activities. *Journal of Gerontological Nursing, 24*(11), 23–30.

CARING FOR THE OLDER ADULT WITH CHRONIC ILLNESS

Most older adults have one or more **chronic illnesses** that they manage on a day-to-day basis. Frequently occurring conditions are arthritis, hypertension, cardiovascular disease, chronic obstructive pulmonary disease, hearing impairment, cataracts, mobility impairments, and diabetes mellitus. These disorders and numerous others are discussed throughout Unit II of this book.

Does the fact that many older adults experience chronic illness mean that the ability to enjoy life is essentially over after age 65? Of course not. What it simply means is that many older adults have alterations in their physical health that they must—and do—manage effectively in order to live full and rich lives. In fact, less than one third of older adults rate their health as "fair" or "poor."

The goal is not to cure a chronic illness, but rather to decrease symptoms, slow illness progression, and improve one's ability to live a full life. By meeting these objectives, an older adult with chronic illness can take control of managing the disorder. Nurses are in an excellent position to assist older adults to meet this goal.

HELPING THE OLDER ADULT MANAGE PAIN

An 80-year-old woman visited her doctor to find out the cause of the pain she was experiencing in her right knee. After a brief physical examination, her physician said to her, "Well, what do you expect? That knee is 80 years old." After a moment of thought, the client remarked to her doctor, "Well, my left knee is 80 years old too, and **it** feels just fine!"

Pain is a signal of tissue damage. Any new onset of pain needs to be explored to determine the cause. With the myriad of **pharmacologic and nonpharmacologic pain treatments** available today, there is no reason why a client of any age needs to experience needless pain. Unfortunately, chronic pain can be difficult to manage. The older adult with chronic pain may need to explore several pain management strategies before finding one that is effective. This section describes pain in the older adult and factors that influence it, and offers strategies for effective pain management.

Pain is a subjective individual experience. Many factors influence someone's perception of pain: culture, past experience with pain, mental status, and others. Although clients may demonstrate objective signs that they are experiencing pain, you cannot decide when a client is or is not experiencing pain. Pain is subjective: if a client complains of pain, then the client is having pain. A widely accepted definition of pain is, "whatever the experiencing person says it is, existing wherever the person says it does" (McCaffery & Beebe, 1989).

Culture and Pain

Culture can affect someone's experience and reporting of pain. In some cultures, reporting pain is viewed as a sign of weakness. An older adult from such a culture may try to act strong and may not admit to experiencing pain in front of his or her family. In other cultures, it is not only accepted to admit the experience and intensity of pain, it is encouraged. An older adult from this culture may cry out verbally and enlist family support in helping to deal with the pain. It would

be a mistake to assume that the first client is not in as much pain as the second one. You need to carefully assess your clients to get a more accurate view of each older adult's experience of pain.

Fear and misconceptions can make the experience of pain worse. Some clients have a fear of becoming addicted to pain medications and therefore will not admit to pain. Other clients may have a fear of what the pain might mean and are reluctant to acknowledge the experience of pain.

In the hospital culture, pain is more accepted. You may find that older adults who have spent more time in the hospital setting are more willing to report pain and accept interventions that you offer.

Acute Versus Chronic Pain

With chronic illness, an older adult may experience **acute pain**, **chronic pain**, or both. Table 4–1 highlights the differences between acute and chronic pain.

Assessment of Pain

Older adults do not experience less pain than younger adults. However, they may be less able to distinguish between different intensities of pain. Pain threshold is higher in the older adult. Pain may be perceived as diffuse rather than localized in the older adult. Older adults may be less likely to report pain.

Because pain is a subjective experience, the older adult must be able to describe dimensions of it to the nurse. If language skills are lacking in an older adult (such as after a cerebrovascular accident), "yes/no" questions may be useful in eliciting presence, location, and characteristics of pain, although it is possible to lead the client to answers. Another approach is to use a visual pain assessment scale whereby the older adult can point to a position on a visual scale to indicate the severity of the pain he or she is experiencing (Fig. 4–2).

If an older adult is cognitively impaired, in addition to being verbally impaired (such as with dementia), you must assess for physical behaviors that may indicate the presence of pain. Physical behaviors that can indicate pain include restlessness, rocking, crying out, grimacing, guarding a body part, or resistance to personal care that involves moving a body part. Some authors recommend

Table 4–1		
ACUTE VERSUS CHRONIC PAIN		
	Acute	**Chronic**
Onset	Sudden	Sudden or insidious
Duration	Hours to weeks	Months to years
Cause	Usually easy to identify	May be known or unknown
Effect on lifestyle	May be unable to carry out regular activities	May lead to radical change in lifestyle
Psychosocial effects	Usually transient or none	Can affect ability to earn a living, enjoy social activities, and maintain self-esteem

Modified from de Wit, S. C. (1998). *Essentials of medical-surgical nursing* (4th ed.). Philadelphia: W. B. Saunders, p. 250.

exploration of several areas when assessing for pain in clients who are unable to recognize and/or communicate the presence of it (Box 4–4). When medicating a cognitively impaired older adult, document the client behaviors that prompted you to administer pain medication.

For the majority of older adults who are cognitively intact and able to communicate, the PQRST formula (Box 4–5) is an easy-to-remember acronym for assessing pain. Although it is especially useful in assessing cardiac pain, this formula is applicable to all forms of pain.

Planning Interventions for Pain Relief

Pain relief measures include both pharmacologic and nonpharmacologic treatments. Our culture,

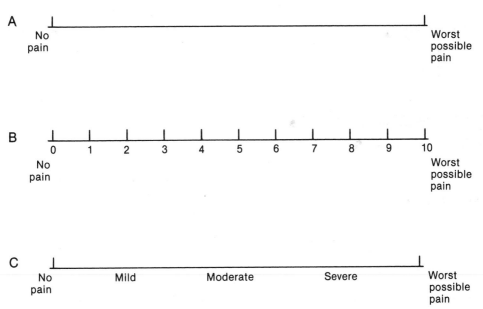

Figure 4–2. Examples of pain assessment scales. *A*, Visual analogue scale. *B*, Numerical rating scale. *C*, Word graphic/rating scale. (From Carrieri-Kohlman, V., Lindsey, A. M., & West, C. M. [Eds.]. [1993]. *Pathophysiological phenomena in nursing: Human responses to illness*, 2nd ed. Philadelphia: W. B. Saunders, p. 315.)

Box 4–4 Components of a Multifaceted Pain Assessment

- Family member or nursing assistant (NA) reports of possible client pain
- Medical diagnoses known to commonly cause pain (e.g., arthritis, cancer, and hip fracture)
- Pain history demonstrated by the use of analgesics
- Aggressive behavior patterns

Adapted from Feldt, K. S., Warne, M. A., & Ryden, M. B. (1998). Examining pain in aggressively cognitively impaired older adults. *Journal of Gerontological Nursing*, 24(11), 14–22.

---

both hospital culture and American culture, is very pharmacologically oriented. According to television advertisements, drugs help you lose weight, allow you to eat spicy foods, alleviate your headache, reverse your hair loss, improve your sexual drive, and more. Consider how drug-oriented we are as a society. Could there be a relationship between this and our society's problems with drug and alcohol dependency?

Ask yourself this: the last time you experienced a headache, what was the first thing you did? Many of you are thinking, "Go straight to the medicine cabinet." What is often forgotten is that

---

Box 4–5 The PQRST Formula for Assessing Pain

P = Provocation: What brings the pain on? What relieves it?

Q = Quality: What does the pain feel like? Is it aching? Burning? Squeezing? Boring? Vise-like? Dull?

R = Region, Radiation: Does the pain radiate to another location?

S = Severity: How intense is the pain using a 0 to 10 scale? (0 = no pain; 10 = the worst pain you could possibly imagine)

T = Timing: When does the pain occur?

Adapted from Monahan, F. D., & Neighbors, N. (1998). *Medical-surgical nursing: Foundations for clinical practice* (2nd Ed.). Philadelphia: W. B. Saunders, p. 188.

---

there are numerous alternatives to drugs. Maybe you did not consider the alternative of having a glass of water or getting some fresh air. Of course, drugs are *very* important in management of pain; however, nurses need to consider non-drug therapies along with drug treatment.

Nonpharmacologic Treatments

Nonpharmacologic measures for reducing pain can be used instead of medications or in addition to medications. When used in combination with pain medications, nonpharmacologic treatments can increase the effectiveness of the drugs and reduce the frequency with which they are needed. Some common nonpharmacologic pain management treatments that can be employed at the bedside are listed in Table 4–2 and Box 4–6.

Other nonpharmacologic measures include hypnosis, acupuncture/acupressure, and transcutaneous electrical nerve stimulation (TENS), which uses low electrical current to block pain impulse transmission. These measures require specific training; use of TENS requires a physician's order.

Table 4–2	
NONPHARMACOLOGIC MEASURES FOR PAIN RELIEF	
Method	**Description**
Sleep	Increases pain tolerance; improves response to analgesia
Heat/warmth	Soothing, increases blood flow to area
	May include compresses, warm blanket, whirlpool, heating pad, and heat lamp
	Use for 15 to 20 minutes only
Cold	Decreases inflammation, reduces joint pain and muscle spasms
	Wrap cold pack in washcloth and use for 10 to 15 minutes only
Distraction	Takes mind off the pain temporarily
	May include television, games, conversation, and music
Relaxation	Conscious relaxation of muscle groups after tensing them
Imagery	Helps client achieve a feeling of comfort; may help during painful procedures
Massage	Relaxes muscles, stimulates circulation, and increases well-being. Do not perform over reddened areas
Binders	Provide support for tissues during movement to decrease pain

Modified from de Wit, S. C. (1998). *Essentials of medical-surgical nursing* (4th ed.). Philadelphia: W. B. Saunders, pp. 248–249.

> ### Box 4-6 Special Alert—Use of Hot and Cold in an Older Adult
>
> The skin of an older adult is thin and susceptible to injury—use hot and cold *with extreme care!*
> - Test the temperature on your wrist or cheek before applying.
> - Carefully assess the skin condition before application and every 5 minutes after.
> - Do not exceed recommended time.
> - Do not use in clients who are unable to inform you of discomfort (e.g., client with speech or language problem).
> - Do not use in clients who may not be able to recognize that they are being burned (e.g., client with dementia or stroke).

Pharmacologic Treatments

Pharmacologic treatments for reducing pain can be extremely effective in alleviating acute pain, and can allow a client with chronic pain to function at a higher level than he or she otherwise would. Pharmacologic measures include both narcotic medications and nonnarcotic medications (Table 4–3).

The nurse can administer pain medication by numerous routes: orally (PO), subcutaneously (SC), intramuscularly (IM), intravenously (IV), sublingually (SL), or rectally (PR). In addition to these traditional routes of medication administration, patient-controlled analgesia (PCA) provides another alternative. With PCA, small doses of intravenous pain medication are administered at intervals chosen by the client by simply pressing a button. This type of medication is ideal in the postoperative setting. For a client with long-term pain management needs (e.g., in cancer care), surgically implantable devices can deliver pain medication.

As discussed in Chapter 3, older adults may be more sensitive to pain medications because of alterations in pharmacokinetics and pharmacodynamics associated with aging. Remember that with this age group, smaller dosages at more frequent intervals usually lead to the best pharmacologic pain strategy for your older adult client.

The nurse plays a key role in helping the older adult with self-care management of pain associated with chronic illness. The nurse can assist the client in understanding the benefits of assuming responsibility for pain management. An important nursing strategy associated with this is client education.

Table 4–3
NARCOTIC AND NONNARCOTIC MEDICATIONS

	Narcotic	Nonnarcotic
Examples	Opiates: morphine, codeine Synthetics: meperidine, methadone	Salicylates (e.g., aspirin) Nonsalicylates (e.g., acetaminophen) Nonsteroidal anti-inflammatory drugs (NSAIDs) (e.g., ibuprofen, celecoxib)
Use	Moderate to severe pain Smaller doses can be found in combination products for less severe pain (e.g., acetaminophen with codeine)	Mild to moderate pain
Other effects	Suppress cough reflex, potentiate anesthetic agents	Reduce fevers NSAIDs and salicylates also reduce inflammation
Adverse effects	Respiratory depression, decreased level of consciousness, nausea, vomiting, constipation, hypotension	Bleeding, tinnitus, nausea, vomiting Allergic reactions Liver failure (acetaminophen)
Contraindications	Head injury, increased intracranial pressure, decreased respiratory reserve, coma	Allergy, surgery Excessive alcohol consumption (acetaminophen)

Data from Hodgson, B. B., & Kizior, R. J. (2001). *Saunders nursing drug handbook.* Philadelphia: W. B. Saunders; Buffum, M., & Buffum, J. C. (2000). Nonsteroidal anti-inflammatory drugs in the elderly. *Pain Management Nursing, 1*(2), 40–50.

Health Promotion Tip

Self-care management of pain:

- Empathizing with the older adult who is experiencing pain
- Creating an environment of trust
- Explaining the physical reason the pain occurs
- Educating the older adult about pharmacologic and nonpharmacologic pain management strategies
- Encouraging the older adult to ask questions
- Encouraging the older adult to decide on specific pain management techniques to implement
- Allowing the older adult to control aspects of the environment such as when to eat, when to sleep, and so forth

CLIENT TEACHING FOR HEALTH PROMOTION

Client teaching is one of the most important aspects of caring for an older adult with chronic illness. By providing the older adult with information about strategies for managing chronic illness, you can help the client take the best possible care of him- or herself, prevent complications, and remain independent as long as possible. Later chapters, which describe various disorders common to older adults, contain client teaching information specific to the disorder discussed. This section describes strategies for adapting the teaching/learning process to the needs of an older adult.

With normal aging, changes to one's memory occur that must be considered in client teaching. In general, although long-term memory, or memory of events in the past, is well preserved, short-term memory may be impaired. This change, often referred to as **age-associated memory impairment** (AAMI), is discussed in Chapter 11. In addition, an older adult may have impairments in special senses, such as vision and hearing, that are important for you to consider. Box 4–7 provides nursing interventions for the teaching/learning session that take into consideration the needs of the older adult.

You must also be aware of fatigue when you are teaching the older adult. Keep teaching/learning sessions relatively short, and schedule rest breaks frequently. Repeat information as needed. In general, older adults benefit more from individualized teaching than from group sessions.

| Box 4–7 | **Strategies for Teaching the Older Adult** |

Before the teaching/learning session

- Make appointment with the client: his/her time is valuable.
- Set goals with the older adult that are easily achievable.
- Determine the best method or methods of presenting the material, based on the topic and the client's needs. Examples include:
  Lecture/discussion
  Presentation
  Demonstration and return demonstration
  Role playing
  Games

At the start of the teaching/learning session

- Make sure glasses are clean and hearing aids are in place and working properly.
- Minimize distractions: close door to the hallway, turn off television, etc.
- Use soft white light to reduce glare.
- Sit at eye level, facing the older adult.
- Provide written material to reinforce the spoken work (large print, if visually impaired).

- Provide opportunity for the older adult to ask questions related to last teaching/learning session (if applicable).

During the teaching/learning session

- Begin with the most important information first.
- Address one topic at a time to avoid information overload.
- Speak loud enough to be heard, but avoid shouting.
- Speak clearly and at a moderate rate.
- Summarize key points at intervals.
- Ask client to rephrase in his or her own words what you have discussed.

At the conclusion of the teaching/learning session

- Summarize the key points presented.
- Ask the older adult, "What questions do you have?" rather than, "Do you have any questions?" (the automatic answer to the latter question is "no").
- Schedule the next session and provide additional opportunity to ask questions.

Summary

- Health-promoting activities include eating nutritious foods, exercising regularly, managing stress, and maintaining an appropriate weight. Nurses can help older adults eliminate unhealthy habits through education and support.
- The Food Guide Pyramid is a guide for promoting nutrition. Nurses should educate the older adult about the benefits of nutrition in preventing chronic disease.
- Culture has a profound effect on dietary habits; this must be taken into consideration during client teaching.
- Activity is an important part of everyday living and has numerous benefits. Nurses can assist the older adult in selecting an exercise program.
- Preventive health measures include regular physical examinations, dental examinations, and immunizations. Nurses should encourage safety habits, such as the use of seat belts and cessation of smoking.
- The goal of caring for the older adult with chronic illness is to manage symptoms and increase the client's ability to live a full life. It is important for an older adult with a chronic illness to take control of his or her health.
- Pain is a subjective individual experience. Any new onset of pain needs to be explored for determination of the cause. Pain associated with chronic illness can be challenging to relieve. Factors that influence someone's experience of pain include culture, past experience with pain, and mental status.
- Acute pain usually is a short-term experience with a sudden onset and a cause that can be corrected. Chronic pain may have a slower onset, may be more difficult to alleviate, and may have negative consequences for a client's lifestyle.
- Older adults may be less able to distinguish between different intensities of pain than younger adults, and they have a higher pain threshold.
- Nonpharmacologic measures for reducing pain can be used instead of medications or in addition to medications; these kinds of treatment can increase the effectiveness of pain medications.

- Pharmacologic measures include both narcotic and nonnarcotic medications. With older adults, smaller dosages at more frequent intervals usually provide the best pharmacologic pain strategy.
- Client teaching is one of the most important components of caring for an older adult with a chronic illness. Provide written material to augment the topic, eliminate distractions, and frequently summarize information. Keep teaching/learning sessions relatively short, and schedule frequent rest breaks.

STUDY QUESTIONS

Multiple-Choice Review

1. The goal for the older adult with a chronic illness is to:
   1. Seek a cure for the illness
   2. Relinquish control to the nurse
   3. Relinquish control to the physician
   4. Decrease symptoms and improve quality of life
2. Pain is:
   1. Present if the client's heart rate and blood pressure are above normal
   2. Present whenever the client says it is
   3. Absent if the client is able to sleep
   4. Impossible to eliminate without the use of medications
3. The culture of an older adult can affect:
   1. The experience and meaning of pain
   2. One's dietary habits and preferences
   3. One's health habits
   4. All of the above
4. The best way to assess a nonverbal, cognitively impaired client for the presence or absence of pain is:
   1. The PQRST formula
   2. A visual pain scale
   3. Asking the client a series of "yes" or "no" questions
   4. Observation for behavior changes
5. Which of the following interventions for pain management is considered a pharmacologic measure?
   1. TENS

2. PCA
3. Biofeedback
4. Touch

Critical Thinking

1. Why does culture affect the health habits of people?
2. Compare your health habits with those described in the chapter. In what ways do your habits promote optimal health? In what ways do your habits discourage good health?
3. What would you say to the older adult who says to you, "I can't start wearing a seat belt now. I've been driving too many years without one"?
4. Describe the optimal setting for a teaching session involving a newly diagnosed client with diabetes mellitus who requires instruction in insulin self-administration.

Resources

Internet Resources

Seniors Online (directory of resources):
   http://www.bev.net/community/seniors/

Seniornet: http://www.seniornet.com/

Arbor Nutrition Guide: http://www.arborcom.com/

National Center for Chronic Disease and Health Promotion:
   http://www.cdc.gov/nccdphp/

Organizations

National Association of Nutrition and Aging Services Program, 2675 44th Street SW, Suite 305, Grand Rapids, MI, 49509. Telephone: (616) 531-9909

National Council on Patient Information and Education, 666 11th Street Northwest, Suite 810, Washington, DC 20001

National Safety Council, 444 North Michigan Avenue, Chicago, IL 60611. Telephone: 1-800-621-7619, ext. 6900. Pamphlet available: Your Home Safety Checklist.

Selected References

Buffum, M., & Buffum, J. C. (2000). Nonsteroidal anti-inflammatory drugs in the elderly. *Pain Management Nursing, 1*(2), 40–50.

Butler, R. N., Davis, L., Lewis, C. B., Nelson, M. E., & Strauss, E. (1998). Physical fitness: Benefits of exercise for the older patient. *Geriatrics, 53*(10), 46, 49–52, 61–62.

Carrieri-Kohlman, V., Lindsey, A. M., & West, C. M. (Eds.). (1993). *Pathophysiological phenomena in nursing: Human responses to illness* (2nd ed.). Philadelphia: W. B. Saunders.

de Wit, S. C. (1998). *Essentials of medical-surgical nursing* (4th ed.). Philadelphia: W. B. Saunders.

DHHS releases latest progress report on prevention—*Healthy People 2000* review, 1995–96 shows progress in almost half of objectives. Centers for Disease Control and Prevention Fact Sheet. CDC Web Site. Available at http://www.cdc.gov/nchswww/releases/96facts/96sheets/hp2knchs.htm. Accessed August 12, 1998.

Feldt, K. S., Warne, M. A., & Ryden, M. B. (1998). Examining pain in aggressively cognitively impaired older adults. *Journal of Gerontological Nursing, 24*(11), 14–22.

Fowler, S. B. (1997). Health promotion in chronically ill older adults. *Journal of Neuroscience Nursing, 29*(1), 39–43.

Hodgson, B. B., & Kizior, R. J. (1999). *Saunders nursing drug handbook.* Philadelphia: W. B. Saunders.

Lusis, S. A. (1996). The challenges of nursing elderly surgical patients. *AORN Journal, 64*(6), 954–962.

Matteson, M. A., McConnell, E. S., & Linton, A.D. (1997). *Gerontological nursing: Concepts and practice* (2nd Ed.). Philadelphia: W. B. Saunders.

McCaffery, M., & Beebe, A. (1989). Pain in the elderly. In M. McCaffery & A. Beebe (Eds.), *Pain: Clinical manual for nursing.* St. Louis: Mosby.

Monahan, F.D., & Neighbors, N. (1998). *Medical-surgical nursing: Foundations for clinical practice* (2nd Ed.). Philadelphia: W. B. Saunders.

Profile of Older Americans: 1999. Administration on Aging. Available at http://www.aoa.dhhs.gov/aoa/stats/profile/default.htm. Accessed 9/14/00.

Resnick, B. (1998). Motivating older adults to perform functional activities. *Journal of Gerontological Nursing, 24*(11), 23–30.

Stone, J. T., Wyman, J. F., & Salisbury, S. A. (1999). *Clinical gerontological nursing: A guide to advanced practice.* Philadelphia: W. B. Saunders.

Tyson, S. R. (1999). *Gerontological nursing care.* Philadelphia: W. B. Saunders.

II

Promotion of Physical Health for the Older Adult

Promoting Activity and Rest

KEY TERMS

Abduction	Muscle wasting
Adduction	Pallor
Atrophy	Patient-controlled analgesia
Cortical bone	Polysomnography
Crepitation	Sarcopenia
Cyanosis	Shearing forces
Débridement	Sleep log
Dyssomnia	Total hip arthroplasty
Erythema	Trabecular bone
Flexion	Tryptophan
Hemiarthroplasty	White noise
Hypertrophy	Xerosis
Kyphosis	

AGE-RELATED CHANGES OF THE MUSCLES, BONES, SKIN, AND HAIR

Muscle

Normal aging leads to changes in the tissues in our bodies. Muscle tissue undergoes **atrophy** and a decrease in the number of muscle fibers. The remaining muscle fibers become smaller in diameter. Once muscle fibers are lost, new ones do not replace them; rather, they are replaced by fibrous connective tissue and adipose tissue. Cell loss depends on many factors, including nutrition, physical activity, heredity, and the condition of the motor neurons that supply the muscle tissue.

Health Promotion Tip

Continued physical activity and proper nutrition are probably the best way to reduce age-associated loss of muscle mass and strength.

As muscle mass is reduced, there is a corresponding decrease in muscular strength. This loss in strength varies from individual to individual; with continued exercise, the loss of strength can be reduced (Fig. 5–1). The mitochondria of muscle cells that are not exercised function less efficiently than mitochondria of exercised muscle cells. This loss of muscle mass and strength is referred to as **sarcopenia**, and can adversely affect the older client's balance, gait, and recovery from falls.

Bones

Aging also leads to changes in the bones of the body. Bone has two major components: the outer, compact type of bone known as **cortical bone**, and the inner, spongy bone known as **trabecular bone**, which has a honeycombed appearance. As one ages, loss of both types of bone occurs, leading to brittle bones in older people. Women experience greater bone loss than men, and it begins at an earlier age. This is the reason why calcium supplements are often recommended for women. Factors involved in bone loss associated with aging are outlined in Box 5–1.

Older adults experience a gradual change in stature. The factors involved include both loss of height of the individual vertebrae of the spinal column and narrowing of the disks between them. Collagen synthesis changes with age, leading to decreased flexibility in tendons and ligaments. Cartilage, on the other hand, continues to grow, as evidenced by the lengthening and broadening of the ears and nose often seen in older people.

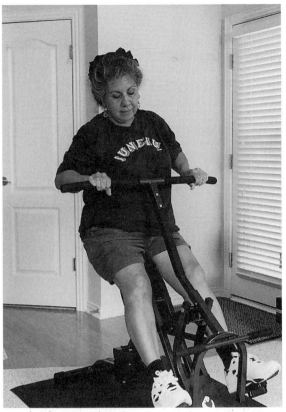

Figure 5–1. Remaining active throughout life is a way to maintain healthy movement in old age. (From Harkreader, H. [2000]. *Fundamentals of nursing*. Philadelphia: W. B. Saunders, p. 463.)

Box 5–1 | Factors Associated with Age-Associated Bone Loss

- Imbalance between osteoblast (bone forming) and osteoclast (breaking down) activity
- Reduced absorption of calcium and vitamin D from the gastrointestinal tract
- Reduced weight-bearing exercise
- Imbalance between calcitonin and parathyroid hormone levels
- Decreased sunlight exposure
- Decreased dietary intake of foods rich in calcium and vitamin D
- Changes in estrogen levels in women

Health Promotion Tip

An active lifestyle with weight-bearing exercise and foods rich in calcium and vitamin D can help offset the age-related loss of bone.

Skin

The most obvious of the normal changes of aging is the changes to the skin. A decrease in the number of elastic fibers and loss of adipose tissue lead to wrinkling and a sagging appearance. Loss of collagen fibers results in skin that is more fragile and slower to heal when injured. The skin is thinner and appears more transparent with aging. A reduction in sebaceous gland activity leads to dryer skin. Reduced sweat gland activity paired with a reduction in subcutaneous adipose tissue makes the older adult less able to physically cope with extremes in environmental temperature.

Health Promotion Tip

The best way to delay aging of the skin is to avoid prolonged sunlight exposure, wear protective clothing, and use sunscreen.

Hair

The graying of hair is another visible sign of the aging process. Hair becomes gray or white from loss of melanocytes. Loss of hair is more common in older men, but can also occur in aging women, and is due to a reduced number of hair follicles. This hair loss and graying occurs on the head but also can be noted in other areas of the body, such as the axillae and the pubic region. Other areas of the body may experience unusual hair growth. Women may notice increased facial hair related to a decrease in estrogen production. Men often experience increased hair growth around the ears, nose, and upper back, along with eyebrows that take on a bushy appearance.

CHANGES TO SLEEP PATTERN WITH AGING

Sleep is important for promotion of one's health. During sleep, restoration and repair of body tissues occur. There are two types of sleep: non–rapid eye movement (NREM) and rapid eye movement (REM). These types of sleep alternate during the night and both are essential for an individual to awaken and have the sensation of being well rested.

During REM sleep, a person's eyes appear to be moving beneath the eyelids. Dreaming occurs during this stage of sleep. It is thought that the brain sorts through information acquired during the day and categorizes, filters, or discards data. Lack of REM sleep can lead to irritability and emotional distress.

Medication Safety Tip

Alcohol and numerous medications, such as hypnotics and sedatives, can interfere with REM sleep.

There are four phases of NREM sleep. Whereas REM sleep is thought to restore the body psychologically, stage IV of NREM sleep is thought to restore the body physically (Table 5–1).

Many people have trouble sleeping as they grow older. Older adults often take a longer amount of time to fall asleep and may awaken more frequently during the night. Less time is spent in the deeper stages of sleep. There is little change in the total number of hours slept per night over the course of one's life, although the older adult may actually spend more time in bed trying to achieve a good night's sleep. Authorities state that older adults generally require only 5 to 6 hours of sleep per night, unless they are in a period of learning or training, such as returning to school.

Older adults often find that they awaken earlier than they did in their younger years. Researchers believe that older adults awaken earlier, in part, because of an alteration in their circadian rhythm. This phase advance of the circadian rhythm can partly explain why some older adults awaken as early as 4:00 or 5:00 AM. Compare this with the typical sleeping habits of a teenager. Teenagers often cannot be pulled out of bed until noon or later, a phase delay of the circadian rhythm. The theory is that these rhythms gradually change over the course of one's lifetime. This may explain why, even if the older adult delays bedtime until later in the evening, he or she may still awaken at 4:00 or 5:00 in the morning (Fig. 5–2).

ASSESSMENT OF MUSCULOSKELETAL AND INTEGUMENTARY SYSTEMS

Head and Neck

To be consistent in your assessment, always assess in the direction from head to toe. Carefully document your assessment and be especially diligent in promptly communicating any abnormalities in your findings to the registered nurse. Beginning with the client's head, inspect the head and neck skin and musculature. Note the presence, distribution, and color of hair. Observe the skin for wrinkling, excessive dryness (**xerosis**), or flaking. Assess the color of the skin. Pale skin, or **pallor**, could indicate anemia, whereas **erythema** could indicate irritation of the skin.

Medication Safety Tip

Erythema or skin rashes are often medication-related and must be reported promptly.

Cyanosis is an indication of poor tissue perfusion. If the older adult is a dark-skinned individual, color can best be observed by inspecting the oral mucous membranes and the conjunctiva beneath the eyes. Observe the muscular development of the head and neck: **hypertrophy** of the neck and upper chest area muscles (the accessory muscles for breathing) could indicate that the older adult has a chronic respiratory impairment.

Table 5–1 STAGES OF NREM SLEEP		
Stage	**Depth**	**Characteristics**
I	Lightest	Person can easily be aroused
II	Somewhat deeper	Deeper stage of relaxation, but still easily aroused
III	Progressively deeper	More difficult to awaken; temperature and heart rate are reduced
IV	Deepest	Body functions are reduced; "restorative sleep"

Adapted from Tyson, S. R. (1999). *Gerontological nursing care.* Philadelphia: W. B. Saunders, p. 190.

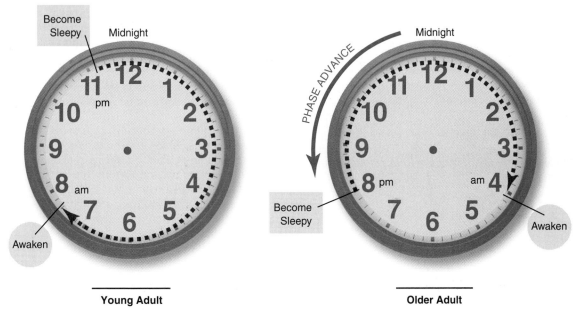

Figure 5–2. Phase advance of the sleep cycle with aging.

Assess the bone structure of the older adult. Observe the neck and upper back area for **kyphosis.** Gently move the neck through its range of motion, but do not force movement. Note any stiffness or limitations in motion.

Chest, Thorax, and Abdomen

Next, observe the skin and musculature of the thorax area. Note hair color and distribution. Assess muscular development. You may observe **muscle wasting** and even visible ribs and clavicles in an older adult with nutritional deficiencies. Loss of muscle tone may be noted in the abdominal area. Assess skin color and note any alterations in skin color, such as bruising, erythema, edema, or pallor. Observe the skin around the genitalia for erythema, rash, or other signs of irritation. Note the color and distribution of hair. Assess the bone structure of the thoracic area; note any abnormalities or the presence of surgical incision sites, old or new.

Arms and Legs

Assess the skin of the extremities carefully. As always, observe for pallor, erythema, or other discolorations. Palmar erythema can indicate liver abnormalities. Skin on the lower arms and hands may have a translucent appearance due to loss of subcutaneous fat. Observe for areas of irritation or dryness. Bruising could indicate injury, including elder abuse, or could simply be a reflection of the increased fragility of the skin and capillaries. Bruising may also be noted if a client is taking anticoagulant medications. Smaller ecchymoses could result from medications such as steroids. Observe and note hair pattern distribution. Hair loss on the lower leg could indicate circulation problems; on the other hand, hair can also be sparse in individuals who have worn knee-length socks for most of their lifetime. Muscular hypertrophy may be observed in the large muscle groups of the arms and legs in an individual who lifts weights. Decreased muscle mass in the large muscle groups can be an indication of a sedentary lifestyle, prolonged bedrest, or poor nutrition.

🍴 Nutrition Tip

Muscle mass is an important indicator of nutritional status in the older adult.

Assess the bone structure of the arms and legs. Note any obvious deformities such as fracture. Gently assess arm and leg movement by evaluating their range of motion.

Health Promotion Tip

The assessment stage is an excellent time to teach health promotion. For example, while performing range of motion, encourage the older adult to perform this activity several times each day.

Hands and Feet

Observe the nails of the hands and feet for thickening, cracking, white appearance (which can indicate fungal infection), or discoloration. Assess the fingernails for a clubbed or flattened appearance, which can indicate problems with oxygenation. Assess with special care the feet of a diabetic older adult. Clients with diabetes mellitus often have decreased sensation in the feet and may be unaware of a lesion or area of irritation. Observe the skin for dryness and cracking, erythema, or signs of a rash. It would be wise to inquire at this point if the older adult uses any over-the-counter products or creams. Assess the bone structure of hands and feet. Note any abnormalities in appearance, such as bony enlargement or erythema associated with arthritis. Gently assess range of motion of the hands and feet, noting any discomfort experienced by the older adult.

Back and Hips

Observe the skin on the back and hips of an older adult. Assess for areas of skin breakdown, especially on an individual confined to bed or wheelchair. Common areas of breakdown include pressure points such as the sacral area, greater trochanter, and scapulae. Note the presence of dryness, erythema, rash, or other visible irritation. Assess the bone structure of the back and hips. Note the presence of any kyphosis, scoliosis, or other alterations.

SLEEP ASSESSMENT

An important component in assessing the sleep quality of an older adult is observation during your initial assessment. Does the client appear alert? Does he or she understand and respond appropriately to questions you are asking? Although an answer of "no" to these questions might indicate other types of problems besides lack of sleep, your initial observations are worthy of consideration in trying to determine if your client may have a sleep disorder.

Ask the client specifically about his or her sleeping patterns. Does he or she feel well rested in the morning? Other questions that can elicit valuable sleep information from the older adult are listed in Box 5–2.

Although this subjective information is very important, objective data are also useful. Instruct the older adult to maintain a **sleep log**, in which he or she can document sleeping aids, bedtime, nighttime awakenings, dreams or nightmares, presence of pain, amount of time slept, how he or she felt upon awakening, naps, and daytime alertness. This log should be kept for at least 1 week.

If the client is experiencing problems with sleep, you can ask a family member to observe whenhe or she is sleeping and note the client's position, movement, restlessness, wakefulness, snoring, apnea, and talking during sleep. Finally, it is important to consider the effect of sleep (or lack thereof) and medications on daytime

---

Box 5–2   Questions to Include in a Sleep Assessment

1. How many hours do you sleep on a typical night?
2. How many times do you usually awaken during the night?
3. Do you nap during the day? How many times? For how long? What time of day do you usually nap?
4. Do you have an exercise routine? What type of activity do you undertake? What time of day?
5. Do you use sleeping medications? What type? How often?
6. Do you drink alcohol?
7. Do you have any bedtime "rituals" (e.g., reading, warm bath, watching television, etc.)?
8. What other medications are you currently taking?
9. What are your eating habits?

functioning. Things to note include morning headaches, irritability, drowsiness, lethargy, short attention span, frequent napping, and complaints of exhaustion.

A sleep study, which is an in-depth assessment of sleep, can be done in a sleep laboratory. In this setting, technicians use **polysomnography** to evaluate the different stages of sleep and to diagnose sleep disorders. This evaluation requires at least an overnight stay, or possibly several days, at the sleep laboratory. If this is viewed as too disruptive for the older adult, home monitoring systems are also available.

DISORDERS COMMON IN THE OLDER ADULT

Osteoporosis

Osteoporosis is a commonly occurring medical condition in the older adult population. The name *osteoporosis* literally means *porous bone;* it is a gradual reduction in bone mass that makes the bone vulnerable to fracture. Osteoporosis is not considered a normal consequence of aging, although it is highly prevalent among older adults because of age-related bone losses. It is more common in older women because older women lose trabecular bone at a faster rate than do older men. Risk factors for the development of osteoporosis can be found in Box 5–3.

Box 5–3 | Risk Factors for the Development of Osteoporosis

- Female
- Asian or white
- Thin, small frame
- Family history of osteoporosis
- Menopause before age 45
- Cigarette smoking
- Diet deficient in calcium or vitamin D
- Sedentary lifestyle/prolonged immobility
- Use of certain medications
- Alcohol abuse
- Excessive caffeine intake

A client with osteoporosis can experience a fracture of any bone in the body; however, the most common areas of fracture are the vertebrae, the femoral neck (hip), and the wrist. These three areas of the body contain more trabecular bone than do other bones in the body. When fractures occur in the vertebral area, the client gradually develops kyphosis or a hunched-over posture; this is commonly referred to as dowager's hump (Fig. 5–3).

A fracture of any kind can lead to impaired mobility, serious health consequences, and potentially the loss of independence for the older adult. The older adult can experience severe back pain due to collapsed vertebrae, as well as decreased height by as much as 6 to 9 inches. Medical treatment of osteoporosis consists primarily of drug therapy (Table 5–2).

Nurses can assist in the prevention of osteoporosis by teaching a healthy diet, exercise, and other health-promoting behaviors to the older adult. Prevention is the best treatment for this disease.

Medication Safety Tip

Medications associated with the development of osteoporosis:

- Corticosteroids
- Anticonvulsants
- Thyroid hormones
- Loop diuretics
- Chemotherapy drugs
- Aluminum-containing antacids
- Heparin
- Cholestyramine
- Cyclosporin A

Adapted from Drugay, M. (1997). Breaking the silence: A health promotion approach to osteoporosis. *Journal of Gerontological Nursing, 23*(6), 38.

Osteoarthritis

Osteoarthritis, sometimes referred to as degenerative joint disease (DJD), is a disorder that affects movable joints. It is characterized by deterioration of the articular cartilage that begins in the 20s and 30s, although symptoms of the disorder usually do not occur until an individual is in the seventh decade of life. It is thought to be the result of wear and tear on the joints and is the most common form of arthritis. Later stages of

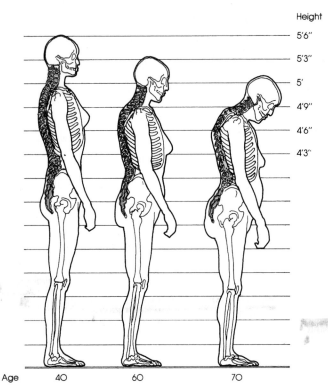

Height

5'6"

5'3"

5'

4'9"

4'6"

4'3"

Age   40   60   70

Figure 5–3. Normal spine at age 40 years and changes brought about by osteoporosis at ages 60 and 70. (From Ignatavicius, D. D., Workman, M. L., & Mishler, M. A. [1999]. *Medical-surgical nursing across the health care continuum* [3rd ed.]. Philadelphia: W. B. Saunders.)

Table 5–2

DRUG THERAPY FOR OSTEOPOROSIS

Category	Function
Estrogen replacement therapy (ERT) or hormone replacement therapy (HRT, consisting of both estrogen and progesterone)	Slows bone loss
Calcium	Aids osteoblast activity to form new bone
Vitamin D	Assists absorption of calcium from the gastrointestinal tract
Calcitonin (Miacalcin)	Decreases number and function of osteoclasts
Alendronate sodium (Fosamax)	Inhibits osteoclast activity, increases bone density
Fluoride	Increases bone mass by stimulating osteoblasts
Raloxifene (Evista)	Increases bone density, similar to estrogen, but without growth-stimulating effects in the breast and uterus

the disease are characterized by pain, stiffness, and joint hypertrophy. Occasionally, **crepitation** is heard with joint movement, due to grating of bone against bone, as articular cartilage is worn away. The joints usually affected are the weight-bearing joints: the knees, hips, and lumbar spine, plus the terminal interphalangeal joints of the hands. Medical treatment of osteoarthritis usually consists of medication, rest, physical therapy, and surgery (Table 5–3).

Pressure Ulcers

Pressure ulcers, also known as decubitus ulcers, are areas of skin breakdown that result from prolonged pressure between the skin and an external object, such as a bed or chair. They usually occur over bony prominences, such as the greater trochanter, sacral area, ankles, heels, elbows, and back. Older adults are at increased risk for the development of pressure ulcers because of the effect of aging on skin, which was described earlier. In addition, an older adult may have additional risk factors that place him or her at greater risk for developing a pressure ulcer (Box 5–4).

An additional factor that can lead to the development of a pressure ulcer in an older adult is friction on the skin, or **shearing forces**. It is

| Box 5–4 | Risk Factors for the Development of Pressure Ulcers |

- Immobility
- Malnutrition
- Cognitive impairment
- Incontinence
- Advanced age
- Impaired sensation

important as you reposition your older client in bed to avoid dragging the client; dragging produces a shearing force that can place him or her at increased risk of developing a pressure ulcer.

The initial appearance of a pressure ulcer may be simply an area of redness. It is important to intervene immediately by providing pressure relief to avoid further breakdown. Superficial pressure ulcers may have a reddened, blistered appearance. Deeper pressure ulcers indicate deep tissue necrosis and may be yellow, white, brown, or black. Pressure ulcers are graded by severity on a scale of I to IV (Table 5–4).

The older adult with a superficial pressure ulcer usually experiences pain. Deep pressure ulcers may result in destruction of pain fibers; however, the edges of the ulcer can be very painful because they are more superficial, and therefore, the pain fibers are intact. However,

Table 5–3
MEDICAL TREATMENTS FOR OSTEOARTHRITIS

Treatment	Examples
Medication	• Salicylates (e.g., ASA) • NSAIDs (e.g., ibuprofen) • Chondroprotective agents (e.g., glucosamine sulfate)
Joint rest	• Minimize weight-bearing on affected joints • Maintain normal joint alignment and motion • Use of cane or crutch • Lose weight if obese
Physical therapy	• Isometric exercise • Walking • Gentle massage over joints • Vigorous massage over muscles
Surgery	• Total joint replacement (arthroplasty) • Joint fusion

ASA, acetylsalicylic acid; NSAIDs, nonsteroidal anti-inflammatory drugs.
Adapted from Matteson, M. A., McConnell, E. S., & Linton, A. D. (1998). *Gerontological nursing: Concepts and practice.* Philadelphia: W. B. Saunders, pp. 209–211.

Table 5–4
GRADING OF PRESSURE ULCERS

Grade	Description
I	• Soft tissue swelling or tissue ulceration lasting 24 hours or longer • Reddened area of skin that does not blanch when pressed
II	• Partial-thickness ulcer penetrating the dermis • Appears superficial, similar to an abrasion, blister, or shallow crater
III	• Full-thickness skin loss with necrosis of the subcutaneous tissue • Appears like a deep crater
IV	• Full-thickness loss of skin demonstrating extensive destruction and tissue necrosis that may involve muscle, bone, or other supporting structures • Bone may be visible

Adapted from Tyson, S. R. (1999). *Gerontological nursing care.* Philadelphia: W. B. Saunders, p. 366.

the absence of pain does not necessarily indicate that the client is improving. The client with deep pressure ulcers may have other signs and symptoms, such as loss of appetite, apathy, dehydration, and signs of infection. Medical treatment of pressure ulcers includes dressing changes, monitoring of fluid and nutrition, and provision of pressure relief. Advanced practice nurses, such as clinical nurse specialists, nurse practitioners, and enterostomal therapists, have expertise in the area of wound care and often are the resource to consult when you are determining the type of dressing appropriate for a particular ulcer. Healing of pressure ulcers occurs from the inside out; with deep pressure ulcers, dressing changes may be required for months in some clients before healing occurs. Deeper stages of ulcers that have a brown or black appearance must be **débrided** by the physician or advanced practice nurse to promote healing.

Nutrition Tip

Good nutrition is of the utmost importance for a client with a pressure ulcer.

Sleep Disorders

Diagnosis of sleep disorders can be difficult in older adults owing to age-related changes. Sleep disorders are more severe than age-related changes. The older adult with a sleep disorder often experiences difficulty falling asleep or staying asleep and excessive daytime drowsiness. In contrast, normal changes of aging may lead to a mild alteration in sleep but should not lead to excessive daytime drowsiness.

An individual with a sleep disorder can be irritable and confused, and may have daytime behavior problems. These difficulties can place enough stress on a family to force them to consider long-term care placement for their loved one. Three major kinds of sleep disorders that affect older adults include **dyssomnias**, medical disorders, and psychiatric disorders (Table 5–5).

To treat a sleep disorder related to a medical condition, the physician may make alterations in the prescription of medications or in other therapies. For example, if arthritis is causing pain that interferes with sleep, a long-acting analgesic medication just before bedtime may be ordered. Drug

Table 5–5
SLEEP DISORDERS AFFECTING OLDER ADULTS

Type	Examples
Dyssomnia	• Obstructive sleep apnea syndrome • Periodic limb movement disorders • Restless leg syndrome
Medical disorders	• Cardiovascular disease • Diabetes mellitus • Gastrointestinal reflux • Arthritis
Psychiatric disorders	• Anxiety disorder • Depression • Cognitive deficits

Adapted from Beck-Little, R., & Weinrich, S. P. (1998). Assessment and management of sleep disorders in the elderly. *Journal of Gerontological Nursing, 24*(4), 22.

therapy and counseling may be prescribed for an older adult with a psychiatric disorder. Dyssomnia treatments are outlined in Table 5–6.

NURSING DIAGNOSES

Nursing diagnoses are derived from the assessment data and are unique to the individual older adult. Although clients with similar diagnoses often experience similar problems, individual differences must be discerned. The focus of a medical diagnosis is the etiology, or cause, of a particular disease; however, a nursing diagnosis focuses on the *client's response* to the health problem.

Table 5–6
MEDICAL TREATMENTS FOR DYSSOMNIAS

Type	Treatments/Medications
Obstructive sleep apnea	• Weight loss • Continuous positive airway pressure (CPAP) mask at night
Periodic limb movement disorder	• Surgery • Clonazepam • Trazodone hydrochloride
Restless leg syndrome	• Benzodiazepines • Vitamin E • Quinine • Low-dose narcotic analgesics

Adapted from Beck-Little, R., & Weinrich, S. P. (1998). Assessment and management of sleep disorders in the elderly. *Journal of Gerontological Nursing, 24* (4), 23.

The North American Nursing Diagnosis Association (NANDA) is a group of nurses who meet yearly to refine and update the list of standardized nursing diagnoses.

Nursing diagnoses are written in a PES format, standing for **P**roblem, **E**tiology (cause), and **S**igns and symptoms. By using the PES format, you are truly tailoring the nursing diagnosis to the client, as well as providing evidence to defend your choice of nursing diagnosis. For example:

impaired skin integrity (P)
related to immobility (E)
as evidenced by 3-cm decubitus ulcer on left greater trochanter (S)

Nursing diagnoses presented throughout this book contain only the first (problem) portion of the nursing diagnosis statement because the second and third portions (etiology and signs/symptoms) are unique to your client and must be determined by your assessment.

Some of the nursing diagnoses (written only as the problem portion) that apply to the older adult experiencing disorders covered in this chapter are included in Table 5–7.

Remember: Not every identified nursing diagnosis is appropriate for every client with a given disorder. Likewise, other nursing diagnoses that were not listed above may be appropriate for your client. For example, the nursing diagnosis *Sensory/Perceptual Alteration: Tactile* may apply to many clients with pressure ulcers. However, not every older adult with osteoporosis will experience pain. It is important to consult the current

list of nursing diagnoses distributed by NANDA and carefully consider each nursing diagnosis when you develop a plan of care for your client.

COLLABORATING ON THE PLAN OF CARE

Although the nursing process (assessment, nursing diagnosis, planning, intervention, evaluation) is primarily the responsibility of the registered nurse (RN), your contribution is invaluable. The professional collaboration between the RN and the licensed practical nurse/licensed vocational nurse (LPN/LVN) is extremely important in ensuring that all assessment data are taken into account, that the nursing diagnoses are accurate, that the outcomes planned for the client are realistic, that the plan makes sense, that interventions are carried out, and that the evaluation occurs. In other words, it is a team approach, and the LPN/LVN is a very important and influential part of the plan of care. Collaboration ensures success of the care plan.

Once you establish the nursing diagnosis, you must set outcomes. It is important to develop outcomes that are realistic, measurable, and tailored to the individual client. An example of a client outcome that is not measurable is: "Client will understand risk factors for osteoporosis." This is not measurable (unless you have psychic abilities). A better way to write this outcome would be: "Client will state two activities that she can undertake to decrease her risk of osteoporosis." One yardstick for determining whether the

Table 5–7				
NURSING DIAGNOSES RELATED TO ACTIVITY AND REST				
	Osteoporosis	Osteoarthritis	Pressure Ulcers	Sleep Disorders
Deficient knowledge	X	X	X	X
Pain	X	X	X	
Disturbed body image	X	X	X	
Risk for injury	X	X		X
Risk for infection			X	
Ineffective tissue perfusion			X	
Impaired skin integrity			X	
Disturbed sleep pattern	X	X	X	X
Impaired physical mobility	X	X	X	
Impaired home maintenance	X	X	X	X

Table 5–8
SAMPLE OUTCOMES FOR AN OLDER ADULT WITH OSTEOPOROSIS

Nursing Diagnosis	Sample Outcomes
Risk for injury	• Client will avoid injury • Client will state environmental modifications he/she can make to increase environmental safety
Pain	• Client will be free from pain
Deficient knowledge: osteoporosis and its treatment	• Client will identify two forms of weight-bearing exercise • Client will name two lifestyle factors that can lead to osteoporosis • Client will list verbally five foods rich in calcium and/or vitamin D

outcome you have written is measurable is this: Can a nurse who has never met your client walk into the client's room with your care plan in hand and immediately evaluate if the client is meeting the outcomes? If the answer is "no," then the planned client outcomes are not measurable. If the answer is "yes," they are.

Based on the previous section, in which nursing diagnoses for osteoporosis were identified, sample outcomes for a client with osteoporosis can be found in Table 5–8. These are samples only because the outcomes that you set must be established with your individual client in mind.

In like fashion, sample outcomes for older adults with nursing diagnoses for osteoarthritis, pressure ulcers, and sleep disorders can be found in Table 5–9.

IMPLEMENTING INTERVENTIONS FOR HEALTH PROMOTION

Interventions to Promote Safety

1. Assess and promote environmental safety. For the older client with osteoporosis, a safe environment is of the utmost importance. The nursing priority is to prevent a fall or other accident that could lead to serious health consequences and the possibility of loss of independence for the client. The nurse must carefully assess the environment and identify obstacles that might pose a threat to the older adult. Items that can be tripped on such as throw rugs, extension cords, and clutter should be eliminated from the environment. The nurse should inquire about and discourage footwear and clothing that might increase the risk for falls, such as long bathrobes and slippery shoes. The nurse should emphasize to the older client the importance of wearing eyeglasses of the current prescription and cleaning them regularly.

2. Assess for toxic effects of medications. Clients with osteoporosis and osteoarthritis may regularly use analgesics to relieve pain associated with these conditions. Signs of toxicity associated with pain medications include tinnitus, hearing loss, nausea, vomiting, anemia, and gastrointestinal bleeding.

🔹 Medication Safety Tip

Owing to age-related changes in hearing, tinnitus may be absent in the older adult who experiences salicylate toxicity. Instead, the nurse must observe for other signs and symptoms, such as dizziness, drowsiness, or excitement.

3. Anticipate and prevent skin breakdown and other hazards of immobility. Nurses must have a clear understanding of the hazards of immobility and methods for preventing them. Older adults who are unable to move independently need to be turned and repositioned frequently. Range-of-motion exercises must be implemented with each position change. Clients who are incontinent must be kept clean and dry.

4. Educate the older adult about exercise safety. Guidelines for exercise safety can be found in Box 5–5.
   Encourage the older adult to select an exercise based on his or her interests. The American Association of Retired Persons (AARP) has information for older adults who are beginning an exercise program; these publications, entitled *Pep Up Your Life with Exercise: The Key to a Good Life* and *Keeping in Shape: Let's Get Moving*, are both available on the Internet.

Table 5–9	
SAMPLE OUTCOMES FOR AN OLDER ADULT WITH OSTEOARTHRITIS, PRESSURE ULCERS, OR SLEEP DISORDERS	
Nursing Diagnosis	**Sample Outcome**
Osteoarthritis	
Impaired physical mobility	• Client will move all joints within their range of motion
Chronic pain	• Client will state that he has temporary relief from pain
Impaired home maintenance	• Client will perform ADLs safely and independently
Pressure Ulcers	
Impaired skin integrity	• Pressure ulcer will decrease by 1 cm in diameter within 2 weeks • No new areas of skin breakdown will be observed
Risk for infection	• Client will verbalize to nurse three signs and/or symptoms of infection and what to do if these are observed/experienced • Client will demonstrate wound care to nurse, observing aseptic technique, within 1 week
Ineffective tissue perfusion: peripheral	• Skin will be pink and warm with capillary refill time <3 seconds
Sleep Disorders	
Disturbed sleep pattern	• Client will report having adequate sleep within 48 hours • Client will obtain restful sleep without the use of medications
Risk for injury	• Client will experience no physical injury
Deficient knowledge	• Client will list verbally the negative effects alcohol has on sleep • Client will identify three measures that can be tried immediately to improve sleep

Interventions to Promote Health Education

1. Under the guidance of the RN, implement a teaching plan specific to the disorder that the older adult is experiencing. For example, the client with osteoporosis should be taught about the relationship between calcium, vitamin D, and bone integrity. Educate the client with osteoarthritis about treatment options prescribed by the physician. Teach the older adult with a pressure ulcer (or the family member, as appropriate) skin care and techniques to prevent further skin compromise. Assist the client with a sleep disorder in understanding how the disorder is different from normal developments of aging, and suggest strategies that might be effective for improving sleep and quality of life.

2. Educate the older adult about the medications being taken for medical disorders: how they work, why they are prescribed, and possible adverse effects to be alert for. The individual with osteoarthritis is helped by acquiring an understanding of the use of pain medications, as well as other nonpharmacologic methods, for managing chronic pain.

| ⟁ Box 5–5 | **Guidelines for Exercise Safety** |

* Before beginning a new exercise program, a medical evaluation should be performed to assess overall health.
* Increase exercises gradually, first incorporating them into everyday activities.
* Breathe evenly and deeply during and between exercises in order to avoid performing the Valsalva maneuver during exercise.
* Always include a warm-up period and a cool-down period.
* Wear comfortable clothing and proper footwear.
* Wear a helmet for bicycle riding.
* Consult a physician for any changes, questions, or concerns.

---

3. Educate the older adult about proper skin care. The skin of the older adult is often dry from the normal changes of aging. Encourage bathing in lukewarm water, as hot water tends to dry the skin. Bathing every other day rather than every day also decreases skin dryness. Regular use of skin moisturizers also helps to alleviate skin dryness.

Interventions to Promote Lifestyle Modification

1. Encourage reduction of excess weight. Weight loss can improve the symptoms of many disorders such as osteoarthritis and sleep apnea.
2. Encourage healthy lifestyle habits. Educate the client about the importance of a diet high in calcium and vitamin D, along with weight-bearing exercise, to improve bone density.
3. Discourage unhealthy lifestyle habits. Teach the client with osteoporosis the negative effects on bone integrity of smoking, alcohol, and excessive caffeine usage. Educate the client who has trouble sleeping about the effects of alcohol on sleep.

Interventions to Promote Mobility

Exercise

In Chapter 1, you learned that one of the objectives of *Healthy People 2010* is to "Increase the proportion of adults who engage regularly, preferably daily, in moderate physical activity for at least 30 minutes per day." We later discussed, in Chapter 4, how exercise is important for the older adult regardless of his or her level of activity. It is important for nurses to encourage regular exercise for the older adult and to assist in selection of an appropriate routine. Regular activity and exercise are important for the management of each of the four disorders discussed in this chapter (Table 5–10).

Physical activity need not be strenuous to provide health benefits. The older adult can notice the improvement in their health when short exercise sessions are undertaken frequently, preferably daily. It is important to keep exercise safety, which was discussed earlier, in mind when you are advising an older adult about physical activity. Many older adults are joining groups of "Mall Walkers" sponsored by Senior Citizen groups.

There are also everyday opportunities for older adults to undertake physical activity. You can encourage the older adult to take the stairs instead of the elevator, walk to the store or post office instead of driving, choose a parking space a little distance away from where he or she is going, and avoid using the remote control to change the television channel. It seems that most of today's technological advances have encouraged individuals to be less active.

Postoperative Interventions for the Client Undergoing Hip Replacement Surgery

Hip replacement surgery may be performed on the older adult who has a fracture in the femoral neck area of the hip. The surgery may be a **total hip arthroplasty** (THA), whereby the femoral head and acetabulum are replaced by a prosthesis, or a **hemiarthroplasty**, in which only a prosthetic femoral head is implanted. For either of these surgeries, there are important nursing and client teaching implications. Nursing interventions can be grouped into the general categories of positioning, promoting mobility, pain management, recognition of complications, and discharge teaching.

It is paramount that proper positioning be maintained for protection of the surgical area. Avoid extremes in range of motion, especially

Table 5–10		
BENEFITS OF EXERCISE FOR SELECTED DISORDERS		
Disorder	**Benefits**	**Comment**
Osteoporosis	• Increased bone mass • Decreased susceptibility to fracture • Improved balance, reduced fall risk	Exercise must be weight-bearing to achieve desired benefit
Osteoarthritis	• Improved flexibility • Increased muscle mass leading to better-supported joints • Weight loss can improve symptoms of disorder	Gentle stretching recommended to reduce stiffness Water exercises may be best tolerated
Pressure ulcer	• Improved tissue perfusion leading to faster healing	Gentle movement only recommended
Sleep disorder	• More restful sleep at night • Weight loss can improve symptoms of disorder	Exercise recommended early in the day

adduction and **flexion** of the joint. The easiest way to avoid adduction is by using a triangle-shaped **abduction** pillow, which keeps the knees apart while the older adult is in bed. Avoid flexion by making certain the hips are never lower than the knees when the client is sitting. Elevated toilet seats are useful in helping the client maintain this position.

Early mobility is important after hip surgery, as after other surgeries; however, it must be assisted. On the first postoperative day, the older adult is assisted from the bed to a chair. Ambulation begins on postoperative day number 2, although full weight bearing is usually not allowed for 6 to 8 weeks.

Pain management is an important part of the postoperative plan. Older adults who have undergone this type of surgery often obtain better pain relief with less confusion using **patient-controlled analgesia** (PCA). PCA uses small intravenous doses of pain medication, such as morphine sulfate, that the client activates by pressing a button. The nurse regularly checks the PCA machine to determine the amount of medication the client has been requesting and receiving. Of course, assessment of the client's level of pain on a regular basis (every 4 hours, or more often as needed) is crucial. As the client becomes more mobile and experiences less pain, the intravenous medication will be changed to an oral

analgesic such as oxycodone, or a nonsteroidal anti-inflammatory medication. Whatever the modality of pain management, however, it is important that the older adult receive pain medication approximately 30 minutes before mobility is undertaken.

The most life-threatening complications that can occur following hip replacement surgery are deep vein thrombosis and pulmonary embolus. Signs and symptoms of these complications, listed in Box 5–6, must be reported immediately.

Other complications of hip surgery include urinary tract infection, confusion, and dislocation of the hip prosthesis. Careful assessment for each of these complications and prompt reporting are essential for safe nursing care of the client undergoing hip replacement surgery.

Discharge teaching about hip precautions consists primarily of reinforcement of activity restrictions and hip movements to be avoided. Suggestions for client teaching are presented in Box 5–7.

Rehabilitative Techniques/Restorative Care

Rehabilitation is the process of restoring an individual's ability to live as normally as possible following a potentially disabling injury or illness. In this chapter, we are primarily concerned with

Box 5–6   Signs and Symptoms of Life-Threatening Complications of Hip Replacement Surgery

Deep vein thrombosis (DVT): usually unilateral, occurring in one leg:

- Pain
- Swelling
- Warmth
- Tenderness

Pulmonary embolus:

- Sudden shortness of breath
- Chest pain
- Tachycardia
- Diaphoresis
- Feeling of fear
- Fever
- Hypoxemia

Adapted from: Yarnold, B. (1999). Hip fracture: Caring for a fragile population. *AJN, 99*(2), 37.

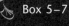

Box 5–7   Discharge Teaching: "Hip Precautions"

Do:

- Keep knees lower than hips when sitting
- Ask for assistance putting on shoes and socks
- Use an elevated toilet seat
- Use an abduction pillow while in bed
- Use a walker or cane for support

Don't:

- Bend at the waist for any reason
- Sit on low chairs, toilets, or stools
- Cross your legs
- Sit with your legs together
- Lean forward when sitting
- Raise your knees when sitting
- Climb on ladders
- Participate in vigorous physical activities

Adapted from Yarnold, B. (1999). Hip fracture: Caring for a fragile population. *AJN, 99*(2), 38.

physical rehabilitation of older adults experiencing musculoskeletal ailments. There is no age limit on rehabilitation: older adults should not be excluded from a plan of rehabilitation simply because of their age. Achievement of goals may take longer, and progress may be slower, but older adults greatly benefit from rehabilitation, in terms of both functional abilities and quality of life.

Expected outcomes of rehabilitation will be different for older adults, when compared with those of young adults. Whereas the outcome for a 35-year-old may be a return to gainful employment, the outcomes for a 75-year-old may include the ability to perform ADL and live independently, prevention of complications, and maintenance of an acceptable quality of life. The basic principles of rehabilitation are outlined in Box 5–8.

Interventions and rehabilitative techniques vary, depending on the older adult's illness or disease process, strengths and abilities, and client interests. For the older adult with osteoarthritis, specialized exercises can help to strengthen muscles that support the affected joints; for example, exercises that strengthen the quadriceps muscle in the leg will also support the knee joint. Exercises also help the older adult to maintain mobility in the joint; for example, an older adult with arthritis in the hands may find that continuing to play the piano or knit helps keep the finger joints limber. Assistive devices, described in the following section, may be useful on a temporary or permanent basis. A plan for rehabilitation is an interdisciplinary process and will include client outcomes, interventions, responsible disciplines, and target dates for reevaluation.

Box 5–8   Principles of Rehabilitation

- Control the underlying illness or disease.
- Develop functional abilities by capitalizing on existing strengths and abilities.
- Prevent secondary disabilities.
- Preserve the dignity of the older adult by promoting self-esteem and self-confidence.

Adapted from Matteson, M. A., McConnell, E. S., & Linton, A. D. (1998). *Gerontological nursing: Concepts and practice*. Philadelphia: W. B. Saunders, p. 888.

Assistive Devices

Assistive devices are important aids for the older adult with impaired mobility. Assistive devices for ambulation include walkers, canes (single or quadripod), and crutches. An important nursing responsibility is to ensure that the client is using the device correctly; a device used incorrectly can actually increase strain on healthy muscles and joints (Fig. 5–4).

The most effective method for teaching a client the proper use of an assistive device is return demonstration: you demonstrate the technique, explaining the rationale for each step; then, the client demonstrates the correct technique back to you. In demonstrating an assistive device for ambulation, the correct technique is as follows: Assistive device ----> weak leg ----> strong leg. If the older adult is unable to correctly or safely use an assistive device, a wheelchair may be the safest alternative for moving about.

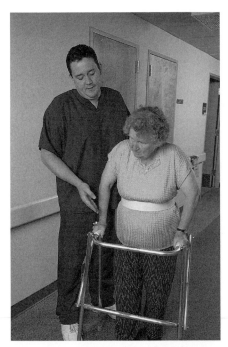

Figure 5–4. Assess the gait of the client learning to use a walker. (From Leahy, J. M., & Kizilay, P. E. [1998]. *Foundations of nursing practice.* Philadelphia: W. B. Saunders, p. 815.)

Interventions to Promote Nutrition

1. Encourage a diet rich in calcium and vitamin D for older adults at risk for osteoporosis. The Recommended Daily Allowance (RDA) for premenopausal women and postmenopausal women taking estrogen is 1 gram of calcium; the RDA for postmenopausal women who are not taking estrogen is 1.5 grams of calcium. Vitamin D assists the gastrointestinal tract in absorbing calcium. The recommended dose for someone with a diet inadequate in vitamin D is 400 IU each day; 15 minutes of sunshine provides the body with approximately the same amount of vitamin D.
2. Encourage a diet rich in protein, vitamin C, and zinc for the older adult with a pressure ulcer. This will assist in tissue repair and promote wound healing.
3. Educate the older adult who is taking aspirin therapy about the possible nutritional depletion of vitamin C and folate that may occur. Encourage foods high in these nutrients.
4. Encourage dietary modifications for older adults with sleep difficulties. These nutritional alterations, which can help nighttime sleep, are discussed in the next section.

Interventions to Promote Rest and Sleep

1. Encourage nutrition that promotes rest and sleep. Heavy meals before bedtime can interfere with sleep, so these should be discouraged in the older adult. However, a light snack with foods containing the essential amino acid **tryptophan** may help promote sleep by increasing the amount of serotonin in the brain (serotonin is a neurotransmitter that influences mood and sleep). Box 5–9 lists common foods containing tryptophan.
2. Discourage the use of caffeine and other stimulants 3 to 4 hours before bedtime. Remind the older adult that caffeine is found not only in coffee and tea, but also in hot chocolate, soft drinks, and medications; it may also be added to prepackaged foods. It is important to check food labels because caffeine is sometimes added to items the average consumer would not consider, such as yogurt, ice cream,

| Box 5–9 | **Foods Containing Tryptophan** |

Corn
Cereal grains
Legumes
Milk and other dairy products
Meat
Eggs
Nuts and seeds

Source: Amino acids: Tryptophan. HealthWorld Online. Available at http://www.healthy.net/hwlibrary-books/haas/amino.trp.htm. Accessed 4/9/99.

desserts, and even some brands of mineral water. The caffeine content of selected foods and drugs is listed in Table 5–11.

3. Encourage weight reduction in overweight clients with osteoarthritis and sleep apnea. It has been shown that weight reduction can help alleviate symptoms of both of these disorders.

4. Minimize nighttime disturbances to the older adult in all care settings. When possible, plan ahead and group activities together so that the older adult may be awakened as few times as possible during the night. For example, it can be helpful if assessments can be performed, vital signs taken, and medications administered at the same visit. It is also a good idea to offer the older adult assistance in getting to the bathroom at this time, so that unnecessary awakening can be avoided.

5. Encourage the older adult with chronic pain to take an analgesic at bedtime. Relief from pain and discomfort may allow the older adult to achieve a deeper state of relaxation and a more restful sleep.

6. Provide support and understanding to the older adult who is experiencing sleep difficulties. Encourage the use of strategies to promote sleep. Some common strategies are listed in Box 5–10.

7. Remind the older adult with osteoarthritis about the importance of rest in minimizing stress on the affected joints.

Table 5–11
CAFFEINE CONTENT OF SELECTED FOODS AND DRUGS

Product	Serving Size (ounces)	Typical Caffeine Content Range (mg)
Coffee (brewed, drip method)	8 ounces	60–180
Instant coffee	8 ounces	30–120
Decaffeinated coffee	8 ounces	1–5
Espresso	1 ounce	30–50
Tea (U.S. brand)	8 ounces	20–90
Tea (imported)	8 ounces	25–110
Tea (instant)	8 ounces	24–31
Some soft drinks	8 ounces	20–40
Cocoa beverage	8 ounces	3–32
Chocolate milk beverage	8 ounces	27
Milk chocolate	1 ounce	1–15
Dark chocolate, semisweet	1 ounce	5–35
Anacin (aspirin) analgesic	1 tablet	32
Dristan (phenylephrine hydrochloride)	1 tablet	16
Excedrin (acetaminophen)	1 tablet	65
Triaminic (phenylpropanolamine hydrochloride)	1 tablet	30

Data from Caffeine safety and labeling of foods and beverages. Available at http://www.ificinfo.health.org/quanda/caflabel.htm. Accessed 4/9/99; and Mitchell, M. K. (1994). *Nutrition across the life span.* Philadelphia: W. B. Saunders, p. 237.

Box 5–10 Strategies to Promote Rest and Sleep

- Establish a consistent bedtime.
- Use the bed for sleep only (not for reading or eating).
- Maintain environment conducive to sleeping.
- Avoid alcohol (more than 1 glass of wine).
- Play "white noise" in the background such as recording of ocean waves.
- Use relaxation techniques.
- Limit fluids after dinner if adequate amounts are consumed during the day.
- Use sleep medications only as a last resort, and only on a short-term basis (4–6 weeks).
- Eat tryptophan-containing snacks 1.5 to 2 hours before bedtime.
- Provide pet therapy.
- Exercise in AM or early afternoon.

GATHERING DATA FOR EVALUATION

Although the RN is officially responsible for evaluation and modification of the plan of care for the client, your contribution with ongoing assessment of client progress is crucial. The data you gather, along with your observation of changes in the client, will ensure that the plan of care continues to be appropriate.

Nursing evaluation should be aimed directly at the outcomes. For example, one expected outcome identified earlier in this chapter for the older adult experiencing a sleep disorder was written, "Client will obtain restful sleep without the use of medications." To evaluate progress toward this outcome, where should you begin? Several sources of information should be consulted. First of all, assess the client. Ask about the quality and quantity of sleep received the prior night. Listen to report from the night shift nurse for any description of wakefulness of the client. Read the progress notes and look for any mention of sleep or nighttime awakenings. Check the medication record for documentation of sleep medications administered on the evening or night shift.

In addition, your evaluation should take into consideration individual interventions employed. For example, if the client states that some nights he or she obtains restful sleep, but other nights he or she does not, inquire about interventions implemented on each of the nights to try and elicit a pattern. The client may state that warm milk at bedtime was effective on Monday night, but hot chocolate on Tuesday night led to insomnia. The difference in effectiveness of interventions may lead directly to opportunities for client education (e.g., the caffeine content of hot chocolate).

In evaluating physical benefits associated with weight-bearing exercises, it may take up to 12 weeks to achieve a noticeable change in function. It is important that repeat assessments be performed to enable comparisons with baseline. Encourage the client to continue the activity program after discharge from health care. Expected outcomes, patterned after the outcomes you have previously written, may include decreased number and severity of falls, improved mobility, and enhanced reports of well-being from the client.

Summary

- Muscle tends to atrophy with age. This process can lead to impairments in strength, balance, and gait. Atrophy is influenced by nutrition and physical activity, and can be reduced by exercise.
- Bones also change with age. Both cortical and trabecular bone experience loss, leading to more brittle bones. Women experience greater bone loss, and it begins earlier. Factors involved include changes in hormone levels with age, sedentary lifestyle, and dietary deficiencies.
- Older adults experience a gradual change in stature due to loss of vertebral height and narrowing of the disks. There is decreased flexibility in tendons and ligaments, while cartilage continues to grow.
- Aging skin is more thin, fragile, and dry, and has a wrinkling and sagging appearance. Hair becomes gray or white from loss of melanocytes, and may become sparse.
- Many older people have trouble sleeping. Older adults often take a longer time to fall asleep, may awaken more frequently, and spend less time in the deeper stages of sleep.
- Always assess in the direction of head to toe, and carefully document and communicate any

abnormalities in your findings to the registered nurse.

- Assess the color of the skin for abnormalities such as pallor, erythema, rashes, jaundice, or cyanosis. Observe muscular development, bone structure, range of motion, and color and appearance of hair and nails. Assess for areas of skin breakdown, especially in an individual confined to bed or wheelchair.

- A sleep assessment begins with observation of client alertness and response. Ask the client about sleep patterns. Objective data can be acquired in a sleep log or by observation. In-depth assessment of sleep can be done in a sleep laboratory.

- Osteoporosis is common in the older adult, especially women. Risk factors include aging, small frame, white or Asian descent, certain medications, and smoking. It results in bones that are vulnerable to fracture, most commonly of the vertebrae, the femoral neck, and the wrist. Treatment consists primarily of drug therapy and weight-bearing exercise.

- Osteoarthritis is a disorder that affects movable joints, and is characterized by deterioration of the articular cartilage. Symptoms include pain, stiffness, and hypertrophy of weight-bearing joints. Medical treatment consists of medication, rest, physical therapy, and surgery.

- Pressure ulcers are areas of skin breakdown that result from prolonged pressure between the skin and an external object, usually over bony prominences. Superficial ulcers have a reddened, blistered appearance. Deep pressure ulcers indicate tissue necrosis. Pressure ulcers are graded by severity on a scale of I to IV. Medical treatment includes dressing changes, monitoring of fluid and nutrition, and pressure relief.

- The older adult with a sleep disorder often experiences difficulty falling asleep or staying asleep and excessive daytime drowsiness, irritability or confusion, or behavior problems. Sleep disorders that affect older adults include dyssomnias, medical disorders, and psychiatric disorders.

- Nursing diagnoses are derived from the assessment data and are unique to the individual. The focus of a medical diagnosis is the cause of a particular disease; a nursing diagnosis focuses on the *client's response* to the health problem. Nursing diagnoses are written in a PES format: **P**roblem, **E**tiology, **S**igns and symptoms.

- Although the nursing process is primariliy the responsibility of the RN, your contribution is invaluable. Once the nursing diagnosis is established, expected outcomes must be set. It is important that the outcomes be realistic, measurable, and tailored to the individual client.

- Interventions to promote safety include the following: assess and promote environmental safety, assess for toxic effects of medications, anticipate and prevent skin breakdown and other hazards of immobility, and educate the older adult about exercise safety.

- Interventions to promote health education include the following: implement a teaching plan specific to the disorder, educate the older adult about the medications being taken, and educate the older adult about proper skin care.

- Interventions to promote lifestyle modification include the following: encourage reduction of excess weight, encourage healthy lifestyle habits, and discourage unhealthy lifestyle habits.

- Interventions to promote mobility include the following: exercise, postoperative interventions for the client undergoing hip replacement surgery, rehabilitative techniques/restorative care, and proper use of assistive devices.

- Interventions to promote nutrition include the following: encourage a diet rich in calcium and vitamin D for older adults at risk for osteoporosis; encourage a diet rich in protein, vitamin C, and zinc for the older adult with a pressure ulcer; educate the older adult on aspirin therapy about possible nutritional depletion of vitamin C and folate; and encourage dietary modifications for older adults with sleep difficulties.

- Interventions to promote rest and sleep include the following: encourage nutrition that promotes rest and sleep, discourage the use of caffeine and other stimulants before bedtime, encourage weight reduction if appropriate,

minimize nighttime disturbances, encourage the older adult with chronic pain to take an analgesic at bedtime, provide support and understanding, and remind the older adult with osteoarthritis about the importance of rest for minimizing stress on the affected joints.
- Nursing evaluation should be aimed directly at the outcomes and should take into consideration the effectiveness of individual interventions.

STUDY QUESTIONS

Multiple-Choice Review

1. Which of the following accurately describes a normal change of aging?
   1. The skin becomes thicker.
   2. Muscles experience gradual hypertrophy.
   3. Bone loss exceeds bone formation.
   4. Sleep time is greater.
2. Which of the following activities would best help to delay age-related changes to the bones?
   1. Swimming
   2. Walking
   3. Washing dishes
   4. Relaxation and imagery
3. Which of the following individuals is at greatest risk for osteoporosis?
   1. Thin white female who smokes and drinks alcohol
   2. Medium-build Asian female aerobics instructor
   3. Large black female body builder
   4. Large white man who is allergic to milk
4. Which of the following is a method of assessing adequacy of a client's sleep?
   1. Observation of general alertness and attention
   2. Client's subjective statement of how well rested he or she feels
   3. Review of the client's sleep log
   4. All of the above
5. Which of the following accurately describes a stage II pressure ulcer?
   1. Reddened area of skin that does not blanch when pressed

2. Appears superficial, similar to an abrasion, blister, or shallow crater
3. Appears like a deep crater
4. Bone may be visible

Critical Thinking

1. What would you say to your older adult client who is asking your advice about having a glass of wine before bedtime to help him sleep?
2. Your 50-year-old female client says to you, "I was diagnosed with osteoporosis. What can I do?" How would you respond to her question?
3. Explain differences between men and women with regard to the aging process of muscles and bones.
4. An older adult woman asks your advice on a new, expensive cosmetic product designed to "take away years" from her aging skin. How would you respond?

Resources

Internet Resources

American Association of Retired Persons (AARP): http://www.aarp.org

American Sleep Disorder Association (web site has both a professional area and a client/public area): http://www.asda.org

Arthritis Foundation: http://www.arthritis.org

National Osteoporosis Foundation: http://www.nof.org

Sleep Disorders ("everything you wanted to know about sleep disorders but were too tired to ask," includes numerous links to research and support groups): http://www.sleepnet.com

Wound Care Communications Network: http://www.woundcarenet.com

Organizations

Arthritis Foundation, 1-800-283-7800

Centers for Disease Control and Prevention

National Center for Chronic Disease Prevention and Health Promotion
Division of Nutrition and Physical Activity, MS K-46
4770 Buford Highway, NE
Atlanta, GA 30341-3724
1-800-CDC-4NRG or 1-888-232-4674

National Institute of Arthritis and Musculoskeletal and Skin Diseases
National Institutes of Health
Bethesda, Maryland 20892-2350

The President's Council on Physical Fitness and Sports
Box SG, Suite 250
701 Pennsylvania Avenue, NW
Washington, DC 20004

Selected References

Amino acids: Tryptophan. HealthWorld Online. Available at http://www.healthy.net/hwlibrarybooks/haas/amino.trp.htm. Accessed 4/9/99.

Beck-Little, R., & Weinrich, S. P. (1998). Assessment and management of sleep disorders in the elderly. *Journal of Gerontological Nursing, 24*(4), 21–29.

Caffeine safety and labeling of foods and beverages. Available at http://www.ificinfo.health.org/quanda/caflabel.htm. Accessed 4/9/99.

Drugay, M. (1997). Breaking the silence: A health promotion approach to osteoporosis. *Journal of Gerontological Nursing, 23*(6), 36–43.

Duffy, J. F., Dijk, D. J., Klerman, E. B., & Czeisler, C. A. (1998). Later endogenous circadian temperature nadir relative to an earlier wake time in older people. *American Journal of Physiology, 275*(5 Pt 2), R1478–R1487.

FDA urged to require caffeine content on food labels. Heart Information Network. Available at http://www.heartinfo.org/news97/fdacaf8597.htm. Accessed 4/9/99.

Jones, J. M., & Jones, K. D. (1997). Promoting physical activity in the senior years. *Journal of Gerontological Nursing, 23*(7), 41–48.

Keeping in shape: Let's get moving. Available at http://www.aarp.org/health/letsgetmoving.html. Accessed 3/30/99.

Kessenich, K. R., & Guyatt, G. H. (1998). Domains of health-related quality of life in elderly women with osteoporosis. *Journal of Gerontological Nursing, 24*(11), 7–13.

Kushner, P. R. (1998). A practical approach to managing osteoporosis. *Hospital Medicine, 34*(6), 15–25.

Matteson, M. A., McConnell, E. S., & Linton, A. D. (1998). *Gerontological nursing: Concepts and practice.* Philadelphia: W. B. Saunders.

Mitchell, M. K. (1994). *Nutrition across the life span.* Philadelphia: W. B. Saunders.

Peckenpaugh, N. J., & Poleman, C. M. (1999). *Nutrition essentials and diet therapy.* Philadelphia: W. B. Saunders.

Pep Up Your Life with Exercise: The Key to a Good Life. Available at http:// www.aarp.org/ programs/pepup/ home.html. Accessed 3/30/99.

Physical activity and health: A report of the Surgeon General. Available at http://www.cdc.gov/nccdphp/sgr/olderad.htm. Accessed 8/23/98.

Rubin, H. Sleep and Aging. Available at http://www.therubins.com/aging/sleep.htm.

Travis, S. T., All, A. C., & Bernard, M. (1999). Remediating the effects of sarcopenia in the elderly client's plan of care. *Home Healthcare Nurse, 17*(3), 167–174.

Tyson, S. R. (1999). *Gerontological nursing care.* Philadelphia: W. B. Saunders.

Yarnold, B. (1999). Hip fracture: Caring for a fragile population. *American Journal of Nursing, 99*(2), 36–40.

Promoting Nutrition and Hydration

OBJECTIVES

After completing this chapter, you will be able to:

- Describe the normal changes of aging of the gastrointestinal tract.
- Identify changes in nutritional requirements with age.
- List the steps in assessment of the gastrointestinal tract.
- Discuss techniques to assess nutrition and hydration in the older adult.
- Compare key clinical features of disorders in the areas of nutrition and hydration commonly affecting older adults.
- Identify nursing interventions for the older adult experiencing disorders related to nutrition and hydration.
- Discuss the nursing process in care planning for the older adult with disorders affecting nutrition and hydration.

CHAPTER OUTLINE

KEY TERMS

Edentulous	Hypodermoclysis
Enteral nutrition	Orthostatic hypotension
Failure to thrive	Parenteral nutrition
Halitosis	Recommended Dietary Allowances
24-Hour recall method	Sepsis
Hypochlorhydria	Xerostomia

CASE STUDY

Miss Williams is a 92-year-old resident of an extended-care facility. She is mentally alert but has decreased vision and hearing. Because of a cerebrovascular accident she experienced 4 years ago, she has limited manual dexterity and needs assistance feeding herself. She has lost 15 pounds over the past 3 months, leaving her 5 foot, 4 inch frame at a mere 90 pounds. Because she has been having dental pain, the doctor changed her diet to a pureed diet. She complains that mealtime is not enjoyable anymore. To make matters worse, there has been inadequate nursing staff on the evening and night shifts. Sometimes, the kitchen staff picks up her dinner tray when she has hardly touched it. Other times, the food is cold and tasteless by the time a nursing assistant arrives to feed her. Still other times, the nursing assistant assigned to feed her combines all the food together—the meat, the vegetable, the fruit, and even the dessert—into oversized spoonfuls and places the spoon in her mouth, making her choke. Although she is often hungry, she has started to dread mealtime. She knows the nurses are very busy, so she does not ask for a drink of water anymore.

If nothing is done, what will become of Miss Williams? How can you save Miss Williams from further decline?

Helping to meet the nutritional needs of the older adult is one of the most crucial nursing interventions in gerontological nursing. Nutrition and hydration are essential to good health, and nurses are the most important health care personnel to help older adults meet their nutrition and hydration needs. Your actions in this area are every bit as life-saving as any other intervention you can implement during your nursing career.

AGE-RELATED CHANGES OF THE GASTROINTESTINAL TRACT

With advancing age, structural and functional changes occur in the gastrointestinal tract. Older adults may lose some or all of their teeth; however, the number of **edentulous** older adults has decreased in recent years owing to better oral hygiene and increased fluoridation. Teeth tend to darken with age, and the gingiva may retract. Salivary glands produce less saliva, which can make food difficult to chew and swallow, and may lead to **xerostomia**. The esophagus does not undergo significant age-related changes. Gastric mucosa atrophies with age. The stomach secretes less hydrochloric acid with age, a condition known as **hypochlorhydria**.

Medication Safety Tip

The decreased acidity of the stomach may affect absorption of certain medications that depend on an acid environment for proper absorption.

The villi of the small intestine undergo a decrease in height and an increase in breadth with aging. The large intestine may have decreased blood flow and slower intestinal motility. Although constipation is common in the older adult, it is not considered to be a normal change of aging. When constipation occurs, it is believed to be related to many other factors, which are be discussed later in this chapter. The pancreas tends to atrophy with age, yet pancreatic enzyme production is unchanged. Cells of the liver decrease in size and are replaced by fibrous tissue. Protein synthesis by the liver is impaired; however, standard liver function test results do not change significantly with age. The liver's functions of storage and clearance slow with aging.

Medication Safety Tip

Metabolism of drugs by the liver can decrease by as much as 30% with aging.

NUTRITIONAL CHANGES WITH AGING

The older adult has only minor changes in nutritional requirements from those of the younger adult. There is a steady decline in caloric requirements because of reduced physical activity, loss of body tissue, and decreased metabolic rate. The **Recommended Dietary Allowances** (RDA) for adults over age 50 are listed in Box 6–1.

Also, certain changes in nutrient absorption occur with aging. Examples of these are outlined in Table 6–1.

In addition, the body may be less able to metabolize glucose efficiently, leading to fluctuations in blood sugar and a greater chance that diabetes mellitus will develop. Zinc has been shown to improve the immune system of the older adult. Folic acid and vitamins B_6 and B_{12} have been shown to decrease the levels of homocysteine in the blood, an event which, according to recent research, may help ward off cardiovascular disease.

The older adult should try to consume a balanced diet, including adequate fluid, fiber, protein, vitamins, and minerals. Because nutritional requirements do not change drastically with age, there is no need for radical change in dietary habits, provided the older adult has been eating a healthy diet all along.

Box 6–1 Recommended Dietary Allowances for Adults Over 50 Years of Age

	MALES	FEMALES
Energy (kcal)	2300	1900
Protein (g)	63	50
Fat-soluble vitamins		
Vitamin A (μg RE)*	1000	800
Vitamin D (μg)†	5	5
Vitamin E (mg α-TE)‡	10	8
Vitamin K (μg)	80	65
Water-soluble vitamins		
Vitamin C (mg)	60	60
Thiamin (mg)	1.2	1.0
Riboflavin (mg)	1.4	1.2
Niacin (mg NE)§	15	13
Vitamin B_6 (mg)	2.0	1.6
Folate (μg)	200	180
Vitamin B_{12} (μg)	2.0	2.0
Minerals		
Calcium (mg)	800	800
Phosphorus (mg)	800	800
Magnesium (mg)	350	280
Iron (mg)	10	10
Zinc (mg)	15	12
Iodine (μg)	150	150
Selenium (μg)	70	55

* 1 RE (retinol equivalent) = 1 μg or 6 μg β-carotene.
† As cholecalciferol. 10 μg cholecalciferol = 400 IU vitamin D.
‡ α-Tocopherol equivalents. 1 mg d-α = 1 α-TE.
§ 1 NE (niacin equivalent) = 1 mg of niacin or 60 mg dietary tryptophan.
From Mitchell, M. K. (1994). *Nutrition across the life span.* Philadelphia: W. B. Saunders, p.322.

Nutrition Tip

It is not too late to encourage proper nutrition in the older adult. After retirement, most adults can expect to live another 20 years or more!

	Table 6–1	
	SELECTED AGE-RELATED CHANGES IN NUTRIENT ABSORPTION AND UTILIZATION	
Nutrient	**Age-Related Change**	**Implication**
Vitamin A	• Decreased clearance by the liver • Possibly increased absorption	Decreased dietary requirement
Vitamin D	• Decreased absorption • Reduced ability to form through skin exposure to sunlight	Increased dietary requirement
Calcium	• Decreased absorption	Increased dietary requirement
Vitamin B_{12}	• Impaired digestion • Bacterial uptake of B_{12} in small bowel	Increased need, especially if older adult has gastritis
Iron	• Decreased losses after menopause	Decreased requirement in older women

From Russell, R. M. Aging as a modifier of metabolism. (Abstract from NIH Workshop: The Role of Dietary Supplements for Physically Active People). Accessed 4/20/99.

ASSESSMENT OF THE GASTROINTESTINAL TRACT

Beginning in a head-to-toe direction, inspect the oral cavity and document your findings carefully. Note the presence or absence of teeth. Observe for the presence of **halitosis**. If the client wears dentures, remove them for the assessment, and inspect the integrity of the dentures. Observe the mucous membranes for any swelling, cracking, redness, or other discoloration such as white patches. Check for areas of irritation or bleeding, especially where the dentures come in contact with the gums. Inspect the tongue for cracking, dryness, or white patches. With a gloved hand, palpate the lips and gums for any areas of tenderness. Use a 2 × 2 gauze pad to grasp the tongue for examination of its sides and base. Direct the client to "stick out your tongue and say ahh," as you use a tongue blade to gently hold the tongue down to examine the throat for redness. You may need to use a penlight for this portion of the assessment. Observe the client's ability to swallow water.

Because most of the gastrointestinal tract is hidden from view, much of your assessment relies on your questions to the client. Questions to include in a gastrointestinal assessment are listed in Box 6–2.

After you have questioned the client, use the techniques of inspection, auscultation, palpation, and percussion to assess the upper and lower gastrointestinal tract. It is very important to auscultate the abdomen prior to palpation or percussion; otherwise, your assessment will not be accurate because you will be creating artificial bowel sounds (Table 6–2).

ASSESSMENT OF HYDRATION AND NUTRITIONAL STATUS OF THE OLDER ADULT

Hydration

Because of age-related decreases in the elasticity of the skin, decreased skin turgor on the back of the hand may not be a valid indicator of dehydration. Testing skin turgor on the forehead or sternum yields more accurate assessment data because the age-related skin changes in these areas are not as dramatic. Examine the tongue and mucous membranes for dryness, cracking, or furrowing, which could indicate dehydration. The presence of **orthostatic hypotension**, also known as postural hypotension, is typically viewed as an indicator of dehydration. In some older adults, however, orthostatic hypotension can exist owing to other reasons, such as medication therapy or

---

Box 6–2 **Questions to Include in a Gastrointestinal Assessment**

- Do you have any disturbances in your sense of taste?
- Do you wear dentures? Are they uppers, lowers, or partials?
- Do you have difficulty in chewing or swallowing?
- Are there any particular foods that upset your digestive tract? If so, which ones?
- How is your appetite? Has it changed in the past month?
- Have you experienced any weight gain or weight loss in the past 12 months?
- Do you experience any of the following symptoms: nausea? heartburn? abdominal cramps? lack of appetite?

- Do you have any of the following signs: vomiting? diarrhea? blood in the stool?
- Do you have any food allergies?
- What are your food preferences and dislikes?
- Do you have any dietary restrictions?
- What do you usually eat on a day-to-day basis?
- When was the last time you visited the dentist?
- Who prepares your meals?
- What is your usual height and weight? Has your weight changed in the past 6 months?

---

disease process. Orthostatic vital sign measurement is described in Box 6–3.

Orthostatic hypotension is defined as a drop in the systolic blood pressure of at least 20 mm Hg, or a drop in the diastolic pressure of at least 10 mm Hg. An increased pulse of at least 10 beats per minute usually accompanies it. The client in Box 6–3 has no orthostatic changes in vital signs. Notice that on the first standing set of vital signs, there is a rise in the pulse rate. Because the pulse did not remain elevated on the second set of standing vital signs, this elevation was probably due to the activity of moving from a sitting to a standing position (Fig. 6–1).

Other signs and symptoms of dehydration include thirst; sudden weight loss; rapid, thready pulse; lightheadedness; and decreased urine output. It is important to assess for and document the presence of any of these signs.

Nutritional Status

History

Gathering a nutritional history is the first step in the assessment of a client's nutritional status. A simple approach that can be used at the bedside is the **24-hour recall method.** The older adult is asked to write down all foods consumed within the past 24-hour period. The nurse and the client analyze the nutritional content of the foods and compare the client's intake with the RDA. Although this is a snapshot approach and may not truly represent your client's normal eating habits, it can yield valuable information for you and the client. A better approach, however, would be to analyze nutritional data from a 3-day period. This can be done either retrospectively via a 72-hour recall or prospectively by instructing the client to write down all foods that are consumed

Table 6–2	
ASSESSMENT OF UPPER AND LOWER GASTROINTESTINAL TRACT	
Inspection	• Assess abdomen for scars, masses, striae, dilated veins, color changes, and lesions
	• Assess shape of abdomen: flat, round, distended
	• Observe abdomen for pulsations and peristalsis
Auscultation	• Listen for bowel sounds with stethoscope in all four quadrants
Percussion	• Tympanic sounds may indicate flatulence
	• Dull sounds may indicate solid organs or constipation
Palpation	• Light palpation can be used to assess for tenderness

Modified from Matteson, M. A., McConnell, E. S., & Linton, A. D. (1998). *Gerontological nursing: Concepts and practice.* Philadelphia: W. B. Saunders, p. 332.

✒ Box 6–3   Measurement of Orthostatic Blood Pressure

Explain procedure to the client.
Instruct the client to recline for 20 minutes.
Measure pulse and blood pressure while the client is lying.
Assist the client to a sitting position; wait 2 minutes.
Repeat pulse and blood pressure measurements.
Assist client to a standing position; wait 2 minutes.
Repeat pulse and blood pressure measurements.
Wait 3 additional minutes.
Repeat pulse and blood pressure measurements.
Document all vital signs and times, noting lying, sitting, standing, repeat
  standing, for example:

#1	#2	#3	#4
10:00 AM	10:02 AM	10:04 AM	10:07 AM
BP 120/84, P74	BP 118/80, P76	BP 110/76, P86	BP 114/78, P80
lying	sitting	standing	repeat standing

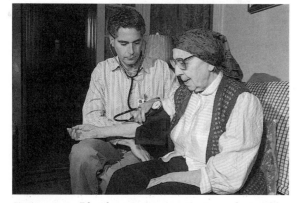

Figure 6–1. Blood pressure monitoring of an older adult in the home environment. (From Leahy, J. M., & Kizilay, P. E. [1998]. *Foundations of nursing practice.* Philadelphia: W. B. Saunders, p. 901.)

during the upcoming 3 days. The risk, of course, of the prospective approach is that the client will consume a different diet than he or she normally would as a result of being studied. It is important to emphasize to the older adult that the more accurate he or she is in providing dietary information, the more accurate you can be in determining his or her nutritional status. Screening tools can be used to elicit nutritional history information, which can indicate an older adult's risk of poor nutrition. One of these tools, the *Determine Your Nutritional Health Checklist*, is described in the following section on malnutrition.

Physical Assessment

An important part of the nutritional assessment of the older adult occurs at the bedside during the physical assessment. As you move from head to toe, numerous areas of the physical assessment can give valuable information regarding the nutritional status of the older adult. Table 6–3 lists

	Table 6–3	
	PHYSICAL ASSESSMENT OF NUTRITIONAL STATUS	
Area of Assessment	Findings Suggesting Good Nutritional Status	Findings Suggesting Poor Nutritional Status
Hair	• Shiny • Strong • No areas of alopecia	• Lackluster • Areas of alopecia • Dull, brittle hair
Eyes	• Bright • Clear • Pink conjunctiva	• Dull • Presence of discharge, redness • Redness or edema of conjunctiva
Mouth	• Evidence of good oral hygiene • Shiny, pink gums • Smooth lips and tongue	• Missing or broken teeth • Ulceration of gums or oral mucosa • Redness or edema of gums • Cracked lips • Furrowed tongue
Skin	• Intact • Normal color	• Broken areas or ulcerations • Pallor • Rashes
Nails	• Intact • Cuticles smooth	• Excessively thick • Cracked or broken cuticles
Musculoskeletal system	• Well-developed muscle tone • Adequate strength	• Poor or flaccid muscle tone • Weakness

physical assessment areas that give information on a client's nutritional status.

Laboratory Data

The physician may order certain laboratory tests to further evaluate the nutritional status of the older adult. These tests can include complete blood count (CBC), serum albumin, total protein, serum glucose, serum electrolytes (especially sodium and potassium), urinalysis, and stool examination for occult blood. Abnormalities in any of these tests may indicate a nutritional deficiency.

Anthropometric Measurement

Anthropometry is the measurement of physical dimensions of the body. It can be used to determine your client's baseline nutritional status before nutritional interventions are employed, or to compare your client with expected norms for his or her height and age. Anthropometry should be performed by a clinician skilled in the use of the tools, whether a nurse, dietitian, or physician. The basic parameters measured in anthropometry are weight, height, upper arm circumference, triceps, and subscapular fatfolds.

DISORDERS COMMON IN OLDER ADULTS

Malnutrition

Malnutrition is a serious problem for older adults. Malnutrition is often referred to as **failure to thrive**, or FTT. Overall, one in four older Americans is considered malnourished; this number is even greater for those in institutions: two in five nursing home residents and *half* of older adults in the hospital population fit into this category (Wellman & Blackburn, 1997). Box 6–4 lists some of the numerous adverse effects of malnutrition on the older adult. In addition, the older

---

Box 6–4 Adverse Effects of Malnutrition on the Older Adult

- Increased susceptibility to infection and disease
- Delayed healing of injuries
- Increased surgical risk
- Longer, more expensive hospital stays
- Greater risk of institutionalization

Source: Wellman, N. S., & Blackburn, G. L. (1997). Incorporating nutrition into health care for the elderly. *Adult Health: Multidisciplinary Approaches To Wellness* 1(1), 2.

---

adult with a nutritional deficiency may have less energy to independently perform activities of daily living (ADL), thereby resulting in a reduced quality of life.

Certain risk factors have been associated with malnutrition. The *Determine Your Nutritional Health Checklist* is a screening tool that attempts to uncover these nutritional risk factors. It uses the acronym **Determine** for the warning signs of **D**isease, **E**ating poorly, **T**ooth loss/mouth pain, **E**conomic hardship, **R**educed social contact, **M**ultiple medicines, **I**nvoluntary weight loss/gain, **N**eeds assistance in self-care, and **E**lder above age 60 (Appendix A).

Signs and symptoms of malnutrition include weight loss of over 5% in a month, or over 10% in 6 months, and decreased laboratory values of serum albumin, total protein, total lymphocytes, and hemoglobin. The malnourished older adult may exhibit muscular weakness and confusion. Medical treatments for malnutrition involve nutritional supplementation. Depending on the type of nutrient deficiency, the physician may order specific nutrient supplementation, such as vitamins, minerals, or increased calories. The physician may also recommend a special diet. For example, a mechanical soft diet may help solve the problem if malnutrition is due to the client's inability to chew solid foods. If the client is extremely malnourished, **enteral** or **parenteral** nutrition may be required to improve the client's nutritional status (Fig. 6–2).

Dehydration

Dehydration is a serious risk for the older adult. With normal aging, total body water decreases, limiting the ability of the older adult to maintain fluid balance and preserve levels of essential body minerals. In addition, the sense of thirst may be decreased with age.

The amount of water required to maintain normal circulation to body organs for the average-sized older adult is 2500 mL per day. Of this 2500, the *minimum* amount of water that should come from fluids is 1500 mL; the balance must come from foods. It has been found that many older adults do not consume the recommended amount of fluid needed each day and are at high risk for dehydration. This can be related to many factors, some of which include decreased thirst, decreased ability to concentrate the urine, fear of incontinence, and physical limitations.

With dehydration, circulation to body organs and tissues is compromised. When organs and tissues receive inadequate perfusion, they are unable to function in a normal manner and may show signs of dysfunction or even failure. For example, decreased perfusion to the brain can impair the thought processes of the older adult, resulting in confusion. Decreased blood flow to the kidneys can lead to decreased urinary output and the possibility of renal failure. Other serious potential consequences of dehydration in the older adult include constipation and fecal impaction,

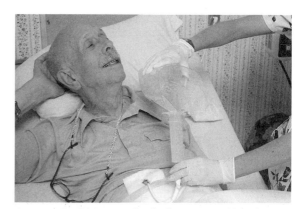

Figure 6–2. Giving a tube feeding to an older client in the hospital environment. (From deWit, S. [2001]. *Fundamental concepts and skills for nursing.* Philadelphia: W. B. Saunders, p. 504.)

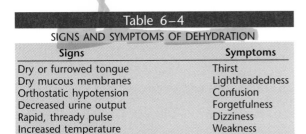

Table 6–4	
SIGNS AND SYMPTOMS OF DEHYDRATION	
Signs	**Symptoms**
Dry or furrowed tongue	Thirst
Dry mucous membranes	Lightheadedness
Orthostatic hypotension	Confusion
Decreased urine output	Forgetfulness
Rapid, thready pulse	Dizziness
Increased temperature	Weakness
Syncope (fainting)	Fatigue

*2500 mL per day
1500 from fluid balance
from food*

loss of the ability to independently perform ADL, infection, risk for falls, and even death. Signs and symptoms of dehydration are outlined in Table 6–4.

Treatment for dehydration consists of replenishing body fluids. This can be accomplished either by the preferred method—oral administration—or by parenteral administration. Parenteral administration usually consists of the administration of intravenous fluids. When fluids are replaced via the intravenous route in an older adult, the client must be monitored very closely to prevent fluid overload. This monitoring includes careful assessment of respiratory rate and auscultation of breath sounds during fluid replacement. Another type of parenteral fluid administration is **hypodermoclysis**. Although this therapy is less frequently used than intravenous therapy, it poses less of a risk of fluid overload and may be the preferred method if insertion of an intravenous line is difficult or undesirable for the client.

Gastrointestinal Esophageal Reflux Disease

Gastrointestinal esophageal reflux disease (GERD) is a disorder that is more common in the older than the younger adult. It is characterized by a reflux of gastric contents upward into the esophagus. Usually the reflux occurs because of a defect in the lower esophageal sphincter, which normally would have kept gastric contents in the stomach. It is a most unpleasant disorder to have because the client experiences heartburn, often associated with eating, exercise, or bending or lying down. Medications used in the treatment of GERD are outlined in Table 6–5.

Medication Safety Tip

Because antacids impair the absorption of many oral medications, it is important that they be administered 1 to 2 hours apart from other oral medications.

Medication Safety Tip

Cimetidine frequently causes neurologic adverse effects in the older adult, including confusion, agitation, anxiety, and hallucinations. Assess carefully for these adverse effects.

Treatment of GERD also consists of advising the older adult to decrease intra-abdominal pressure by avoiding tight clothing, refraining from lifting or straining, and sleeping with the head of the bed elevated. Surgical procedures for GERD are not commonly done; but if symptoms are severe, they can be done.

Constipation

Constipation is the change in bowel habits, resulting in the passage of hard, dry stools at a frequency less than usual (typically fewer than three bowel movements per week). Constipation is not a normal change of aging. Age-related changes, however, place the older adult at greater risk for constipation than the young adult; these changes

Table 6–5		
MEDICATIONS USED IN THE TREATMENT OF GASTROINTESTINAL ESOPHAGEAL REFLUX DISEASE		
Category	**Action**	**Examples**
Antacid	Decreases acidity of gastric contents	• Magnesium and aluminum (Maalox) • Magnesium, aluminum, and simethicone (Mylanta)
Histamine-2 receptor antagonist	Blocks gastric acid secretion	• Cimetidine (Tagamet) • Ranitidine (Zantac) • Famotidine (Pepcid)
Proton pump inhibitor	Blocks secretion of gastric acid by the parietal cells	• Omeprazole (Prilosec)

include decreased motility in the gastrointestinal tract. The older adult may also be less able to sense rectal fullness, leading to postponement of defecation and possible constipation. Risk factors for constipation are outlined in Box 6–5.

> ### Health Promotion Tip
>
> The best way to prevent constipation is to get regular exercise, drink plenty of fluids, and include adequate fiber in the diet.

Symptoms can include a sensation of abdominal or rectal fullness, abdominal discomfort, headache, diminished appetite, and nausea. Treatment of constipation usually consists of promoting a regular time of day for bowel evacuation, increasing the consumption of fiber and fluids, and physical activity. Laxatives may be used occasionally, as overuse can lead to dependence.

Hemorrhoids

Hemorrhoids are enlarged or varicose veins of the mucous membrane inside or just outside of the rectum. When they are located inside, they are called internal hemorrhoids; when they protrude outside the rectum, they are called external hemorrhoids. Older adults may get hemorrhoids, especially if prone to constipation.

The cause of hemorrhoid formation is increased pressure on the veins of the anus. This pressure can be related to straining at the stool, prolonged sitting, and hard, dry stools that are difficult to pass. Usually, the first sign of hemorrhoid formation is bleeding during defecation. Symptoms include pain, pruritus, and a sensation of pressure. Treatment consists of local application of cold, sitz baths and avoidance of constipation. Severe hemorrhoids may require surgical intervention, such as cryosurgery or hemorrhoidectomy.

NURSING DIAGNOSES

As was discussed in Chapter 5, nursing diagnoses are derived from the assessment data and are unique to the individual client. Again, remember that a nursing diagnosis focuses on the client's response to the health problem.

Common nursing diagnoses (written only as the "problem" portion of the PES nursing diagnosis statement) that apply to the older adult experiencing disorders covered in this chapter are found in Table 6–6.

As stated before, not every nursing diagnosis identified is appropriate for every client with a given disorder. Likewise, other nursing diagnoses that were not listed above may be appropriate for your client. For example, not every client with GERD experiences a sleep pattern disturbance because of it. Carefully consider every nursing diagnosis to individualize a plan of care for the older adult with disorders related to nutrition and hydration.

COLLABORATING ON THE PLAN OF CARE

Once the nursing diagnosis is established, expected outcomes must be set. Remember to write outcomes that are realistic, measurable, and tailored to the individual client. Based on the previous section on nursing diagnoses, sample client outcomes for malnutrition can be found in Table 6–7. These are samples only because the outcomes that you set must be established with your individual client in mind.

In like fashion, sample outcomes for older adults with nursing diagnoses for the conditions of dehydration, GERD, constipation, and hemorrhoids can be found in Table 6–8.

IMPLEMENTING INTERVENTIONS FOR HEALTH PROMOTION

Interventions to Promote Safety

1. Reinforce teaching specific to reducing the risk of aspiration from GERD. These include

---

Box 6–5	Risk Factors for Constipation

Drug therapy
Dehydration
Decreased activity
Laxative abuse
Neurologic or endocrine disorders
Inadequate dietary fiber
Depression

Table 6–6
NURSING DIAGNOSES RELATED TO NUTRITION AND HYDRATION

	Malnutrition	Dehydration	GERD	Constipation	Hemorrhoids
Imbalanced nutrition: less than body requirements	X		X	X	
Risk for infection	X	X		X	X
Constipation	X	X		X	X
Diarrhea	X	X			
Urinary retention				X	
Ineffective tissue perfusion: gastrointestinal				X	X
Deficient fluid volume		X		X	
Risk for aspiration			X		
Fatigue	X	X			
Disturbed sleep pattern			X		
Knowledge deficit	X	X	X	X	X
Nausea	X	X	X	X	
Impaired comfort			X	X	X

GERD, gastrointestinal esophageal reflux disease.

Table 6–7
SAMPLE OUTCOMES FOR AN OLDER ADULT WITH MALNUTRITION

Nursing Diagnosis	Sample Outcomes
Imbalanced nutrition: Less than body requirements	• Client will consume 2000 kcal per day • Client will eat 80% of all meals served • Client's weight will increase by 2 kg within a month*
Deficient knowledge: Nutrition	• Client will select three foods high in protein from a list of foods • Client will identify three foods high in potassium from a list of foods • Client will state two benefits of eating nutritious foods
Risk for infection	• Client will state the importance of handwashing • Client will show no signs or symptoms of infection

* Body weight is more appropriate as a long-term, rather than a short-term goal when related to nutrition. Day to day fluctuations in body weight are more often due to changes in fluid status, not true nutritional status.

measures such as maintaining the head of the bed elevated at 30 degrees and restricting foods and fluids 2 hours before bedtime.

2. Always check tube placement before instituting a nasogastric feeding or administering medications via this route. It is critical that the nasogastric tube be exactly in the place where it belongs. Reassess tube placement at the beginning of your shift, and whenever the client is turned or repositioned. Methods to determine placement of the tube are described in Box 6–6.

3. When a client is on continuous tube feedings, check the residual every 4 hours, or according to institutional policy. This prevents overfilling of the stomach and the possibility of aspiration. Add food coloring to the feeding if the client is at risk for aspiration. If a client coughs (or is suctioned) "sputum" the same color as the added coloring, aspiration has likely occurred. If, on the other hand, client secretions are white, but the tube feeding is blue, aspiration has probably not occurred.

4. Use aseptic technique when providing enteral and parenteral nutrition. Both tube feedings and parenteral nutrition are excellent media for bacterial multiplication. Bacterial multiplication

Table 6–8

SAMPLE OUTCOMES FOR AN OLDER ADULT WITH DEHYDRATION, GERD, CONSTIPATION, OR HEMORRHOIDS

Nursing Diagnosis	Sample Outcomes
Dehydration	
Constipation	• Client will explain, in simple terms, why constipation presents a risk of dehydration • Client will consume 2000 mL of fluids each day • Client will have regular, formed bowel movements, at least three times per week, and consistency of stool will not be hard
Deficient fluid volume	• Client will demonstrate no orthostatic changes in vital signs • Skin turgor on sternum and/or forehead will be elastic (not "tenting") • 24-hour intake will be ≥24-hour output • Mucous membranes will be pink and shiny
Deficient knowledge: Importance of fluids	• Client will describe (in general terms) the role of fluids in maintaining body homeostasis • Client will state the recommended amount of fluids to consume every day
GERD	
Risk for aspiration	• Client will not aspirate
Balanced nutrition: Less than body requirements	• Client will achieve his or her optimal weight • Client will follow prescribed dietary recommendations
Deficient knowledge: Symptom management	• Client will identify foods that increase symptoms • Client will explain the rationale for sleeping with head of bed elevated • Client will state three measures to decrease the risk of complications
Constipation	
Deficient knowledge: Laxative and enema use	• Client will describe two negative effects of chronic laxative use • Client will become less dependent on the use of laxatives and enemas as evidenced by requiring laxatives or enemas less than 2 times per week
Constipation	• Client will have regular, formed bowel movements, at least 3 times per week, and consistency of stool will not be hard • Client will state the role of fluid and dietary fiber in preventing constipation
Deficient knowledge: Methods to promote bowel motility	• Client will describe the effect of activity on gastrointestinal motility • Client will identify three foods high in fiber • Client will state the recommended fluid intake to help prevent constipation
Hemorrhoids	
Deficient knowledge: Contributing factors	• Client will describe two contributing factors to the development of hemorrhoids (i.e., dietary habits, prolonged sitting) • Client will describe the effect of straining at the stool on the development of hemorrhoids
Constipation	• Client will describe the relationship between constipation and hemorrhoids • Client will have regular, formed bowel movements, at least 3 times per week, and consistency of stool will not be hard • Client will state the roles of fluid and dietary fiber in preventing constipation
Impaired comfort	• Client will describe actions that reduce pain or discomfort • Client will be free from pain

GERD, gastrointestinal esophageal reflux disease.

with tube feedings can lead to diarrhea in the tube-fed client. The risks of bacterial multiplication for a client receiving parenteral nutrition are even greater. Because of the high sugar content of the fluid and the central access, infection can easily lead to an overwhelming systemic infection, or **sepsis**, which poses the risk of death. Other aseptic practices to employ with enteral and parenteral nutrition procedures are outlined in Box 6–7.

5. Encourage the older adult to change positions gradually. This will reduce the risk of falls associated with dehydration.

6. Carefully monitor all vital signs of the older adult. If you suspect fluid volume deficit, assess for orthostatic changes.

| Box 6–6 | Methods to Determine Placement of Nasogastric Tubes |

- "Swoosh of air": Instill 5 mL of air through a nasogastric tube while listening to the stomach with a stethoscope.
- Gastric aspiration: Aspirate fluid from the tube and analyze for decreased pH.
- X-ray: Radiography is usually used to determine placement of small, flexible tubes that extend into the small intestine (such as Keofeed feeding tubes).

Data from *Saunders manual of nursing care*. (1997). Philadelphia: W. B. Saunders, p. 1263.

7. Monitor and record intake and output for the older adult in an acute or subacute care setting, when ordered by the physician or registered nurse.
8. Keep careful bowel records for older adults, and report constipation to the registered nurse. Untreated constipation can be very serious and may lead to the development of fecal impaction, which can have serious consequences, such as stercoral ulceration, or pressure necrosis of the bowel.

Interventions to Promote Health Education

1. Under the guidance of the registered nurse, implement a teaching plan specific to the disorder that the older adult is experiencing. For example, the client with malnutrition needs education regarding nutritious foods. The older adult with GERD requires education regarding medications used to manage the disorder, including instructions on their use and possible adverse effects for which to observe.
2. Teach the older adult who consumes oil-based laxatives about the potential loss of fat-soluble vitamins if the laxatives are taken near mealtimes.
3. Reinforce teaching about the recommended daily fluid intake. By consuming approximately 2000 mL of fluid each day, the older adult will be less likely to experience dehydration and constipation.
4. Reinforce teaching about the role of dietary fiber in maintaining a formed stool. Adequate fiber intake is important in the treatment and prevention of constipation; fiber can be found in a variety of fruits, vegetables, and whole grains. The National Cancer Institute recommends consumption of 20 to 30 grams of fiber each day. One caution, however: it is important to teach the older adult to consume

| Box 6–7 | Aseptic Practices to Employ with Enteral and Parenteral Nutrition Procedures |

Enteral Nutrition

- Change tubing and equipment per institutional policy (e.g., every 24 hours).
- Label the feeding and all equipment with the date and time prepared, and your initials.
- Use clean technique when entering the system, when assembling equipment, when connecting to gastric or enteral tube, and when adding liquid nutrition.
- Do not leave more than 4 to 6 hours' worth of nutrition in the feeding bag at any time.

Parenteral Nutrition*

- Change tubing every 24 hours.
- Label the solution and all equipment with the date and time hung, and your initials.
- Use strict aseptic technique when changing system, adding bag, or performing site care.
- Do not "piggyback" any substance other than lipids into the parenteral nutrition line.
- Do not interrupt the system unnecessarily.
- Follow hospital policy carefully when performing dressing changes and site care.

*Refer to your state's Nurse Practice Act to determine the role of practical/vocational nurses with regard to parenteral nutrition in your state. Also, refer to your individual hospital's policies and procedures.

Table 6–9
FIBER CONTENT OF SELECTED FOODS

Food	Serving Size	Total Fiber (g)
Banana	1	1.8
Strawberries	1/2 cup	1.3
Orange	1	2.2
Avocado	1/2	3.8
Carrot	1/2 cup	1.9
Green beans	1/2 cup	1.5
Sweet potato (peeled)	1/2 cup	1.9
Spinach	1/2 cup	2.3
Artichoke	1	6.4
Corn flakes	1 cup	1.2
40% Bran flakes	1 cup	5.5
Oatmeal cookie	1 large	0.9
Black beans	1/2 cup	2.8
Popcorn	1 cup	0.8
Flour tortilla	1	0.9
Hominy	3/4 cup	3.0
Bagel	1/2 small	1.0

From Peckenpaugh, N. J., & Poleman, C. M. (1999). *Nutrition essentials and diet therapy.* Philadelphia: W. B. Saunders, pp. 552–569.

adequate fluid along with the fiber because increased fiber intake without increased fluid intake can lead to constipation (Table 6–9).
5. Reinforce teaching about the role of physical activity in promoting bowel motility. This can prevent constipation in clients who are otherwise prone to it.
6. Collaborate with the registered nurse to arrange visits for the client with professionals from other disciplines, such as a diabetes educator, as appropriate.

Interventions to Promote Lifestyle Modification

1. Encourage weight loss in overweight older adults. Reduction of excess weight decreases intra-abdominal pressure, thereby reducing the symptoms of GERD. In addition, weight reduction can decrease the chance that the client will develop hemorrhoids, by decreasing pressure in the rectal area.
2. Encourage the older adult to maintain a balanced diet (Fig. 6–3). Increased amounts of fresh fruits and vegetables instead of refined sugars and fats not only benefit the malnourished individual, but also help those with

constipation and hemorrhoids. Dietary guidelines developed by the U.S. Department of Agriculture in collaboration with the U.S. Department of Health and Human Services (USDHHS) are reviewed in Box 6–8.

Interventions to Promote Mobility

1. Encourage the older adult to engage in physical activity. Virtually any type of physical activity is helpful for the older adult who is experiencing disorders related to nutrition and hydration. Symptoms of many of the disorders reviewed in this chapter may be minimized or eliminated by physical activity. Even bedridden clients benefit from position changes and range of motion performed every 2 hours. Table 6–10 summarizes the benefits of physical activity in improving symptoms from selected disorders.
2. Collaborate with the registered nurse to arrange visits for the client with staff members from physical therapy (PT), occupational therapy (OT), and recreation therapy, as appropriate.

Interventions to Promote Nutrition

1. Encourage regular oral hygiene and annual visits to the dentist. Selected objectives from *Healthy People 2010* that address oral health are listed in Box 6–9.
   It is very important that nurses encourage oral hygiene for older adults in institutional settings because many of these clients depend on nurses to help them meet their hygiene needs. In institutional settings, oral hygiene often falls to a low level of priority for reasons such as inadequate staffing, lack of client cooperation, and lack of perceived importance on the part of responsible staff.

🚴 Health Promotion Tip

It is crucial for the LPN/LVN to take a leadership role in promoting oral hygiene for the older adult by both role modeling and reminding other staff of its importance.

Modified Food Pyramid for 70+ Adults

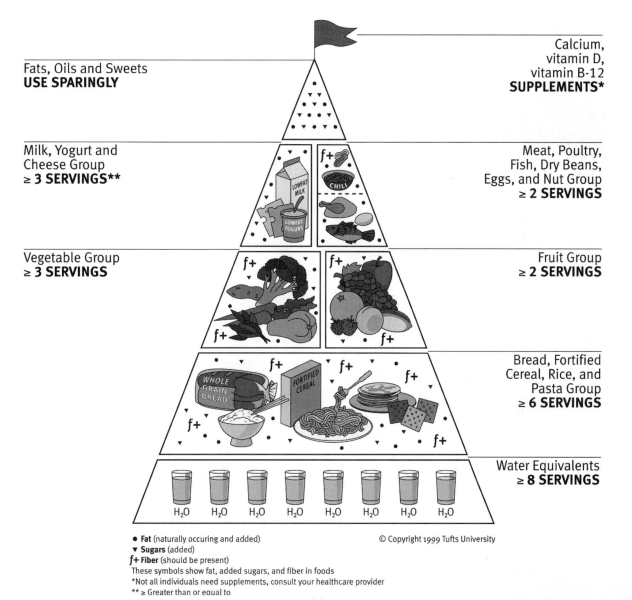

Figure 6–3. Modified Food Pyramid for 70+ Adults. (From Tufts University School of Nutrition Science and Policy, Medford, MA, © 1999.)

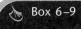

Box 6–8   **Dietary Guidelines for Americans**

- Eat a variety of foods.
- Balance the food you eat with physical activity—maintain or improve your weight.
- Choose a diet low in fat, saturated fat, and cholesterol.
- Choose a diet with plenty of grain products, vegetables, and fruits.
- Choose a diet moderate in sugars.
- Choose a diet moderate in salt and sodium.
- If you drink alcoholic beverages, do so in moderation.

Source: U.S. Department of Agriculture, Agriculture Research Service, Dietary Guidelines Advisory Committee (1995). Available at http://www.nal.usda.gov/fnic/dga/dguide95.html.

Box 6–9   **Selected *Healthy People 2010* Oral Health Objectives**

- Reduce the proportion of older adults who have had all their natural teeth extracted.
- Reduce periodontal disease.
- Increase the proportion of oral and pharyngeal cancers detected at the earliest stage.
- Increase the proportion of long-term care residents who use the oral health care system each year.

Provide mouth care before and after meals for the older adult who is unable to meet his or her own hygiene needs. Oral care for older adults with physical limitations and for older adults with dentures is described in Boxes 6–10 and 6–11, respectively.

2. Encourage the older adult to limit the quantity of fried foods they consume, as these are more difficult to digest.
3. Encourage the older adult to stay physically active. Remember that mobility promotes motility.
4. Educate the older adult who is living alone about nutritional support services and programs

available in the community. Some older adults may be reluctant to obtain services for many reasons. Some may believe receipt of such services is a sign of "getting old" or admitting that they are unable to care for themselves; reassurance and pointing out the benefits of receiving a nutritious meal may help to combat this fear. Other older adults may be reluctant to seek out such services owing to monetary fears. Inform clients that many of these programs are free or have a nominal cost. Popular nutritional programs and services are listed in Table 6–11.

5. Strive as nurses to improve staffing in long-term care facilities. Low staffing continues to be a serious problem that has an adverse impact on client nutrition. The primary

Table 6–10
BENEFITS OF PHYSICAL ACTIVITY IN IMPROVING SYMPTOMS OF SELECTED DISORDERS

Disorder	Benefit
Constipation	• Improvement of intestinal motility • Toning of abdominal muscles
Hemorrhoids	• Reduction of pressure in anal and rectal veins from sitting in one position for long periods • Prevention of constipation
GERD	• Reduction of weight • Decreased intra-abdominal pressure

GERD, gastrointestinal esophageal reflux disease.

Box 6–10   **Oral Care for Older Adults with Physical Limitations**

- Wash your hands.
- Assemble equipment at bedside: oral suction, emesis basin, wash cloth, toothbrush, toothpaste, dental floss, rinse agent (mouthwash or plain water), clean gloves.
- Position client upright with chin resting on padded table (if possible) to prevent jaw fatigue.
- Don clean gloves.
- Carefully brush and floss all teeth, taking care at the back of the mouth not to elicit a gag reflex.
- Assist client to rinse debris and expectorate into emesis basin (use oral suction if client unable).
- Offer client clean, dry wash cloth.

Box 6–11 Oral Care for Older Adults with Dentures

- Wash your hands.
- Assemble equipment at bedside: oral suction, emesis basin, wash cloth ×2, toothbrush, toothpaste, rinse agent (mouthwash or plain water), clean gloves.
- Place clean wash cloth in sink to be used (to decrease the chance of breakage if dentures are dropped).
- Don gloves.
- Remove client's upper dentures and place in denture cup.
- Remove client's lower dentures and place in denture cup.
- Offer client rinse agent of 1/2 mouthwash and 1/2 plain water.
- Assist client to rinse debris and expectorate into emesis basin (use oral suction if client unable).
- Offer client clean, dry wash cloth.
- Rinse denture cup with water.
- Using toothbrush, toothpaste, and running lukewarm water, clean all surfaces of dentures, taking care not to drop dentures.
- Replace dentures in denture cup.
- Fill denture cup with warm water and product such as Efferdent, if preferred by the client.
- Label with client name and room number.

---

responsibility of feeding long-term care residents usually falls on the nursing assistant; when there is inadequate staffing, client nutrition suffers. Meal trays are often removed before a client who eats slowly has a chance to finish the meal; staff may assist and feed an independent but slow eater to save time, thus turning an independent eater into someone requiring assistance, or a "feeder." It has been suggested that what has traditionally been viewed as an eating problem of older adults in long-term care facilities is really a staffing problem (Kayser-Jones, 1997). In addition to striving for additional staffing, we as nurses must make ourselves available and help nursing assistants with their monumental task of feeding several residents (Fig. 6–4).

6. Consider the use of quiet music at mealtime for the agitated client. Studies suggest that certain agitated behaviors in cognitively impaired clients may be reduced in this way. Certainly, any environmental manipulation that creates a less clinical and more comfortable, homelike setting is likely to relax the older adult and make mealtime a more pleasant experience.

Table 6–11
NUTRITIONAL SUPPORT PROGRAMS AND SERVICES

Program/Service	Restriction	Description
Meals on Wheels	Over age 60	Home-delivered lunch (sometimes supper) delivered to homebound client. Eligibility and payment requirements vary
Food stamps	Low income	Used to purchase groceries or pay for meals at certain restaurants. Special considerations for older adults
Senior Center	Over age 60	Nutritious lunch for over age 60 and spouse; payment voluntary
Soup kitchens, food banks, emergency food pantries	People in need	Privately run; provide groceries or cooked meal
Homemaker, home health aide	Low income	Shopping, cooking, homemaking services
Food shopping assistance		Federally funded and privately run services that help individuals with shopping for groceries
Adult day care	Older adults	Meals and daytime care

Adapted from Tyson, S. R. (1999). *Gerontological nursing care.* Philadelphia: W. B. Saunders, p. 137.

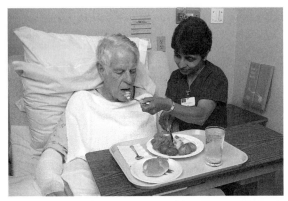

Figure 6–4. Nurse assisting an older client with feeding. (From deWit, S. [2001]. *Fundamental concepts and skills for nursing.* Philadelphia: W. B. Saunders, p. 487.)

7. Ensure proper positioning during and for 30 minutes following mealtime. During the meal, the optimal position is sitting in a chair. If this is physically impossible, high Fowler's position in bed is imperative. Be careful, however: unless the older adult is assisted ("boosted up") before the bed is raised to a high Fowler's position, it is quite possible for the **bed** to be in high Fowler's but the **client** to be slumped. This slumped position both increases the difficulty of eating and poses a risk for aspiration. In addition, the tray should be at a level low enough that the older adult can see the food clearly and easily manipulate utensils. This usually requires that a side rail be lowered and the nurse stay with the client. Following the meal, the older adult who is sitting in a chair should stay in an upright position for 30 minutes to facilitate digestion. The client in bed should also remain in an upright position, but the head of the bed can be lowered safely to a semi-Fowler's position.

Interventions to Promote Rest and Sleep

1. Raise the head of the bed by 30 to 45 degrees for sleep. In this way, gravity helps to alleviate symptoms of the disorder and decreases the likelihood that the older adult will awaken with indigestion during the night.
2. Discourage heavy meals before bedtime. Although a light snack may be beneficial, heavy meals should be consumed earlier in the day to allow adequate time for digestion.

3. Reinforce teaching about adequate intake of water and fluids. The older adult may wish to restrict fluids during the evening hours in an attempt to minimize the number of awakenings during the night. This is an acceptable practice, so long as adequate fluids are consumed earlier in the day to make up the deficit.

GATHERING DATA FOR EVALUATION

As was stated earlier, your contribution to the evaluation portion of the nursing process is crucial and may make the difference in the ultimate success or failure of the care plan. Direct your nursing evaluation at the outcomes. One outcome identified earlier in this chapter for the older adult experiencing dehydration was written, "Client will consume 2000 mL fluid per day." To evaluate progress toward this outcome, accurate intake and output records must be kept. With accurate documentation, evaluation of this outcome will be easy. Other outcomes may require careful evaluation from several sources. For example, consider one outcome previously identified for an older adult with constipation, which was written, "Client will become less dependent on the use of laxatives and enemas as evidenced by requiring laxatives or enemas less than 2 times per week." Although this outcome seems wordy, the "as evidenced by. . ." portion makes it extremely measurable. (In fact, sometimes adding an "as evidenced by. . ." when developing outcomes can save you unnecessary aggravation later during the evaluation phase of care planning.) To evaluate this outcome, you can consult a few sources. First of all, you can question the client about laxative or enema use. You can also question any caregivers, both staff and family members, involved in the care of the older adult. In addition, you can check available documentation, such as intake and output records, medication records, and progress notes.

Your evaluation should also take into consideration individual interventions employed. For example, if the progress notes indicate that prune juice is as effective as a stool softener in promoting bowel evacuation for the client, this not only provides a powerful evaluation of interventions employed, but also gives important information for modification of the plan of care. In this way, the evaluation helps set a new direction for nursing interventions.

Summary

- Changes in the gastrointestinal tract with aging are numerous. In the mouth and stomach there is tooth loss/darkening, gingival retraction, decreased saliva production, gastric mucosal atrophy, and hypochlorhydria. In the small intestine, villi have decreased height and increased breadth. The large intestine may develop decreased blood flow and slower motility, although constipation is not a normal change of aging.
- A steady decline in caloric requirements occurs in the older adult, due to reduced physical activity, body tissue, and metabolic rate. The older adult should try to consume a balanced diet, with adequate fluid, fiber, proteins, vitamins, and minerals.
- Perform assessment of the gastrointestinal tract in a head-to-toe direction, beginning with the oral cavity. Observe the mucous membranes and tongue for any swelling, cracking, redness, or discoloration. Palpate the lips and gums and examine the sides and base of the tongue. Assess the client's ability to swallow water. Question the client about appetite, weight gain or loss, and gastrointestinal symptoms. Use inspection, auscultation, palpation, and percussion to assess the upper and lower GI tract.
- In assessing hydration, test skin turgor on the forehead or sternum. Examine the tongue and mucous membranes for dryness, cracking, or furrowing. Assess for orthostatic hypotension, thirst, sudden weight loss, rapid and thready pulse, lightheadedness, and decreased urine output.
- A thorough nutritional assessment involves a physical assessment, laboratory data, and anthropometric measurements.
- Malnutrition can lead to increased susceptibility to infection and disease, inability to perform ADL, and reduced quality of life. Signs and symptoms of malnutrition include weight loss, altered laboratory values, muscular weakness, and confusion. Medical treatments involve nutritional supplementation, including enteral or parenteral nutrition.
- Dehydration is a serious risk for the older adult. With normal aging, total body water decreases and the sense of thirst may decrease. Many older adults do not consume adequate fluid and are at risk for dehydration. With dehydration, circulation to body organs and tissues is compromised, which can lead to organ dysfunction or failure. Other risks of dehydration include constipation and fecal impaction, inability to perform ADL, infection, risk for falls, and death. Treatment for dehydration consists of replenishing body fluids, either by oral or parenteral administration.
- In GERD, there is reflux of gastric contents upward into the esophagus. Medications used to treat GERD include antacids, histamine-blocking agents, and proton pump inhibitors. Treatment also consists of advising the older adult to avoid tight clothing, refrain from lifting or straining, and sleep with the head of the bed elevated.
- Constipation is not a normal change of aging, although there are age-related changes that place the older adult at greater risk, such as decreased GI motility. Drug therapy, dehydration, and decreased activity are among the common risk factors for constipation. Signs and symptoms include fewer stools; dry, hard stools; a sensation of abdominal or rectal fullness or discomfort; and diminished appetite. Treatment usually consists of promoting a regular time of day for bowel evacuation and increasing fiber, fluids, and physical activity. Laxatives are used occasionally.
- Hemorrhoids are enlarged or varicose veins of the mucous membrane inside or just outside the rectum. The cause is increased pressure on the anal veins, related to straining at the stool, prolonged sitting, or constipation. Signs and symptoms include bleeding, pain, pruritus, and a sensation of pressure. Treatments include application of cold, sitz baths, avoidance of constipation, cryosurgery, and hemorrhoidectomy in severe cases.
- Nursing diagnoses are derived from the assessment data and are unique to the individual client. Once the nursing diagnosis is established, outcomes must be set, which must be <u>realistic, measurable, and individualized.</u>
- Interventions to promote safety include the following: reinforce teaching to reduce the

risk of aspiration; check tube placement before feeding via nasogastric tube; check residual every 4 hours; use aseptic technique with enteral or parenteral nutrition; encourage the older adult to change positions gradually; record vital signs and bowel activity; and report constipation to the RN.

- Interventions to promote health education include the following: reinforce teaching about the potential loss of fat-soluble vitamins if oil-based laxatives are taken near mealtimes; and teach about the role of fiber, fluid, and physical activity in promoting bowel motility.

- Interventions to promote lifestyle modification include the following: encourage weight loss in overweight older adults, and encourage the older adult to maintain a balanced diet.

- Interventions to promote mobility include encouraging the older adult to engage in physical activity.

- Interventions to promote nutrition include the following: encourage regular oral hygiene and annual visits to the dentist; encourage the older adult to limit fried foods; encourage physical activity; educate the older adult about nutritional support services and community programs; strive to improve staffing in long-term care facilities; consider the use of quiet music at mealtime for the agitated client; and ensure proper positioning during and for 30 minutes following mealtime.

- Interventions to promote rest and sleep include the following: raise the head of bed by 30 to 45 degrees; discourage heavy meals before bedtime; and educate the client about adequate fluid intake.

- Nursing evaluation should be aimed directly at the outcomes. Your evaluation should also take into consideration the effectiveness of interventions, and can set a new direction for nursing interventions.

STUDY QUESTIONS
Multiple-Choice Review

1. Which of the following is considered a normal age-related change of the gastrointestinal tract?
   1. Increased secretion of hydrochloric acid
   2. Increased motility
   3. Gastric mucosal atrophy
   4. Increased secretion of saliva

2. Which of the following is the best statement regarding nutritional requirements with aging?
   1. Older adults need more calories than younger adults do.
   2. The older adult should try to consume a balanced diet.
   3. Older adults should consult the advice of a nutritionist because numerous adjustments should be made to the diet to meet their changing nutritional needs.
   4. Older women have an increased need for iron.

3. Which of the following would be the best way to assess the nutritional status of an older adult?
   1. 24-hour recall method
   2. Determine Your Nutritional Health Checklist
   3. 72-hour recall method
   4. Physical examination, laboratory data, and anthropometic measurement

4. The recommended daily fluid intake for the older adult is:
   1. 1000 mL
   2. 1500 mL
   3. 2000 mL
   4. 2500 mL

5. Which of the following individuals is at greatest risk of developing hemorrhoids?
   1. An underweight 90-year-old man who is bed-bound
   2. An overweight 70-year-old man who is confined to a wheelchair
   3. A medium-build 80-year-old woman who enjoys needlecraft
   4. An overweight 60-year-old woman who walks her dog every day

Critical Thinking

1. Why is it important that auscultation be performed before palpation during assessment of the gastrointestinal tract?

2. What advice would you give to an older adult who is asking about nutritional requirements with aging?

3. A 70-year-old woman tells you, "I am worried about my bowels. I don't have a bowel movement every day." How would you respond to her statement?

4. What are some interventions you could employ, as an individual, to promote nutrition for older adults in your community?

Resources

Internet Resources

Nutrition Science News
http://www.nutritionsciencenews.com

Mayo Clinic Health Oasis
Consumer information on health
http://www.mayohealth.org

National Digestive Diseases Information Clearinghouse
Information on a variety of digestive disorders
http://www.niddk.nih.gov

Nutrition Navigator
A Rating Guide to Nutrition Websites
Tufts University Center on Nutrition Communication, School of Nutrition Science and Policy
http://www.navigator.tufts.edu/focuson/

Organizations

Nutrition Screening Initiative (NSI)
1010 Wisconsin Avenue, NW
Suite 800
Washington, DC 20007
(202) 625-1662
Literature available on: food/drug interactions; effect of nutrition on oral and mental health

National Dairy Council
Dairy and Nutrition Council
6300 North River Road
Rosemont, IL 60018
Literature available on nutrition

Selected References

Bonnel, W. B. (1999). Meal management strategies of older adult women. *Journal of Gerontological Nursing, 25*(1), 41–47.

Denney, A. (1997). Quiet music: An intervention for mealtime agitation? *Journal of Gerontological Nursing, 23*(7), 16–22.

Eckler, J. A. L., & Fair, J. M. S. (1996). *Pharmacology essentials.* Philadelphia: W. B. Saunders.

Fortes, C., Forastiere, F., Agabiti, N., et al. (1998). The effect of zinc and vitamin A supplementation on immune response in an older population. *Journal of the American Geriatrics Society, 46*(1), 19–26.

Gaspar, P. M. (1999). Water intake of nursing home residents. *Journal of Gerontological Nursing, 25*(4), 23–29.

Healthy People 2010 Nutrition Objectives. Available at http://www.health.gov/healthypeople/Document/tableof contents.htm Accessed 11/9/00.

Healthy People 2010 Oral Health Objectives. Available at http://www.health.gov/healthypeople/Document/tableof contents.htm Accessed 11/9/00.

Kayser-Jones, J. (1997). Inadequate staffing at mealtime: Implications for nursing and health policy. *Journal of Gerontological Nursing, 23*(8), 14–20.

Matteson, M. A., McConnell, E. S., & Linton, A. D. (1998). *Gerontological nursing: Concepts and practice.* Philadelphia: W. B. Saunders.

Peckenpaugh, N. J., & Poleman, C. M. (1999). *Nutrition essentials and diet therapy.* Philadelphia: W. B. Saunders.

Russell, R. M. Aging as a modifier of metabolism. (Abstract from NIH Workshop: The Role of Dietary Supplements for Physically Active People) Available at http://www.healthy.net/hwlibrarybooks/nihdietarysupplements/aging.htm Accessed 4/20/99.

Saunders manual of nursing care. (1997). Philadelphia: W. B. Saunders.

Stone, J. T., Wyman, J. F., & Salisbury, S. A. (1999). *Clinical gerontological nursing: A guide to advanced practice.* Philadelphia: W. B. Saunders.

Tyson, S. R. (1999). *Gerontological nursing care.* Philadelphia: W. B. Saunders.

Wellman, N. S., & Blackburn, G. L. (1997). Incorporating nutrition into health care for the elderly. *Adult Health: Multidisciplinary Approaches to Wellness, 1*(1), 1–14.

Worobec, F., & Brown, M. K. (1997). Hypodermoclysis therapy in a chronic care hospital setting. *Journal of Gerontological Nursing, 23*(6), 23–28.

Promoting Adequate Excretion, Reproductive and Regulatory Well-Being

OBJECTIVES

After completing this chapter, you will be able to:

- Discuss the normal changes of aging that affect excretion, and reproductive and regulatory well-being.
- Describe the sequence of assessment and areas of importance in assessing genitourinary/reproductive and endocrine systems.
- Compare the key clinical features of disorders commonly affecting older adults in the areas of excretion, and reproductive and regulatory well-being.
- Examine the nursing process in care planning for the older adult with disorders of benign prostatic hyperplasia, urinary incontinence, urinary tract infection, and diabetes mellitus.

CHAPTER OUTLINE

KEY TERMS

Afferent arteriole

Bladder training

Creatinine clearance

Diuresis

Dysuria

Gangrene

Glomerular filtration rate

Habit training

Homeostasis

Hyperglycemia

Hyperkalemia

Hypernatremia

Hyponatremia

Nephrotoxic

Nosocomial infection

Pelvic exercises

Pelvic floor electrical stimulation

Polydipsia

Polyphagia

Polyuria

Septicemia

Transurethral resection of the prostate

Urgency

Urinary incontinence

Urinary retention

Urinary tract infection

CASE STUDY

Mrs. B. is a 78-year-old widow on a limited income who lives in rural Oklahoma. She lives alone and is self-sufficient with her activities of daily living (ADL) and instrumental activities of daily living (IADL). One morning, while putting away the dishes, Mrs. B. slips on a wet floor and falls to the ground. She pulls herself to the telephone to call for help. Instead of dialing 911, Mrs. B. accidentally calls a neighbor. The neighbor, an LPN named June, recognizes Mrs. B.'s voice and instructs her to stay still and wait for help. After calling 911 and Mrs. B.'s daughter, June goes to Mrs. B.'s house to help until emergency personnel arrive. June discovers Mrs. B. attempting to remove old newspaper from her undergarments. Although June cautions Mrs. B. to lie still until help arrives, Mrs. B. frantically tells her, "Please help me to get this mess out of my underwear—I don't want to let my daughter see me this way!" Mrs. B. explains that she is unable to control her urine and cannot afford pads or protective undergarments. What should June do?

AGE-RELATED CHANGES IN THE GENITOURINARY/REPRODUCTIVE AND ENDOCRINE SYSTEMS

The kidney is an important body organ in promoting normal **homeostasis** of the body. With normal aging, some changes take place that affect the body's ability to maintain homeostasis. These changes are not usually noticed in day-to-day activities but rather in times of stress, such as environmental stress, the stress of illness, or stress on the kidneys imposed by medications.

The kidney decreases in size and weight by as much as one fourth by the age of 80. Renal blood flow can be compromised owing to age-related sclerosis of the **afferent arteriole,** which brings blood to the kidney. Glomeruli can become sclerosed, which affects their ability to filter out toxic substances from the body. The rate of this filtering of substances is referred to as the **glomerular filtration rate,** or GFR; it decreases from age 30 onward at a rate of approximately 10% per decade. The GFR can be estimated with the use of a diagnostic test called **creatinine clearance.**

Physicians often use this test to determine appropriate dosages of medications for older clients.

Medication Safety Tip

The decreased ability of the glomeruli to filter substances with aging explains the older adult's reduced ability to metabolize many medications.

The kidney tubules also change in their ability to perform various homeostatic functions, such as managing body concentrations of sodium and potassium and maintaining the body's acid-base balance. Older adults are more susceptible to **hyperkalemia** and are less able to conserve sodium when the need arises, which can lead to **hyponatremia**. On the other hand, the older adult is also less able to excrete excess sodium, which can lead to **hypernatremia**. Total body water decreases with age; this effect is more pronounced in women because of their increased proportion of fat to lean body tissue. The older adult has a decreased ability to handle large water loads or to tolerate water deprivation. The latter of these two phenomena partially explains why, during heat waves, the older adult is at increased risk of hyperthermia and death.

In addition, the renal threshold for glucose is elevated as aging occurs; in other words, an older adult will sustain higher blood glucose values before spilling sugar into the urine than will a younger adult. This is one reason why blood glucose monitoring is preferable to urine glucose monitoring in the older adult. A summary of changes in kidney homeostasis associated with aging can be found in Box 7–1.

The bladder may also undergo changes with aging, including replacement of smooth muscle and elastic tissue with fibrous connective tissue. This can explain the decreased bladder capacity experienced by some older adults. On the other hand, bladder muscles can weaken, leading to **urinary retention** and a risk for **urinary tract infections** (UTIs), and urine pH increases, thus increasing the risk for UTIs. **Urinary incontinence** is <u>not</u> a normal change of aging (this is discussed later in the chapter).

The older woman experiences many age-related changes in the vaginal area, generally as a result of decreased estrogen. Age-related genitourinary and reproductive changes in men

---

Box 7–1 Changes in Kidney Homeostasis Associated with Aging

Decreased glomerular filtration rate
Decreased tubular function

- Increased susceptibility to development of hyperkalemia
- Decreased ability to excrete a sodium load
- Decreased ability to conserve sodium
- Decreased ability to excrete an acid load

Abnormal water metabolism

- Decrease in thirst
- Decreased ability to concentrate the urine

Data from Beck, L. H. (1998). Changes in renal function with aging. *Clinics in Geriatric Medicine: Genitourinary Problems, 14*(2), 199.

---

and women are listed in Box 7–2. These normal age-related changes can have an effect on sexual activity; for example, they can cause vaginal dryness in the older woman and less-firm erections in the older man. Sex, however, remains an

---

Box 7–2 Age-Related Genitourinary and Reproductive Changes in the Older Woman and Man

Woman

- Atrophy of genitalia
- Narrowing and shortening of the vagina
- Flattening of labia
- Decreased external hair
- Decreased tissue elasticity
- Diminished lubrication

Man

- Hyperplasia of prostate tissue
- Decreased fat in area surrounding penis and scrotum
- Decreased elasticity in tissues supporting scrotum
- Decreased blood flow to penis

Data from Tyson, S. R. (1999). *Gerontological nursing care*. Philadelphia: W. B. Saunders, p. 420.

important and pleasurable activity for the older adult. Sexual activity and the older adult is discussed in greater detail in Chapter 12.

Changes to the endocrine system also occur with aging. The endocrine system consists of various organs and glands that secrete hormones, which regulate numerous body processes. The locations of the major endocrine glands can be seen in Figure 7–1.

The hormones released by endocrine glands act by stimulating other glands or tissues, thereby influencing cellular processes. For example, the endocrine tissues called the islets of Langerhans (specifically the beta cells) release a hormone called insulin in response to an elevated blood sugar. Insulin stimulates body cells, which allows sugar to enter the cells for fuel, a process that leads to lowering of the blood sugar. A list of major endocrine glands, the hormones they secrete, and age-related changes is presented in Table 7–1.

ASSESSMENT OF THE GENITOURINARY/REPRODUCTIVE AND ENDOCRINE SYSTEMS

It is very important that the health care professional provide privacy and demonstrate sensitivity to the older adult client undergoing an assessment. The older adult may not be comfortable with a nurse of the opposite gender performing the assessment. Allowing the older adult choices regarding who is to perform the assessment is an appropriate approach. Assessment of the genitourinary system begins with inspection. Inspect the external genitalia, observing for discharge, abnormal skin growth or lesions, skin discoloration, or signs of irritation. You will observe normal age-related changes, such as graying and thinning of pubic hair, decreased fat tissue, and decreased elasticity. Note whether the male client is circumcised or uncircumcised. Inspect for erythema, edema, or discharge, especially in the uncircumcised male client. You need to document and report these assessment findings because they are not normal age-related findings. Note the general state of genital hygiene of the older adult.

Observe and document the presence of any urinary devices, such as a Foley catheter or an external catheter, and note the use of protective undergarments. Observe and accurately document the amount and overall appearance of urine on the intake and output (I&O) sheet. Communicate any unusual findings to the registered nurse (RN). Ask the older adult about his or her usual voiding patterns. Examine the abdomen for distention. If you suspect the older adult is retaining urine after voiding, palpate the abdomen. You will hear dull sounds if the bladder is full when percussed. If your facility has one, a bladder scanner provides a quick, noninvasive means of estimating the amount of urine present in the bladder. If you use a bladder scanner, check your institution's policy; you may be required to catheterize the client if the amount of urine present exceeds a particular volume.

Ask the client how frequently he or she visits the rest room, including how many times during the night, and if he or she experiences episodes of urinary incontinence.

As stated earlier, the endocrine system regulates numerous body processes. When a client has a disorder of the endocrine system, he or she experiences either a decrease in gland activity

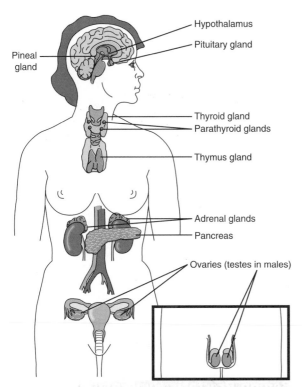

Figure 7–1. Organs of the endocrine system. (From Hansen, M. [1998]. *Pathophysiology*. Philadelphia: W. B. Saunders, p. 798.)

Pineal gland

Hypothalamus

Pituitary gland

Thyroid gland

Parathyroid glands

Thymus gland

Adrenal glands

Pancreas

Ovaries (testes in males)

Table 7–1
SELECTED ENDOCRINE GLANDS, HORMONES SECRETED, AND AGE-RELATED CHANGES

Endocrine Gland	Hormones Secreted	Age-Related Changes
Pituitary gland	Anterior pituitary: • Growth hormone • Adrenocorticotropic hormone (ACTH) • Thyroid-stimulating hormone (TSH) • Follicle-stimulating hormone (FSH) • Luteinizing hormone (LH) • Prolactin Posterior pituitary: • Antidiuretic hormone (ADH) • Oxytocin	• Decreased size and weight • Decreased cell mass • Atrophy • Fibrosis • Decreased vascularity
Adrenal glands	Adrenal cortex: • Cortisol • Aldosterone • Sex hormones Adrenal Medulla: • Epinephrine • Norepinephrine	• Aldosterone secretion may be decreased
Thyroid gland	• Thyroxine (T_4) • Triiodothyronine (T_3) • Calcitonin	• Gland fibrosis and infiltration of leukocytes • Decreased level of T_3 • Decreased basal metabolic rate
Pancreas (islets of Langerhans)	• Insulin • Glucagon • Somatostatin	• Decreased insulin secretion • Increased resistance to insulin at target organs
Ovaries	• Estrogen • Progesterone	• Reduced estrogen production during and after menopause • Reduced progesterone production after menopause
Testes	• Testosterone	• Decreased testicular volume • Impaired spermatogenesis • Decreased secretion of testosterone
Parathyroid glands	• Parathormone (PTH)	• Increased interstitial fatty tissue in the gland • Increased PTH levels

Adapted from Matteson, M. A., McConnell, E. S., & Linton, A. D. (1997). *Gerontological nursing: Concepts and practice.* Philadelphia: W. B. Saunders, pp. 356–358.

⚠ **Signs and Symptoms Tip**

Urinary incontinence is sometimes the only sign of UTI in an older adult.

(hypofunction) or an increase in gland activity *(hyperfunction)*. For example, an older adult with decreased activity of the thyroid gland is said to have hypothyroidism. Your assessment of the endocrine system is indirect in that you cannot usually inspect, palpate (except perhaps an enlarged thyroid gland), auscultate, or percuss an endocrine gland. Instead, you perform a head-to-toe physical examination as usual, but keeping a keen eye on signs and symptoms in the older adult that might indicate endocrine dysfunction. As can be seen in Table 7–2, signs of endocrine dysfunction can appear throughout your physical assessment. This pervasiveness of signs in nearly every body system demonstrates the importance of careful, complete documentation of your physical examination.

In addition, laboratory tests can validate or rule out an endocrine disorder. Laboratory and diagnostic tests that may be ordered for the older adult suspected of having an endocrine disorder are listed in Box 7–3.

DISORDERS COMMON IN OLDER ADULTS

Benign Prostatic Hyperplasia

Benign prostatic hyperplasia, or BPH, is a disorder that affects many men as they age. This

Table 7–2		
SELECTED ASSESSMENT CLUES TO ENDOCRINE DYSFUNCTION		
Assessment Parameter	**Abnormal Finding**	**Possible Endocrine Influences**
Vital signs	Increased or decreased temperature	• Thyroid • Ovaries
	Increased or decreased pulse	• Thyroid • Adrenal medulla • Adrenal cortex • Ovaries • Islets of Langerhans • Posterior pituitary
	Increased or decreased blood pressure	• Adrenal medulla • Adrenal cortex • Thyroid • Posterior pituitary
Skin, hair, nails	Brittle nails, dry skin, lackluster hair	• Thyroid • Pituitary
Skin	Abnormal (increased or decreased) pigmentation	• Adrenal cortex • Thyroid
Musculoskeletal system	Decreased muscle mass	• Islets of Langerhans • Thyroid
Genitourinary system	Large urine output	• Posterior pituitary • Islets of Langerhans
Overall appearance	Fatigue Weight loss Mental status changes Skin changes (pruritus, rash)	• Thyroid • Adrenal cortex • Islets of Langerhans

disorder, which occurs in as many as 80% of men older than age 60, is an enlargement of the prostate gland. Some sources refer to the disorder as benign prostatic *hypertrophy* because there is hypertrophy of the prostate gland; however, the

correct terminology for the pathologic process is *hyperplasia* because the disorder involves an increase in the *number*, rather than the *size*, of cells (Fig. 7–2).

As the prostate gland enlarges, it grows in an inward and upward direction, thereby encroaching on both the bladder opening and the urethra. The result is that the older man experiences difficulty with urination. The build-up of pressure that results from inability to empty the bladder can lead to hypertrophy of the longitudinal muscles of the bladder; left untreated, this pressure back-up can extend in an ascending direction to the ureters and even the kidneys, causing tissue damage. The exact cause of BPH is unknown, although there is a strong correlation with advanced age. Other factors, such as diet, metabolic characteristics, and atherosclerosis, have also been studied as possible risks for the development of BPH. Signs and symptoms of the disorder are outlined in Box 7–4.

It is interesting to note that the severity of symptoms does not necessarily positively correlate with the severity of gland enlargement. In other words, it is possible for an older man to have severe urinary symptoms with minimal or no gland

---

Box 7–3 Selected Endocrine Laboratory and Diagnostic Tests

Blood studies
• Serum electrolytes
• Serum glucose
• Serum hormone levels
• Hematology
• Serum osmolality

Urine studies
• Urine osmolality
• Urine electrolytes

Other
• Hormone stimulation tests
• Glucose tolerance test
• X-rays
• CT scan

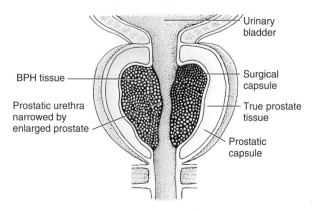

Figure 7–2. Benign prostatic hyperplasia (BPH) grows inward, causing narrowing of the urethra. (From Ignatavicius, D. D., Workman, M. L., & Mishler, M. A. [1999]. *Medical-surgical nursing across the health care continuum* [3rd Ed.]. Philadelphia: W. B. Saunders, p. 2022.)

enlargement; on the other hand, one can have relatively minor symptoms with quite advanced prostatic hyperplasia. Symptoms are usually graded using a scale such as that presented in Figure 7–3.

Medical treatment of BPH in the early stages depends primarily on the level of discomfort and the preferences of the client. The client may delay intervention until his symptoms become bothersome enough that he elects to undergo treatment. During this time, however, he is monitored annually by the physician or advanced practice nurse for cancer, renal dysfunction, and UTI. This approach is described as watchful waiting. If the client decides to pursue treatment, both medical and surgical options are available (Fig. 7–4).

These options, along with nursing implications, are summarized in Tables 7–3 and 7–4, respectively.

Urinary Incontinence

Urinary incontinence, or UI, refers to the involuntary loss of urine. It affects as many as one third of older adults who live at home, and up to half of those who reside in long-term care facilities; it is twice as common in women than in men. UI is not a normal change of aging, and most older adults who become incontinent experience only mild incontinence. Numerous risk factors are associated with urinary incontinence; many of these are outlined in Box 7–5.

Medication Safety Tip

Medications that can lead to incontinence in the older adult:

- Antihypertensive medications
- Antipsychotic medications
- Anticholinergics
- Calcium channel blockers
- Sedatives
- Antidepressants
- Antispasmodics
- Antiemetics
- Antiarrhythmics
- Anticonvulsants

Data from O'Connell, H. E., & McGuire, E. J. (1996). Assessing and managing urinary incontinence in primary care. *Medscape Women's Health, 1*(12), 1–11. Available at http://www.medscape.com/Medscape/WomensHealth/journal/1996/v01.n12/w151.o'connell/w151.o'connell.html

---

Box 7–4 Signs and Symptoms of Benign Prostatic Hyperplasia

Signs
- Decreased urinary stream
- Dribbling after voiding
- Hematuria
- Urinary frequency
- Bladder distention

Symptoms
- Hesitancy
- Frequency
- Nocturia

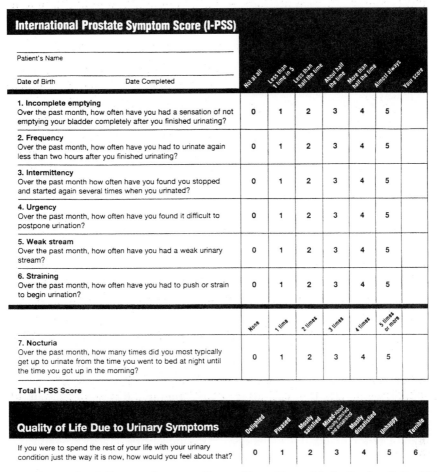

Figure 7–3. International Prostate Symptom Score. (From Barry, M. J., Fowler, F. J., O' Leary, M. P., et al. (1992). The American Urological Association symptom index for benign prostatic hyperplasia. *Journal of Urology, 148*: 1549.

An older adult may experience acute or chronic incontinence. Acute or temporary incontinence may occur with the onset of a new illness or medication, and it usually subsides when the underlying problem is resolved. Examples of conditions that can cause temporary incontinence include vaginal and urinary tract infections, adverse effects of medication, and constipation. Chronic incontinence may also be reversible, but treatment may be lengthier and may involve multiple treatment modalities.

There are four different types of chronic urinary incontinence: stress, urge, overflow, and functional. Each has different signs and symptoms with a different pathophysiology underlying

the disorder; therefore, different treatments are prescribed. These are outlined in Table 7–5.

As you can see from the table, the majority of treatments for UI are interventions that nurses can employ. Urinary incontinence is a disorder with numerous treatment options, but the older adult may be unaware of the treatments available and may assume falsely that he or she must live with this uncomfortable and embarrassing problem. It is important that health care professionals understand the stigma and embarrassment for older clients associated with this condition. The older adult may live in fear of an embarrassing episode of incontinence or with the fear of

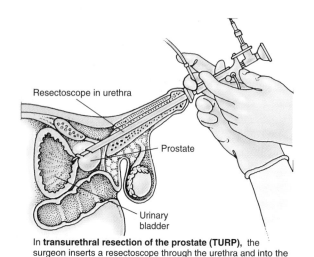

Figure 7–4. Transurethral resection of the prostate (TURP). (From Ignatavicius, D. D., Workman, M. L., & Mishler, M. A. [1999]. *Medical-surgical nursing across the health care continuum* [3rd Ed.]. Philadelphia: W. B. Saunders, p. 2025.)

In **transurethral resection of the prostate (TURP)**, the surgeon inserts a resectoscope through the urethra and into the bladder and removes pieces of tissue from the prostate gland.

producing an odor. He or she may avoid important social situations for fear of an accident. When caring for the older adult with urinary incontinence, the health care professional must be extremely sensitive to these very personal fears and feelings. When assisting a client with daily care, for example, NEVER refer to adult undergarments as "diapers." This term is humiliating and degrading to the older adult. Role model the appropriate terminology for other staff members. Always treat the older adult with dignity and respect.

Urinary Tract Infection

Urinary tract infection, or UTI, is an umbrella term that includes infections of the urethra (*urethritis*), the urinary bladder (*cystitis*), and the kidneys (*pyelonephritis*). These infections are more common among older adults because of the age-related physical changes described earlier in the chapter, and because of other age-associated risk factors, which are summarized in Box 7–6.

Bacteria usually enter the urinary tract through the urethra. If a UTI develops and is left untreated, it will usually progress in an ascending manner: urethritis, cystitis, then pyelonephritis. Pyelonephritis is a serious situation that can lead to life-threatening **septicemia** in the older adult.

The organism usually responsible for a UTI is *Escherichia coli*, or *E. coli*. Urinary tract infection is the most common type of **nosocomial infection;** older adults who either are hospitalized or are living in institutional settings have higher rates of UTI than do those who live at home. The older

Table 7–3			
MEDICAL TREATMENT FOR BENIGN PROSTATIC HYPERPLASIA			
Drug Category	**Example**	**Mechanism of Action**	**Nursing Implications**
5-alpha reductase inhibitor	finasteride (Proscar)	Blocks the conversion of testosterone to dihydrotestosterone, leading to decreased prostate size	• Do not handle tablets if you are, or may become, pregnant (can damage male fetus) • Adverse effects may include decreased libido or impotence (3% to 4%) • Client must take medication for 6 months before symptoms improve
Alpha-adrenergic antagonist	terazosin (Hytrin)	Relieves obstruction by blocking alpha$_1$ receptors in the prostate capsule	• Symptom improvement usually seen in weeks • Monitor for orthostatic hypotension, dizziness, and fatigue

Data from Gerber, G. S. (1998). Benign prostatic hyperplasia in older men. *Clinics in Geriatric Medicine: Genitourinary Problems, 14*(2), 323–325; Hodgson, B. B., & Kizior, R. J. (1999). *Saunders nursing drug handbook.* Philadelphia: W. B. Saunders.

Table 7–4		
SURGICAL TREATMENT FOR BENIGN PROSTATIC HYPERPLASIA		
Procedure	**Description**	**Nursing Implications**
Transurethral resection of the prostate (TURP)	A resectoscope is passed through the urethra to excise and cauterize excess prostatic tissue. Viewed by physicians as the "gold standard" for BPH treatment	• Short recovery time because there is no incision and no general anesthesia • Postprocedure care: continuous bladder irrigation • Monitor for infection, hemorrhage, and confusion
Transurethral electrovaporization of the prostate	Same equipment as with TURP, except roller electrode is used to heat and vaporize prostate tissue	• Bleeding is usually less than with TURP • Urinary catheter is left in for less time • Shorter hospital stay
Transurethral needle ablation (TUNA)	Low-level radio frequency waves are delivered to the prostate through needles, to heat and destroy tissue	• Minimal or no anesthesia (local) • Done in clinic setting • Decreased risk of incontinence and sexual dysfunction compared with TURP
Transurethral microwave therapy (TUMT)	Heating of prostate using probes and either low or high energy	• Low energy is less painful but may be less effective • High energy requires sedation or anesthesia and closer nursing observation • High energy: greater urethral iritation; client may require catheterization for 1–3 wk

Data from Gerber, G. S. (1998). Benign prostatic hyperplasia in older men. *Clinics in Geriatric Medicine: Genitourinary Problems, 14*(2), 326–328; Issa, M. M., Myrick, S. E., & Symbas, N. P. (1998). The TUNA procedure for BPH: Review of the technology. Available at http://www.medscape.com/SCP/IIU/1998/v.11n04/u3086.issa.html Accessed 8/23/98.

adult may present with the classic signs and symptoms of a UTI, with an atypical presentation, or with no signs and symptoms whatsoever. Traditional signs and symptoms of a UTI are listed in Table 7–6.

> **Box 7–5 Risk Factors for Urinary Incontinence**
>
> • Decreased bladder capacity
> • Benign prostatic hyperplasia
> • Decreased estrogen levels
> • Obesity
> • Chronic constipation
> • Smoking
> • Cognitive impairment
> • Immobility
> • Self-care deficits
> • Neurologic impairment
> • Certain medications
> • Gynecologic or urologic surgery
> • Environmental factors

> **Signs and Symptoms Tip**
>
> Atypical presentation of urinary tract infection:
>
> • Anorexia
> • Nausea and vomiting
> • Confusion
> • Urinary incontinence
> • Blunted fever response
> • Falls
> • Tachypnea, hypotension

The intended outcomes of treatment for an older adult with a UTI are to rid the urinary tract of the invading organism and to prevent the recurrence of infection. To this end, the physician or advanced practice nurse may prescribe antibiotic therapy. Occasionally, topical antibiotics applied to the external meatus may be added to the treatment plan. If the older adult experiences severe discomfort from **dysuria**, a urinary anesthetic

Table 7–5

SIGNS AND SYMPTOMS OF URINARY INCONTINENCE

Type	Pathophysiology	Signs/Symptoms	Treatments
Urge	• Uninhibited bladder contractions • Can be related to neurologic disorders or genitourinary conditions	• **Urgency** • Leakage of large volumes of of urine	• Bladder training • Habit training • Pelvic muscle exercises with biofeedback • **Pelvic floor electrical stimulation** • Drug therapy: anticholinergic agents, smooth muscle relaxants
Overflow	• Obstruction of urinary outlet: can be related to stricture of urethra, benign prostatic hyperplasia (BPH) • Atonic bladder: can be related to neuropathy, spinal cord lesions, or anticholinergic medications	• Straining to void • Leakage of small volumes of urine	• Surgical repair of obstruction • Drug therapy for BPH • Urinary catheterization • Incontinence ring (women) if obstruction is due to pelvic organ prolapse • Scheduled voiding
Stress	• Sphincter insufficiency • Pelvic floor weakness	• Occurs with cough, sneeze, or exercise owing to increased intra-abdominal pressure • Loss of small volumes of urine	• Pelvic muscle exercises with or without biofeedback • Cone-shaped vaginal weights • Electrical stimulation • Drug therapy: alpha-adrenergic agonists, estrogen • Surgery
Functional	• Otherwise continent clients who cannot reach the toilet because of barriers such as: physical: immobility pharmacologic: diuretics, sedatives psychological: dementia, depression environmental: restraints, location of facilities	• Inability to toilet • Variable volume of urine loss	• Manipulation of medication dosages or schedules • Treatment of depression • Removal of environmental barriers • Provision of assistive devices (commode, urinal) • Provision of protective undergarments

Source: Busby-Whitehead, J., & Johnson, T. M. (1998). Urinary incontinence. *Clinics in Geriatric Medicine, 14*(2), 285–295.

such as phenazopyridine (Pyridium) may be prescribed to relieve symptoms.

🔖 Medication Safety Tip

Although phenazopyridine (Pyridium) relieves the dysuria associated with UTI, it has no therapeutic effect regarding treatment of the infection and must NEVER be used in lieu of antibiotics.

Diabetes Mellitus

Diabetes is a disorder of the metabolism of glucose by the body. Diabetes mellitus is characterized by an abundance of glucose in the bloodstream that is unable to enter the body cells to be used as fuel. This inability of the glucose to enter the cells is related to one of two factors—either a lack of the hormone insulin (usually the defect with type 1 diabetes mellitus) or a resistance to insulin at the cellular or tissue level (the primary problem with type 2 diabetes mellitus).

The endocrine pancreas secretes the hormone insulin. Insulin allows glucose to enter body cells to provide energy. Think of the cell wall as a locked door with insulin as the key. In type 1 diabetes mellitus, it is as if you have no key. In type 2 diabetes, you have keys, but the locks have changed. Either way, glucose

> **Box 7–6 Risk Factors for Urinary Tract Infections**
>
> - Urinary retention
> - Increased urinary pH
> - Catheterization
> - Shorter urethra in women
> - Decreased estrogen level after menopause
> - Increased vaginal pH
> - Sexual activity
> - Institutionalization
> - Diseases: diabetes mellitus, cerebrovascular accident
> - Decreased functional status
> - Decreased mental status

accumulates in the bloodstream, leading to **hyperglycemia.**

The three classic signs and symptoms of diabetes mellitus are the "3 P's": **polyuria, polydipsia,** and **polyphagia;** all are related to the hyperglycemia associated with this disorder. The glucose molecule is a heavy osmotic particle in the vasculature; as blood sugar levels rise, polyuria ensues as an osmotic **diuresis.**

> **Signs and Symptoms Tip**
>
> Because of age-related changes in thirst sensation, the older adult with diabetes mellitus may not exhibit the sign of polydipsia.

This diuresis leads to fluid volume deficit, which manifests as polydipsia. Polyphagia results because cells send a message to the brain that fuel is needed for the body.

> **Signs and Symptoms Tip**
>
> Polyuria can manifest as incontinence in the older adult.

Type 1 diabetes mellitus (formerly called juvenile-onset diabetes) is more common in young adults and children, whereas type 2 diabetes mellitus (formerly called adult-onset diabetes) is more common in the older adult. As was mentioned earlier in the chapter, the tendency toward insulin resistance by cells and tissues with age explains the increase in type 2 diabetes mellitus among older adults. However, aging also causes somewhat decreased insulin production. Hence, many older adults with type 2 diabetes may develop both insulin resistance and decreased amounts of insulin.

Diabetes appears to accelerate the aging process; physiologically, a client with diabetes mellitus is approximately 10 years older than his or her chronological age. Similarities between diabetes mellitus and the aging process are outlined in Box 7–7.

In diabetes mellitus, glucose cannot enter the cell owing to a lack of insulin; it therefore remains in the bloodstream and increases to a dangerous level. The body must obtain fuel for energy from other sources, such as the breakdown of fat. Brain cells, however, rely exclusively on glucose for energy; when they are starved for glucose, the client exhibits signs of confusion. Elevated blood glucose also has serious detrimental effects on the body over time, including damage to the blood vessels leading to disorders such as coronary artery disease, peripheral vascular disease, and many others. Hence, both acute and chronic complications of diabetes mellitus can pose serious risks to the health and wellness of

Table 7–6	
TRADITIONAL SIGNS AND SYMPTOMS OF URINARY TRACT INFECTION	
Signs	**Symptoms**
Small urine volumes	Urinary frequency
Foul-smelling urine	Urinary urgency
Hematuria	Dysuria
Elevated temperature	Suprapubic or back pain
Elevated white blood cell count (if severe)	Sensation of incomplete bladder emptying

---

Box 7–7 Similarities Between Diabetes Mellitus and Aging

- Alteration in DNA unwinding rate
- Increased collagen cross-linkage
- Increased free radical activity
- Increased capillary basement membrane thickening
- Cataracts
- Atherosclerosis
- Decreased functional status

Source: Morley, J. E. (1999). An overview of diabetes mellitus in older persons. *Clinics in Geriatric Medicine: Advances in the Care of Older People with Diabetes, 15(2), 211–212.*

---

the older adult. Table 7–7 outlines the causes, signs and symptoms, and treatment options for acute complications of diabetes mellitus.

 Health Promotion Tip

It is crucial that smoking cessation be encouraged in the client with diabetes mellitus, as smoking worsens several of the chronic complications associated with diabetes.

Table 7–8 outlines several chronic complications associated with diabetes mellitus.

 Signs and Symptoms Tip

Clients with diabetes mellitus often experience **no chest pain**, even in the face of a myocardial infarction, owing to peripheral neuropathy.

Table 7–7

ACUTE COMPLICATIONS OF DIABETES MELLITUS

Disorder	Causes	Signs/Symptoms	Treatment Options
Acute hypoglycemia	• Decreased/delayed food intake following insulin administration • Overdose of insulin or oral hypoglycemic medications • Excessive exercise without carbohydrate consumption	• Blood glucose <60 • Headache • Weakness • Diaphoresis • Blurred vision • Anxiety • Nausea • Tremulousness • Pallor • Tachycardia • Palpitations	• (Only if alert) 10–20 grams of simple carbohydrate (30–50 calories) orally, repeat every 15 minutes until blood sugar within normal range. *Examples:* orange juice, candy, glucose gel/paste • Glucagon IM or SC • 50% dextrose IV
Diabetic ketoacidosis (DKA)	• More common with type 1 diabetes • Deficiency of insulin • May be initial presentation of illness for new client with diabetes mellitus	• Blood glucose elevated to 250 to 800, or higher • Dehydration • Polyuria • Polydipsia • Fatigue • Kussmaul's respirations • Acetone breath	• IV fluid replacement • IV insulin replacement • IV electrolyte replacement (potassium, sodium) • Hourly blood sugar measurement
Hyperosmolar nonketotic coma (HHNK)	• More common with type 2 diabetes • Deficiency of insulin • Often related to stress of new illness (e.g., infection, pneumonia)	• Elevated blood sugar: higher than DKA (often >1000) • Severe dehydration • Tachycardia, hypotension • Onset over days; history of polyuria and polydipsia • No acetone breath • Altered mental status	• IV fluid replacement: up to 10 L depending on deficit • IV insulin replacement • IV electrolyte replacement (potassium, sodium) • Hourly blood sugar measurement • Treatment of underlying disorder that precipitated event (e.g., pneumonia)

Table 7–8

SELECTED CHRONIC COMPLICATIONS OF DIABETES MELLITUS

Complication	Description	Treatment Options/ Preventive Strategies
Retinopathy	Damaged retinal blood vessels related to prolonged blood glucose elevation; can lead to blindness	• Annual eye examinations • Careful blood glucose control • Laser surgery
Nephropathy	Damaged renal blood vessels related to prolonged blood glucose elevation; can lead to renal failure	• Careful blood glucose control • Dialysis (peritoneal or hemodialysis)
Neuropathy	Damaged peripheral nerves, more commonly in lower extremities; can be associated with decreased sensation, hypersensation, or burning sensation	• Careful blood glucose control • Daily foot care • Protective footwear • Podiatry consultation • Daily inspection of feet with mirror to detect irritations or areas of possible breakdown that cannot be felt
Coronary artery disease (CAD)	Damaged blood vessel endothelium, twice as common in clients with diabetes mellitus; can lead to myocardial infarction	• Careful blood glucose control • Reduction in other cardiac risk factors, such as by smoking cessation, consuming a low-fat diet, and exercise
Peripheral vascular disease (PVD)	Damaged blood vessel endothelium, 30 times more common in clients with diabetes mellitus; can lead to amputation of limbs (usually lower extremities)	• Careful blood glucose control • Smoking cessation • Podiatry consultation
Cerebrovascular disease	Damaged blood vessel endothelium; can lead to cerebrovascular accident	• Careful blood glucose control • Reduction in other cerebrovascular accident risk factors, such as by smoking cessation and consuming a low-fat diet
Sexual dysfunction	Poorly understood; probably related to similar blood vessel damage	• Careful blood glucose control • Smoking cessation • Inflatable devices • Medications such as prostaglandin E_1

One very serious risk associated with diabetes is amputation of extremities (usually lower extremities) from **gangrene**. This usually begins innocently enough with foot ulceration. For several reasons, persons with diabetes mellitus are at very high risk for developing foot ulcerations: compromised circulation from vascular disease, lack of sensation from peripheral neuropathy, and lack of pain fibers. What might begin as a minor irritation from an unnoticed rock in one's shoe can lead to ulceration, infection, gangrene, and loss of a toe, a foot, or the lower leg. Recent research has shown that African Americans and Mexican Americans experience a higher frequency of diabetes-related lower extremity amputations (Lavery et al., 1999).

Because loss of limbs is a huge price to pay, preventive approaches such as daily foot care are paramount in the treatment of clients with diabetes mellitus. Reduction of foot ulcers in clients with diabetes mellitus is one of the *Healthy People 2010* objectives. Other *Healthy People 2010* objectives that pertain to clients with diabetes mellitus are listed in Box 7–8.

The older adult who is living at home must be taught to perform daily foot inspections with a mirror. For those residing in extended-care facilities, the American Diabetic Association and the

---

Box 7–8 Selected *Healthy People* 2010 Objectives Related to Diabetes Mellitus

- Increase the proportion of persons with diabetes who receive formal diabetes education.
- Prevent diabetes.
- Reduce diabetes-related deaths among persons with diabetes.
- Reduce deaths from cardiovascular disease in persons with diabetes.
- Reduce the frequency of foot ulcers in persons with diabetes.
- Reduce the rate of lower extremity amputations in persons with diabetes.
- Increase the proportion of adults with diabetes who have an annual dilated eye examination.
- Increase the proportion of adults with diabetes who have at least an annual foot examination.
- Increase the proportion of persons with diabetes who have at least an annual dental examination.
- Increase the proportion of adults with diabetes who perform self–blood glucose monitoring at least once daily.

Source: *Healthy People 2010* website. Available at http://www.health.gov/healthypeople/Document/tableof contents.htm Accessed 11/13/00.

American Association of Diabetes Educators recommend both daily foot care and weekly inspections under the direction of a registered nurse; this recommendation is based on the fact that extended-care facility residents with diabetes undergo a significantly greater number of amputations than do their counterparts in the community. Many facilities do not allow licensed nurses to trim or cut the toenails of a client with diabetes because the risk of infection is so great. Instead, podiatrists are employed to perform these procedures.

Treatment options for diabetes mellitus include medications, diet, and exercise. Medication used for the treatment of type 1 diabetes mellitus consists primarily of insulin replacement therapy, usually in the form of subcutaneous injection (Fig. 7–5). Medications used for the treatment of type 2 diabetes mellitus include oral hypoglycemic agents, most of which act on cell

receptors, thereby allowing insulin to perform its function. Occasionally, as clients with type 2 diabetes mellitus grow older, they may also require insulin replacement. Medications for type 1 and type 2 diabetes mellitus are summarized in Tables 7–9 and 7–10, respectively.

NURSING DIAGNOSES

As was discussed in earlier chapters, nursing diagnoses are derived from assessment data and are unique to the individual client. Also, you may recall that a nursing diagnosis focuses on the *client's response* to the health problem.

Common nursing diagnoses (written only as the problem portion of the *Problem, Etiology,* and *Signs and symptoms* [PES] nursing diagnosis statement) that apply to the older adult experiencing disorders covered in this chapter are listed in Table 7–11.

As was discussed earlier, not every identified nursing diagnosis is appropriate for every client with a given disorder. Likewise, other nursing diagnoses than those listed in Table 7–11 may be appropriate for your client. For example, not every client with urinary incontinence experiences social isolation because of it. Carefully consider every nursing diagnosis as you individualize a plan of care for the older adult with disorders related to excretion, and reproductive and regulatory well-being.

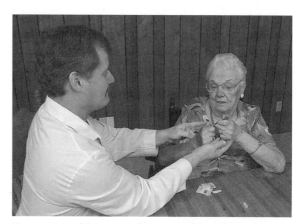

Figure 7–5. Nurse teaching an older client how to draw up insulin. (From deWit, S. [2001]. *Fundamental concepts and skills for nursing.* Philadelphia: W. B. Saunders, p. 125.)

Table 7–9

MEDICATIONS FOR TYPE 1 DIABETES MELLITUS

Insulin	Onset of Action	Peak Effect	Duration	Comments
Lispro	10–15 min	30–90 min	<5 hr	Newest form
Regular	30 min	2–5 hr	5–8 hr	Most commonly used for changing insulin needs (e.g., infection)
NPH/Lente	1–3 hr	6–12 hr	16–24 hr	Can be mixed with Regular, if ordered
70/30, 50/50	30 min	7–12 hr	16–24 hr	Pre-mixed NPH with Regular
Ultralente	4–6 hr	8–20 hr	24–36 hr	Ensures regular food intake or can lead to prolonged hypoglycemia

Adapted from Tyson, S. R. (1999). *Gerontological nursing care.* Philadelphia: W. B. Saunders, p. 376.

COLLABORATING ON THE PLAN OF CARE

Once the nursing diagnosis is established, expected outcomes must be set. Remember to write outcomes that are realistic, measurable, and tailored to the individual client.

Sample outcomes for a client with benign prostatic hyperplasia can be found in Table 7–12. These are samples only because the outcomes you set must be established with your individual client in mind.

In like fashion, sample outcomes for older adults with nursing diagnoses for the conditions of urinary incontinence, UTI, and diabetes mellitus can be found in Tables 7–13, 7–14, and 7–15, respectively.

IMPLEMENTING INTERVENTIONS FOR HEALTH PROMOTION

Interventions to Promote Safety

1. Encourage fluid intake in the older adults following any diagnostic procedure in which contrast dye is used. Use of a contrast agent in the dehydrated older adult can lead to

Table 7–10

MEDICATIONS FOR TYPE 2 DIABETES MELLITUS

Category	Generic Name	Brand Name(s)	Comments
Sulfonylurea agents (first generation)	Tolbutamide	Orinase	
	Chlorpropamide	• Diabinese	Not recommended for older adults (long duration; 60 hr)
	Tolazamide	Tolinase	
	Acetohexamide	Dymelor	
Sulfonylurea agents (second generation)	Glipizide	Glucotrol Glucotrol XL	Second-generation agents newer; generally preferred
	Glyburide	DiaBeta Micronase Glynase	
	Glimepiride	Amaryl	
Biguanides	Metformin	Glucophage	Contraindication: liver or renal disease
Alpha-glucosidase inhibitors	Acarbose	Precose	Frequently causes GI upset, diarrhea
Thiazolidinediones	Troglitazone	Rezulin	Monitor for signs of infection
	Rosiglitazone maleate	Avandia	FDA-approved 5/29/99
Meglitinides	Repaglinide	Prandin	Take only with meals

Data from Avandia for Diabetes: An Alternative to Rezulin? *Drug Infoline, 1999.* Available at http://www.pharminfo.com/pubs/druginfoline/druginfol_13.html; Hodgson, B. B., & Kizior, R. J. (1999). *Saunders nursing drug handbook.* Philadelphia: W. B. Saunders; Tyson, S. R. (1999). *Gerontological nursing care.* Philadelphia: W. B. Saunders, p. 376.

Table 7–11

NURSING DIAGNOSES RELATED TO EXCRETION, REPRODUCTIVE AND REGULATORY WELL-BEING

	Benign Prostatic Hyperplasia	Urinary Incontinence	Urinary Tract Infection	Diabetes Mellitus
Imbalanced nutrition: more than body requirements				X
Imbalanced nutrition: less than body requirements				X
Risk for infection	X	X	X	X
Impaired urinary elimination	X	X	X	X
Stress urinary incontinence		X	X	X
Reflex urinary incontinence	X	X	X	X
Reflex urinary retention	X	X	X	X
Altered tissue perfusion			X	X
Risk for imbalanced fluid volume	X	X	X	X
Risk for impaired skin integrity		X		X
Social isolation	X	X		X
Sexual dysfunction	X			X
Risk for peripheral neurovascular dysfunction				X
Sleep pattern disturbance	X	X	X	X
Deficient knowledge	X	X	X	X
Anxiety	X	X	X	X

Table 7–12

SAMPLE OUTCOMES FOR AN OLDER ADULT WITH BENIGN PROSTATIC HYPERPLASIA

Nursing Diagnosis	Sample Outcomes
Anxiety related to impending surgical procedure	• Client will verbalize questions regarding postoperative concerns • Client will describe methods of pain control available to him postoperatively • Client will acknowledge reduction in anxiety level
Risk for infection	• Client will verbalize the desired daily PO fluid intake • Client will exhibit no signs/ symptoms of infection
Impaired urinary elimination	• Client will regain bladder control as evidenced by a decrease in urinary frequency and nocturia • Client will experience improved bladder emptying as evidenced by intake and output records

Table 7–13

SAMPLE OUTCOMES FOR AN OLDER ADULT WITH URINARY INCONTINENCE

Nursing Diagnosis	Sample Outcomes
Risk for impaired skin integrity	• Client will state the importance of good skin hygiene following each incontinent episode • No areas of skin irritation will be observed
Social isolation	• Client will verbalize supplies needed for short outings • Client will not isolate self in home environment
Sleep pattern disturbance	• Client will report having adequate sleep within 48 hours • Client will obtain restful sleep without the use of medications • Client will demonstrate daytime alertness

acute renal failure, as contrast dyes tend to be **nephrotoxic**. Older adults are more prone to this complication because of the age-related changes that occur in the kidneys.

2. Encourage annual gynecologic examinations in the older female client. The older adult may have a misconception that gynecologic examinations are only for younger people; however, health promotion strategies such as preventive screening for disease are vitally important in helping to keep the older members of our community functioning at their optimal health status.

3. Encourage annual digital rectal prostate examinations in the older male client. As with the older female adult, preventive screening is vitally important for the older men in the community. The incidence of prostate cancer increases with advancing age, and treatment options are available.

4. Remove barriers that are obstacles to self-care in the client with urinary incontinence. This begins with assessment of the environment. Important nursing interventions in this arena include clearing pathways to the restroom, assisting with ambulation as needed, providing for privacy, providing adequate lighting for elimination, and providing adequate space for elimination.

5. Periodically review the medications taken by the older adult, and assess for potentially nephrotoxic medications or medication combinations. Remember that age-related changes in the kidneys leave the older adult vulnerable to the nephrotoxic effects of many medications.

6. Under the guidance of the RN, educate the client with diabetes mellitus regarding daily foot care (Box 7–9). Review and reinforce foot care with the older adult at every opportunity.

Table 7–14
SAMPLE OUTCOMES FOR AN OLDER ADULT WITH URINARY TRACT INFECTION

Nursing Diagnosis	Sample Outcomes
Deficient knowledge: Treatment of urinary tract infection (UTI)	• Client will state the correct administration of medications: how many tablets for how many days • Client will state the recommended oral fluid intake • Client will verbalize the basic actions and special instructions for each medication prescribed
Deficient knowledge: Strategies for risk reduction for future urinary tract infections	• Client will state the recommended oral fluid intake • Client will state 3 strategies for UTI risk reduction (such as voiding after sex, wiping front to back, and good perineal hygiene)
Ineffective tissue perfusion: Renal	• Vital signs will remain within normal limits • Urine output will remain >30 mL/hr

---

Table 7–15
SAMPLE OUTCOMES FOR AN OLDER ADULT WITH DIABETES MELLITUS

Nursing Diagnosis	Sample Outcomes
Deficient knowledge: Daily foot care	• Client will describe the daily foot care that he or she must perform (or request assistance with) • Client will state the rationale regarding the importance of daily foot care • Client will state the rationale for daily foot inspection with mirror
Deficient knowledge: Signs/symptoms and treatment of acute hypoglycemia	• Client will list 4 signs and/or symptoms of acute hypoglycemia • Client will state immediate action to undertake in the event of acute hypoglycemia • Client will verbalize the importance and rationale for not skipping meals while taking antidiabetic medications
Imbalanced nutrition: Greater than body requirements	• Client will verbalize benefits of weight reduction and exercise in management of diabetes mellitus • Client will adhere to 2000-calorie diet • Client will demonstrate safe, gradual weight loss of 3 pounds per month

Box 7–9 Diabetic Foot Care

Always protect the feet:

- Wear sturdy, supportive, well-fitting, closed-toed shoes.
- Always wear socks.
- Test bathwater temperature with wrist or elbow before placing feet into tub.
- Do not fall asleep with feet near fireplace.
- Avoid using electric blankets or hot water bottle to heat the feet.
- Do not go barefoot.

Regularly inspect feet and shoes:

- Inspect inside of shoes prior to each wearing.
- Change shoes every 5 hours.
- Buy shoes that fit—never depend on them to stretch.
- Inspect feet daily, using a mirror to visualize the undersurface.
- Undergo inspection by podiatrist at least every 3 months.

Provide good hygiene and skin care to the feet:

- Wash thoroughly with soap and water.
- Do not soak feet—can lead to tissue maceration.
- Clean carefully between the toes.
- Dry thoroughly with soft cloth.
- Use emollient cream, but not between toes.

Promote optimal circulation:

- Do not cross legs or feet.
- Do not smoke.
- Avoid tight socks or garters.
- Perform leg exercises 2 to 3 times each day.

Box 7–10 Continuous Bladder Irrigation

For continuous bladder irrigation (CBI), do the following:

- Use normal saline for the bladder irrigant, unless otherwise ordered by the physician.
- Adjust the rate of irrigant according to the physician's order. Keep the registered nurse informed of your adjustments. The physician generally orders a rate that will keep the output clear and free of clots.
- Monitor the color, consistency, and amount of output.
- Check the drainage tubing frequently for kinking or other external obstructions.
- Monitor the client for signs of internal obstruction, such as clots, low urine output, and bladder spasms. Report any unusual findings to the registered nurse.
- If the urinary catheter is obstructed, turn off the CBI and irrigate with 30 to 50 mL of normal saline, under the direction of the registered nurse.
- Notify the registered nurse immediately if the obstruction does not resolve with hand irrigation, or if urinary return has the appearance of ketchup.
- Monitor intake and output (I&O).

Adapted from: Ignatavicius, D. D., Workman, M. L., & Mishler, M. A. (1999). *Medical-surgical nursing across the health care continuum.* Philadelphia: W. B. Saunders, p. 2030.

7. Encourage the older adult with diabetes mellitus to have annual eye examinations. In this way, signs of retinopathy can be discovered at the earliest opportunity, appropriate treatments can be recommended, and blindness can be prevented.

8. Implement appropriate postoperative nursing interventions for the client who has undergone transurethral resection of the prostate (TURP). Include in the nursing care the monitoring of continuous bladder irrigation (Box 7–10) and assessment for any complications such as infection, hemorrhage, bladder spasm, and confusion (a sign of electrolyte imbalance related to the irrigant).

9. After each incontinent episode, provide careful skin care for the client with urinary incontinence, to prevent skin breakdown.

10. Monitor for superinfection the older adult who is on antibiotic therapy for the treatment of a UTI. Owing to age-related changes in the immunologic system, superinfections are more common in older adults who are taking antibiotics.

11. Maintain strict aseptic practices when caring for the older adult with a urinary catheter. Periurethral care with soap and water (or per facility protocol) should be performed at least two times each day. Maintain the integrity of the closed system of drainage, and position

the drainage bag so that no obstruction is present. Role model for other staff members by stressing the importance of wearing gloves when working with the drainage system, and of thorough handwashing before and after manipulation of the urinary drainage system.

Interventions to Promote Health Education

1. Encourage monthly breast self-examinations (BSE). Again, preventive health care practices remain important throughout one's life, not just during the reproductive years.
2. Provide emotional support and teaching for chronic disease management (Fig. 7–6). Older adults with chronic urinary incontinence or benign prostatic hyperplasia have specific educational and supportive needs regarding excretion and regulatory well-being. The older client with diabetes mellitus has a myriad of educational needs, both on initial diagnosis and over the long term. Refer to Chapter 4 for a more thorough discussion regarding chronic pain management, including encouragement of healthy lifestyle habits and tips for teaching the older adult.
3. Provide education that urinary incontinence is not a normal change of aging. Encourage any

older adult experiencing this disorder to seek medical evaluation for treatment options. Many older adults have a common misconception that incontinence is a normal change of aging—fueled, in part, by the numerous television advertisements for incontinence aids. Although these ads provide a valuable service in encouraging the older adult with incontinence to "get back into life" and live an active life, they may leave some with the impression that incontinence is both inevitable with aging and untreatable, except for the use of adult undergarments. It is neither.
4. Educate the older adult with urge or stress incontinence about the correct performance of Kegel exercises to strengthen perineal muscles and promote continence. These **pelvic exercises** involve tightening or contraction of the vaginal and anal muscles to increase strength and tone, thus improving bladder control by increasing the closing force of the urethra. They can be done at any time of day and in any position. An easy-to-use instruction for Kegel exercises can be found in Box 7–11.
5. Educate the older adult about risk factor reduction for UTI. These instructions are summarized in Box 7–12.

Interventions to Promote Lifestyle Modification

1. Encourage the reduction of weight, if appropriate. Weight reduction can have beneficial effects on overweight older adults with diabetes mellitus type 2 and stress or functional urinary incontinence.
2. Encourage exercise to your client's level of tolerance. Exercise can lower the need for medications in a client with diabetes mellitus. Physical activity promotes circulation, which is beneficial for the client with diabetes mellitus. Physical activity also prevents urinary stasis, thereby lowering one's risk of UTI.
3. Educate the client who has undergone TURP about postoperative dietary restrictions. Items to avoid in the immediate postoperative period (because they can overstimulate the bladder) include alcohol, caffeine, and spicy foods.
4. Educate the older adult with incontinence about treatment options such as **bladder training** or reeducation, and **habit training.**

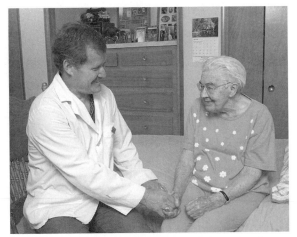

Figure 7–6. It is important to provide emotional support to an older client with diabetes. (From deWit, S. [2001]. *Fundamental concepts and skills for nursing.* Philadelphia: W. B. Saunders, p. 85.)

Box 7–11 Kegel Exercises

1. Lie on back with hips and knees bent. Tighten stomach and buttock muscles; then flatten back on bed. Hold for count of 5, relax.
2. Same position. Lift head, hold for count of 5, relax.
3. Lie on back with legs out straight and ankles crossed. Tighten buttocks, anus, and vagina. Hold for count of 5, relax. Try this exercise while sitting and standing.
4. Get onto all four extremities. Let the back sway. Tighten stomach, buttocks, anus, and vagina, and raise back up in the air like a cat. Hold for a count of 5, relax.
5. Perform the Kegel exercise while urinating: try to stop the flow of urine by tightening the buttocks, anus, and vagina.

   Practice these exercises four times each day, doing five repetitions of each step. Work up to ten times each day for each exercise.

Adapted from: Lentz, S. S., & Homesley, H. D. (1998). Gynecologic problems in older women. *Clinics in Geriatric Medicine: Genitourinary Problems, 14*(2), 304.

Box 7–12 Risk Reduction for Urinary Tract Infections

- Wear cotton underclothes.
- Consume 2 to 3 L of fluid each day to discourage bacterial growth and encourage bladder washout.
- Void whenever necessary so that stagnant urine does not remain in the bladder.
- After having a bowel movement, wipe in the direction of front to back. Bacteria in the feces can contaminate the urethra and increase one's chance of developing a urinary tract infection.
- Practice thorough perineal hygiene.
- Void after sexual intercourse to expel microorganisms from the urethra. Consuming fluids prior to intercourse can also help to encourage this.
- If you have a chronic urinary drainage device, wash your hands before and after catheter care and use aseptic technique when performing irrigations.

Bladder training is scheduled voiding by the client without response to the desire to void between scheduled times. (The interval between voids is gradually extended.) Habit training is scheduled voiding by the client along with voiding between scheduled times if the desire to void occurs. See Table 7–16 for a summary of behavioral strategies for urge and stress incontinence.

5. Implore the older adult with diabetes mellitus who smokes to quit. As was discussed earlier, smoking accelerates most, if not all, of the chronic complications associated with diabetes mellitus.

Health Promotion Tip

Clients with type 2 diabetes mellitus can often reduce and occasionally eliminate their need for oral hypoglycemic medications by engaging in a regular exercise program.

6. Refer the client with diabetes mellitus to a Certified Diabetes Educator (CDE). The CDE can assist the older adult in developing strategies to facilitate lifestyle change.

Health Promotion Tip

Recent research studies show that positive client outcomes are associated with diabetes education programs that focus on self-management, emphasize behavioral strategies, and provide culturally relevant information.

Source: Whittemore, R. (2000). Strategies to facilitate lifestyle change associated with diabetes mellitus. *Journal of Nursing Scholarship, 32*(3), 225–232.

Interventions to Promote Mobility

1. Encourage the older adult with urinary incontinence to be as mobile as possible and to avoid social isolation. The use of protective undergarments may help the older adult avoid isolation while more definitive treatment measures are being explored.
2. Encourage the individual with functional urinary incontinence to wear garments that are easy to manipulate.

Table 7-16

BEHAVIORAL TECHNIQUES FOR MANAGEMENT OF URGE AND STRESS URINARY INCONTINENCE

Technique	Description
Bladder training bladder reeducation, bladder drill	Voiding is scheduled for every 2 hr. Interval for voiding is gradually increased to every 3 to 4 hr. If urge to void occurs between scheduled times, client is encouraged to resist
Habit training	Client voids according to a timetable, but is not discouraged to void if urge occurs between scheduled times
Prompted voiding	Similar to habit training, plus a caregiver checks for wetness at scheduled intervals and prompts the client to void
Pelvic muscle exercises (Kegel exercises)	Periodic tightening and relaxation of pelvic, perivaginal, and anal muscles

Data from Busby-Whitehead, J., & Johnson, T. M. (1998). Urinary incontinence. *Clinics in Geriatric Medicine: Genitourinary Problems, 14*(2), 291–292; Steeman, E., & Defever, M. (1998). Urinary incontinence among elderly persons who live at home. *The Nursing Clinics of North America: Advances in Geriatric Nursing, 33*(3), 449–450.

3. Encourage the older male client who has undergone TURP to get out of bed and start moving as soon as possible postoperatively, but discourage strenuous activities for 2 to 3 weeks after surgery.
4. Encourage physical activity because inactivity can lead to urinary stasis and an increased risk for UTI.

Interventions to Promote Nutrition

1. Under the guidance of the RN, implement dietary teaching for the older adult with diabetes mellitus.
2. Promote optimal nutrition, including plenty of protein, zinc, and vitamin C, for the older adult with impaired skin integrity. This category of clients includes postoperative older men who have undergone TURP, as well as clients with urinary incontinence who are at high risk for skin breakdown.

3. Encourage the drinking of 12 to 14 glasses of water per day, early in the day, for the postoperative TURP client. These clients also should avoid foods that tend to constipate, and should consume plenty of fiber to decrease the risk of constipation.
4. Encourage the client with urinary incontinence to avoid caffeine because it is a bladder irritant.
5. Encourage the older adult who is prone to UTI to consume 2 to 3 liters of fluid per day.
6. Educate the older adult who is prone to UTI about the potentially beneficial effects of vitamin C and cranberry juice in preventing UTIs. These promote an acidic urine environment and may prevent a UTI from developing by preventing adherence of *E. coli* to urinary tract walls. One word of caution, however: although these may help ward off a UTI, they should NEVER be considered as an alternative to appropriate medical evaluation and treatment once a UTI has developed.

Interventions to Promote Rest and Sleep

1. Encourage the client with a UTI to try a sitz bath to relieve discomfort before bedtime and to promote restful sleep.
2. Discuss the restriction of fluids before bedtime with the client who experiences urinary incontinence. Acknowledge that this is acceptable, but only if the recommended quantities of fluid are consumed earlier in the day.

GATHERING DATA FOR EVALUATION

Although the RN is officially responsible for evaluation and modification of the plan of care for the client, your contribution is crucial. The data you gather, along with your observation of changes in the client, often make the difference in whether or not the plan of care is successful.

Nursing evaluation should be aimed directly at client outcomes. Many of the outcomes identified earlier in this chapter are straightforward and objective, often requiring that the client list, state, or verbally acknowledge learned information. For example, one outcome identified for the older adult experiencing a UTI reads, "Client will state the correct administration of medications: how many tablets for how many days." The nurse should evaluate this outcome not only by listening to the older adult as he or she states the correct administration, but also by watching as the client demonstrates the correct selection of the medication being discussed.

Evaluation of other outcomes may require additional investigation. For example, one outcome for the older adult with benign prostatic hyperplasia reads, "Client will exhibit no signs/symptoms of infection." Evaluation of this outcome requires assessment and nursing judgment and may require you to consult various sources of information. Don't forget to evaluate not only the typical signs and symptoms of a UTI but also the *atypical* signs and symptoms. The most obvious way to begin is by evaluating the client's vital signs for abnormalities. Next, because the type of infection for which this client is most at risk is a UTI, you must assess the color and clarity of the urine output. If the client has a urinary drainage device, examine the area where the tubing meets the meatus. If you are caring for the client in an acute care setting and have access to recent laboratory data, a white blood cell count or culture results can also provide important data. One final source not to be forgotten is other personnel, who can communicate helpful information to you. As you gather data, this involves recording information from nursing reports and reading progress notes from other personnel. The progress notes can be extremely useful for the detection of atypical signs and symptoms that other staff members might not have associated with a UTI, such as confusion, falls, loss of appetite, nausea, or incontinence.

In addition, your evaluation should take into consideration individual interventions that have been employed. Consider the nursing diagnosis, "Anxiety related to impending surgical procedure" for the older male client with benign prostatic hyperplasia. You will find that interventions effective in reducing one person's anxiety will not be effective for all anxious clients. Some clients respond favorably to therapeutic touch; others are offended by it. Some clients enjoy verbalizing their anxiety; others prefer the quiet approach. Your written evaluation will be very helpful to other nurses as they too implement the care plan.

Summary

- Age-related changes in the kidney include decreased size and weight, decreased renal blood flow, and reduced GFR. Tubules become less able to regulate sodium and potassium. Total body water declines, especially in women. The ability to handle fluid volume deprivation or overload decreases.

- The bladder may undergo replacement of smooth muscle and elastic tissue with fibrous connective tissue. Bladder muscles can weaken, leading to urinary retention. Urinary incontinence is not a normal part of the aging process. The older woman experiences age-related atrophic changes in the vaginal area; changes in the pubic region of the older male adult include decreases in fat tissue, elasticity, and blood flow. Many endocrine glands undergo atrophy and exhibit diminished hormone secretion.

- Begin your assessment with a thorough examination and documentation of your findings. Question the client about voiding patterns and the use of urinary devices or protective undergarments. Examine the abdomen for distention. Ask the client about rest room use frequency, including visits at night, and any episodes of urinary incontinence.

- BPH affects many older men. The prostate gland enlarges and compresses the bladder opening and urethra, leading to difficulty with urination. Left untreated, renal damage can occur. The exact cause is unknown. Signs and symptoms include urinary hesitancy, frequency, and dribbling, and bladder distention. Medical treatment varies with the level of discomfort and client preferences; it can range from watchful waiting to the use of various medical and surgical options, including TURP.

- Urinary incontinence, or UI, refers to the involuntary loss of urine. It affects many older adults, and is twice as common in women. UI is not a normal change of aging and is associated with numerous risk factors. Temporary incontinence may occur with the onset of a new illness or medication and is reversible. Chronic incontinence may also be reversible, but treatment may be lengthier.

- Urinary tract infections, or UTIs, include infections of the urethra, bladder, or kidneys. The older adult is at risk owing to age-related body changes. Left untreated, a UTI progresses in an ascending manner: urethritis, cystitis, then pyelonephritis, which can lead to septicemia. Institutionalized clients have higher rates of UTI. The older adult may present with the classic signs and symptoms, with an atypical presentation, or with no signs and symptoms whatsoever. Treatment goals are to destroy the invading organism, usually with antibiotics, and to prevent the recurrence of infection.

- Diabetes mellitus is a disorder of glucose metabolism, characterized by an abundance of glucose in the bloodstream that is unable to enter the cells. This inability is related to one of two factors—either a lack of the hormone insulin (type 1) or a resistance to insulin at the cellular or tissue level (type 2). The three classic signs and symptoms of diabetes mellitus are polyuria, polydipsia, and polyphagia. Type 1 diabetes mellitus is more common in young adults and children, whereas type 2 diabetes mellitus is more common in the older adult.

- Both acute and chronic complications are associated with diabetes mellitus. Acute complications of diabetes include acute hypoglycemia, diabetic ketoacidosis (DKA), and hyperosmolar nonketotic coma (HHNK). Chronic complications include vascular disorders, retinopathy, neuropathy, and nephropathy. Treatment options for diabetes mellitus include medications, diet, and exercise. Medication used for the treatment of type 1 diabetes mellitus consists primarily of insulin; medications used for the treatment of type 2 diabetes mellitus include oral hypoglycemic agents, which act on cell receptors, thereby allowing insulin to perform its function.

- Nursing diagnoses are unique to the individual client. Your contribution to the nursing process is invaluable. Once the nursing diagnosis is established, outcomes must be set. It is important that they be realistic, measurable, and tailored to the individual client.

- Interventions to promote safety include the following: encourage fluid intake following diagnostic procedures in which contrast dye is used; encourage annual gynecologic examinations in the older woman and prostate examinations in the older man; review medications taken by the older adult; educate the client with diabetes mellitus regarding daily foot care and annual eye examinations; implement postoperative interventions for the post-TURP client; provide skin care for clients with urinary incontinence; monitor for superinfection clients who are taking antibiotics; maintain strict aseptic practices.

- Interventions to promote health education include the following: encourage monthly BSE; provide support and teaching for chronic disease management; provide education that urinary incontinence is not a normal part of the aging process; teach Kegel exercises; educate the older adult about risk factor reduction for UTIs.

- Interventions to promote lifestyle modification include the following: encourage weight reduction, if appropriate; encourage exercise; educate the postoperative TURP client about postoperative dietary restrictions; educate the older adult with incontinence about treatment options; implore the older adult with diabetes mellitus who smokes to quit.

- Interventions to promote mobility include the following: encourage the older adult with urinary incontinence to avoid social isolation; encourage this client to wear garments that are easy to manipulate; encourage the older man who has undergone TURP to get out of bed as soon as possible postoperatively, but prohibit strenuous activities for 2 to 3 weeks; encourage physical activity because inactivity can lead to urinary stasis.

- Interventions to promote nutrition include the following: provide dietary teaching for the client with diabetes mellitus; promote nutrition for the older adult with impaired skin integrity; encourage 12 to 14 glasses of water per day for the client who has undergone TURP; encourage the client with urinary incontinence to avoid caffeine; encourage the older adult who is prone to the development of UTIs to consume 2 to 3 liters of fluid per day and inform him or her about the potentially beneficial effects of urine-acidifying foods.
- Interventions to promote rest and sleep include the following: encourage the client with a UTI to try a sitz bath; discuss fluid restriction prior to bedtime with the client who experiences urinary incontinence.
- Nursing evaluation should be aimed directly at the planned outcomes, and should take into consideration the effectiveness of individual interventions.

STUDY QUESTIONS

Multiple-Choice Review

1. Which of the following are age-related changes that may occur in the genitourinary system?
   1. Fibrous tissue in the bladder is replaced with smooth muscle and elastic tissue.
   2. Bladder muscles undergo hypertrophy.
   3. The client experiences urinary incontinence.
   4. Bladder capacity is decreased.
2. Assessment of the genitourinary and endocrine systems involves which of the following assessment parameters?
   1. Physical examination
   2. Laboratory and diagnostic data
   3. Intake and output records
   4. All of the above
3. Which of the following is an accurate statement regarding benign prostatic hyperplasia?
   1. Symptoms are dependent on the size of the prostate gland.

2. Because most afflicted men are too old for surgical intervention, the treatment of choice is watchful waiting.
   3. Left untreated, benign prostatic hyperplasia can lead to prostate cancer.
   4. Left untreated, benign prostatic hyperplasia can lead to renal damage.
4. Which of the following behavioral therapies would **not** be beneficial for a client with urge incontinence?
   1. Bladder training
   2. Habit training
   3. Kegel exercises
   4. Negative reinforcement after each incontinent episode
5. Your client, Mr. Hewitt, is a 75-year-old gentleman with diabetes mellitus. He smokes two packs of cigarettes each day, and spends much of the day at the mall, where his retirement interest was to open an ice cream shop. His 5'7" frame holds 125 pounds of body weight. He takes his diabetes medications religiously and performs a fingerstick on himself each morning and night, although he does admit to "cheating" on his diet occasionally. He asks your advice about management of his illness. If you could convince him to do one thing to reduce his risk of complications, what would it be?
   1. Reduce his weight.
   2. Stop "cheating" on the diabetes diet.
   3. Stop smoking.
   4. Gain weight.

Critical Thinking

1. When are you likely to observe the effects of normal aging on the kidneys? Describe some of these circumstances.
2. Compare and contrast the normal changes of aging noted in the genitourinary tract in older male and older female clients.
3. Describe some of the psychosocial effects of urinary incontinence and identify the nursing interventions you can implement to help the older adult manage these psychosocial effects.
4. If you were June, the LPN in the Case Study presented at the beginning of the chapter, how would you proceed to assist Mrs. B., while helping to protect her dignity?

5. Why is it important for you to encourage monitoring of blood glucose in the older client with diabetes mellitus?

Resources

Internet Resources

Agency for Health Care Policy and Research Information for caregivers of incontinent individuals and health care professionals
http://www.ahcpr.gov/clinic/

Fastats on Diabetes
http://www.cdc.gov/nchswww/fastats/diabetes.htm

Medicine Net
Information provided by physicians for educational use
http://www.medicinenet.com

Organizations

American Association of Diabetes Educators
444 North Michigan Avenue, Suite 12340
Chicago, IL 60611
(800) 338-3633

American Diabetes Association
1600 Duke Street
P.O. Box 25757
Alexandria, VA 22314
(800) 232-3472

Bladder Health Council
c/o American Foundation for Urologic Disease
300 West Pratt Street, Suite 401
Baltimore, MD 21201
(410) 727-2908

National Association for Continence
P.O. Box 8310
Spartanburg, SC 29305
1-800-BLADDER

Wound, Ostomy, and Continence Nurses Society
2755 Bristol Street, Suite 110
Costa Mesa, CA 92626
(714) 476-0268

Selected References

Avandia for Diabetes: An Alternative to Rezulin? *Drug Infoline, 1999*. Available at http://www.pharminfo.com/pubs/druginfoline/druginfo1_13.html

Beck, L. H. (1998). Changes in renal function with aging. *Clinics in Geriatric Medicine: Genitourinary Problems, 14*(2), 199–209.

Busby-Whitehead, J., & Johnson, T. M. (1998). Urinary incontinence. *Clinics in Geriatric Medicine: Genitourinary Problems, 14*(2), 285–295.

Funnell, M. M. (1999). Care of the nursing-home resident with diabetes. *Clinics in Geriatric Medicine: Advances in the Care of Older People with Diabetes, 15*(2), 413–422.

Gerber, G. S. (1998). Benign prostatic hyperplasia in older men. *Clinics in Geriatric Medicine: Genitourinary Problems, 14*(2), 317–331.

Gilden, J. L. (1999). Nutrition and the older diabetic. *Clinics in Geriatric Medicine: Advances in the Care of Older People with Diabetes, 15*(2), 371–385.

Healthy People 2010 Web Site. Available at http://www.health.gov/healthypeople/Document/tableofcontents.htm. Accessed 11/13/00.

Hodgson, B. B., & Kizior, R. J. (1999). *Saunders nursing drug handbook.* Philadelphia: W. B. Saunders.

Ignatavicius, D. D., Workman, M. L., & Mishler, M. A. (1999). *Medical-surgical nursing across the health care continuum.* Philadelphia: W. B. Saunders.

Issa, M. M., Myrick, S. E., & Symbas, N. P. (1998). The TUNA procedure for BPH: Review of the technology. Available at http://www.medscape.com/SCP/IIU/1998/v.11n04/u3086.issa.html Accessed 8/23/98.

Jacobs, A. M., & Appleman, K. K. (1999). Foot-ulcer prevention in the elderly diabetic patient. *Clinics in Geriatric Medicine: Advances in the Care of Older People with Diabetes, 15*(2), 351–369.

Lavery, L. A., Van Houtum, W. H., Ashry, H. R., Armstrong, D. G., & Pugh, J. A. (1999). Diabetes-related lower-extremity amputations disproportionately affect Blacks and Mexican Americans. *Southern Medical Journal, 92*(2), 593–599.

Lentz, S. S., & Homesley, H. D. (1998). Gynecologic problems in older women. *Clinics in Geriatric Medicine: Genitourinary Problems, 14*(2), 297–315.

Matteson, M. A., McConnell, E. S., & Linton, A. D. (1998). *Gerontological nursing: Concepts and practice.* Philadelphia: W. B. Saunders Company.

Morley, J. E. (1999). An overview of diabetes mellitus in older persons. *Clinics in Geriatric Medicine: Advances in the Care of Older People with Diabetes, 15*(2), 211–224.

Mulvihill, C. J. (1999). Why cranberry juice works for UTI prevention. Available at http://www3.pitt.edu/~cjm6/s99cranberry.html Accessed 7/26/99.

O'Connell, H. E., & McGuire, E. J. (1996). Assessing and managing urinary incontinence in primary care. *Medscape Women's Health, 1*(12), 1–11. Available at http://www.medscape.com/Medscape/WomensHealth/journal/1996/v01.n12/w151.o'connell/w151.o'connell.html

Overview: Urinary incontinence in adults, clinical practice guideline update. Rockville, MD: Agency for Health Care Policy and Research, March 1996. Available at http://www.ahrq.gov/clinic/uiovervw.htm Accessed 11/13/00.

Steeman, E., & Defever, M. (1998). Urinary incontinence among elderly persons who live at home. *The Nursing Clinics of North America: Advances in Geriatric Nursing, 33*(3), 441–453.

Sulzbach-Hoke, L. M., & Schanne, L. C. (1999). Using a portable ultrasound bladder scanner in the cardiac care unit. *Critical Care Nurse, 19*(6), 35–39.

Tyson, S. R. (1999). *Gerontological nursing care.* Philadelphia: W. B. Saunders.

Vinik, A. I. (1999). Diagnosis and management of diabetic neuropathy. *Clinics in Geriatric Medicine: Advances in the Care of Older People with Diabetes, 15*(2), 293–320.

Whittemore, R. (2000). Strategies to facilitate lifestyle change associated with diabetes mellitus. *Journal of Nursing Scholarship, 32*(3), 225–232.

Promoting a Healthy Heart and Peripheral Vascular System

OBJECTIVES

After completing this chapter, you will be able to:

- Discuss the normal changes of aging that affect the heart and peripheral vascular system.
- Describe the sequence of assessment and areas of importance in assessing the heart and peripheral vascular system.
- Compare the key clinical features of disorders commonly affecting the heart and peripheral vascular system of older adults.
- Examine the nursing process in care planning for the older adult with disorders of coronary artery disease, congestive heart failure, hypertension, and peripheral arterial disease.

KEY TERMS

Angina	Intermittent claudication
Atherosclerosis	Intima
Atrophy	Ischemia
Body mass index	Maximum heart rate
Capillary refill time	Myocardium
Cardiac output	Necrosis
Contractility	Rubor
Cyanosis	Sinoatrial node
Homocysteine	Stroke volume
Hypertension	Thready
Hypertrophy	

AGE-RELATED CHANGES OF THE CARDIOVASCULAR SYSTEM

The overall size of the heart does not change with age. The left ventricle, which is responsible for the majority of the heart's pumping action, does however increase in thickness. Like any other body muscle, the heart may **atrophy** with age if it is not used to its capacity on a regular basis. This is one reason why exercise is important in maintaining a healthy heart. If the heart is constantly challenged to excess by disease, such as **hypertension,** the heart may **hypertrophy** from the constantly increased workload.

Many of the age-related changes that occur in the heart are not noticeable during ordinary activities, but can be observed during times of stress when one needs to call upon body reserves. The resting heart rate and **stroke volume** remain unchanged with aging, and cardiac output is not significantly changed during ordinary circumstances. However, aging does alter other parameters, which relate to the heart's ability to adequately cope with stress. For instance, the **maximum heart rate** is decreased with age; this becomes noticeable as the older adult tries to ward off infection or illness.

⚠ Signs and Symptoms Tip

An older adult trying to fight off infection may not exhibit the usual sign of tachycardia.

With aging, the heart becomes somewhat less efficient as a pump, owing to the increased stiffness of the cardiac muscle. This may lead to decreased **cardiac output** in some individuals, although many believe that this age-related change can be modified by regular exercise.

The valves of the heart tend to thicken and stiffen with age, a change that is in part related to deposits of calcium. Because of this, murmurs are commonly heard in the older adult. There is some cell loss in the **sinoatrial node** (SA node), or pacemaker, which partly explains why some older adults have an irregular heartbeat.

Blood vessels of the body become less distensible with age, and undergo some degree of **atherosclerosis**. This happens to some degree in most people, but is more pronounced in people with high dietary cholesterol intake, people who smoke, and those with diabetes mellitus. Systolic blood pressure may increase slightly with age; however, the definition of high blood pressure, hypertension, remains the same as for young people.

ASSESSMENT OF THE CARDIOVASCULAR SYSTEM

Cardiovascular assessment should begin with the accurate measurement of vital signs. Temperature, pulse, blood pressure, and respiration measurements are called "vital" signs, meaning that they are signs that life is present. In the older adult, the ranges of what is considered normal are the same as in the younger adult, except for temperature, which may run as low as 96.4°F (Fig. 8–1).

While palpating and auscultating the pulse, take special care to notice any irregularities, remembering the age-related changes associated with the sinoatrial node. If any irregularities are detected, the apical pulse measurement must be taken for a full minute. In addition, try to determine if the pulse is regularly irregular—that is, it exhibits a pattern you can detect—or is irregularly irregular, having no such pattern. Accurately record the value, and report the irregularity next to the value on the vital signs sheet, using the notation "irreg." In addition, report this finding to the registered nurse (RN).

At times, an irregular pulse is also a fast pulse, making it all the more difficult to measure. When a pulse is irregular and fast, it is often **thready**, or very weak and thin, again providing you with another layer of difficulty. If you find that the pulse is so quick that you are unsure of the value you are obtaining, start over. You may have to begin again two or three times before you obtain

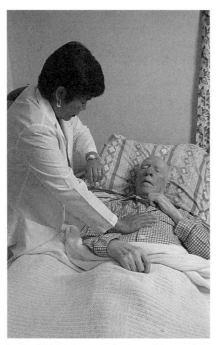

Figure 8–1. Measuring vital signs in an older adult. (From deWit, S. [2001]. *Fundamental concepts and skills for nursing.* Philadelphia: W. B. Saunders, p. 357.)

an accurate pulse. It is not accurate to count until the end of the minute and think, "105, but I missed a few beats." When the heart rate is rapid, you may have missed 20 or 30 beats—indicating a possible medical emergency. If the pulse you obtain is above 110, you should complete measurement of the other vital signs; then stop your assessment and report these findings to the RN immediately before resuming the remainder of your assessment.

Next, measure orthostatic vital signs (review instructions in Chapter 6). Document and report all values obtained. Before assisting your client to a different position for the remainder of the assessment, note the color of the lower extremities in the dependent position. If a client has a vascular disorder, you will often see dependent **rubor**. Document and report this finding to the RN.

After measurement of vital signs is complete, begin a cardiovascular assessment moving in a head-to-toe direction. Assess the head and face, observing skin color. Document color, being certain to communicate any unusual findings, such as a ruddy appearance, pallor, or **cyanosis.** Cyanosis can indicate a problem either with perfusion or with oxygenation (see Chapter 9). In a darker-skinned older adult, the color of the oral mucous membranes and the sclera should be assessed and documented. Also, note any increased facial vascularity, such as erythema or broken blood vessels on the nose or around the eyes.

Next, auscultate heart sounds anteriorly after instructing your client to breathe normally. The apical pulse may be easier to hear at the lower left area of the client's chest. Also, observe the chest and abdominal area for any visible pulsations.

Search the upper and lower extremities for edema or bruising. Bruising may be observed if the client is taking certain medications, such as aspirin or prednisone, but it can also be a sign of elder abuse. Observe the pattern of hair growth in the lower extremities. Hair loss in the lower extremities can be a sign of vascular insufficiency, although there are other factors that may account for absence of hair in the lower extremities as well, such as cultural variations, or a lifetime of wearing knee-length socks. Observe and document pallor or cyanosis of the extremities. Also, note the appearance of thin, shiny skin. Document the presence of thickened nails. Compare the temperature of the extremities bilaterally, and document.

Palpate peripheral pulses—radial in the upper extremities—comparing strength of the pulse bilaterally. If the pulse feels thin and weak, it can be described as "thready." If the pulse feels very strong, it can be described as "bounding." Also note whether the pulse is regular or irregular in rhythm. For the lower extremities, palpate the posterior tibial and the dorsal pedal pulses on each foot. If you have difficulty locating any of these pulses, document their absence and notify the RN immediately following your assessment. In some facilities, a Doppler device may be available to assess weak or absent pulses. If the pulses are absent to palpation, but audible to Doppler, the pulse can be charted, "Doppler +" followed by the location of the pulse being assessed.

If your client's feet had dependent rubor, note whether this has disappeared with the lower extremities no longer in a dependent position. Next, assess and document **capillary refill time** (CRT). To do this, gently press (blanch) the nail of the great toe and quickly release. Perform this maneuver on each foot. Assess the amount of time required for the skin to return to its pink color. A normal capillary refill time is less than or equal to 3 seconds. This can be charted, "CRT ≤3 sec bilat." Capillary refill time can be very difficult to assess in an older adult because thick toenails may prevent you from seeing the skin color underneath; also, pale or dark skin can be difficult to evaluate. In these cases, locate the pinkest part of the great toe (often the medial aspect), and perform the assessment at that location.

DISORDERS COMMON IN OLDER ADULTS

Coronary Artery Disease

Coronary artery disease, or CAD, is the leading cause of death in the United States. It begins with the process of atherosclerosis, which narrows the lumen of the coronary arteries and interferes with the flow of oxygen and blood through the coronary arteries to the **myocardium**. The process of atherosclerosis can begin early in life and is influenced by a variety of risk factors (Box 8–1).

Box 8–1 Risk Factors for Coronary Artery Disease

- Increased body mass index
- Increased blood pressure
- Increased low-density lipoprotein cholesterol levels
- Increased triglyceride levels
- Cigarette smoking
- Elevated plasma homocysteine levels
- Insulin resistance syndrome
- Increased levels of C-reactive protein (present with chronic inflammation)
- Infection with *Chlamydia pneumoniae*
- Loss of estrogen after menopause (women)

Data from Confronting aging and disease: CVD and estrogen. *Women's Health Treatment Updates*, 1999, *Medscape*. Available at http://cardiology.

medscape.com/Medscape/WomensHealth/Treatment Update/1999/tu01/tu01–10.html; Gaziano, J. M. (1998). When should heart disease prevention begin? *New England Journal of Medicine, 338*(23), 1690–1692; Graham, I. M., Daly, L. E., Refsum, H. M., et al. (1997). Plasma homocysteine as a risk factor for vascular disease: The European Concerted Action Project. *Journal of the American Medical Association, 277*(22), 1775–1781; Homocysteine, fibrinogen, Lp(a), small dense LDL, oxidative stress, and C pneumoniae infection: How important are they? Online coverage from the American College of Cardiology 48th Annual Scientific Session, March 7–10, 1999. Available at http://www.medscape.com/Medscape/CNO/1999/ACC/eng/03.10/0251.chan/0251.chan.htm

---

The process starts with the development of fatty streaks on the **intima** portion of the vessel wall. These fatty streaks can develop into an atherosclerotic plaque that grows and matures, thereby limiting blood flow. The plaque can become irregular in shape, which attracts platelets to adhere to its surface. Tears or breaks in the plaque can lead to small hemorrhages. Either of these two processes further increases the size of the atherosclerotic plaque and reduces the lumen of the coronary artery (Fig. 8–2).

Once the lumen is more than 70% obstructed, the heart may be unable to respond to the body's increased need for oxygen and to its metabolic demands; symptoms of coronary artery disease then appear. These symptoms appear whenever there is an imbalance between oxygen supply and oxygen demand (Box 8–2).

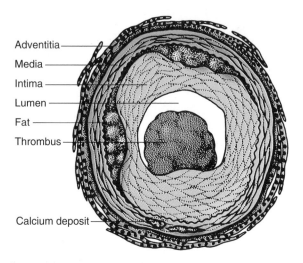

Adventitia

Media

Intima

Lumen

Fat

Thrombus

Calcium deposit

Figure 8–2. A cross-section of an atherosclerotic coronary artery. (From Ignatavicius, D. D., Workman, M. L., & Mishler, M. A. [1999]. *Medical-surgical nursing across the health care continuum* [3rd Ed.]. Philadelphia: W. B. Saunders, p. 902.)

Symptoms of CAD reflect the lack of blood flow and therefore the reduction in oxygen being supplied to the heart muscle. The chest pain experienced in coronary artery disease is referred to as **angina**. If reduced oxygen occurs for a short time, the result is tissue **ischemia**. In stable angina, the symptoms appear with exertion or other increase in cardiac workload; they subside with rest or with administration of the medication nitroglycerin. Unstable angina occurs at lower and lower levels of activity, eventually occurring at rest, and it occurs with increasing frequency and may not respond to

rest or nitroglycerin. The client experiencing unstable angina is at high risk of experiencing a myocardial infarction, or MI ("heart attack"), characterized by tissue death, or **necrosis,** of the heart muscle. Emergency medical attention is required.

Some older adults experiencing a myocardial infarction do not have the classic sign of chest pain. Clients more likely to have an atypical presentation of MI include older adults, African Americans, women, and people with diabetes mellitus. This is important to understand so you can assess for other signs and symptoms when you suspect that a cardiac event is taking place.

⚠ Signs and Symptoms Tip

Atypical signs and symptoms of myocardial infarction:

- Pain in a site other than the chest
- Dyspnea
- Nausea
- Vomiting
- Fatigue
- Fainting

Data from Lee, H. (1997). Typical and atypical clinical signs and symptoms of myocardial infarction and delayed seeking of professional care among blacks. *American Journal of Critical Care, 6*(1), 7–13.

Numerous treatments for coronary artery disease are available. Reduction of risk factors is an important component of medical treatment. *Healthy People 2010* includes objectives related to cardiac disease (Box 8–3).

Current research suggests that an elevated plasma **homocysteine** level can be reduced by increased intake of folate, vitamin B_6, and vitamin B_{12}. Following a low-fat, low-cholesterol diet and exercising regularly can reduce cholesterol levels. In addition, antioxidant vitamins may provide cardioprotection.

🍴 Nutrition Tip

Antioxidants include vitamins A, C, and E, beta-carotene, flavonoids, and folic acid.

Box 8–2 | Symptoms of Coronary Artery Disease

- Pain: chest, epigastric area, jaw, neck, arms, or scapular area, which may be described as squeezing, tight, stabbing, heaviness, or a dull ache
- Indigestion
- Shortness of breath
- Dyspnea on exertion (DOE)

All of the information presented here reveals that a balanced diet may go a long way in protecting heart health.

> ### Health Promotion Tip
>
> Reduction of risk factors for cardiac disease:
>
> - If you are obese, reduce weight.
> - If you are a smoker, stop smoking.
> - Try to reduce stress in your life.
> - If you have a sedentary lifestyle, incorporate 30 minutes of physical activity into your daily schedule.
> - Eat a nutritious, balanced diet, including plenty of folic acid, vitamin B_6, and vitamin B_{12}.
> - Eat a low-fat, low-cholesterol diet.
> - If you have diabetes mellitus, manage your blood sugar carefully.

Other medical treatments for coronary artery disease include pharmacologic interventions. Numerous drugs have been developed that may be used alone or in combination with other drugs.

Medications commonly used to treat coronary artery disease are listed in Table 8–1.

In addition, various surgical and nonsurgical interventions (Table 8–2) are available for the treatment of coronary artery disease.

> ### Medication Safety Tip
>
> Beta-blockers, calcium channel blockers, and diuretics can have additive hypotensive effects in the older adult. Monitor your client carefully if he or she is taking more than one category of these medications.

Congestive Heart Failure

Congestive heart failure, or CHF, is a state in which the heart fails to pump an adequate amount of blood to meet the metabolic needs of the body. CHF can result from damage to the heart muscle itself, such as that associated with a myocardial infarction, or it can be caused by a constantly increased workload for the heart, such as occurs with hypertension. Common causes of CHF are listed in Box 8–4.

Approximately 4.7 million Americans experience CHF; it is the most frequent cause of hospitalization among persons age 65 or older. Half of those diagnosed with CHF die within a 5-year period. Health care professionals have noted with interest that differing disease patterns and differing responses to treatment appear to be related to racial/ethnic group and gender of the patient; this theory is now beginning to be researched. For example, the disease disproportionately affects African Americans, but in one study, African Americans had lower posthospitalization mortality rates than their white counterparts (Alexander et al., 1999). The study of racial and gender differences in this disorder is likely to be the focus of continued research.

Signs and symptoms of CHF, which are outlined in Box 8–5, reflect the ineffectiveness of the heart as a pump and the resultant sluggish circulation.

One of the objectives of *Healthy People 2010* is to "reduce hospitalizations of older adults with congestive heart failure as the principal diagnosis" (*Healthy People 2010* website). The mainstays of treatment for CHF involve medical interventions, although surgical options are available for patients in whom the underlying cause can be surgically treated. For mild heart failure, dietary

Table 8–1

DRUGS USED IN THE TREATMENT OF CORONARY ARTERY DISEASE

Category	Examples	Mechanism of Action	Nursing Implications
Antilipidemics	• atorvastatin (Lipitor) • simvastatin (Zocor) • pravastatin sodium (Pravachol)	Interfere with cholesterol synthesis	• Contraindicated in liver disease • Encourage low-cholesterol diet
Nitrates	• nitroglycerin (Nitrostat) • isosorbide dinitrate (Isordil)	Act directly on smooth muscle of coronary vessels to produce vasodilation	• May cause headache or dizziness • Keep sublingual tablets in cool, dry, dark place
Beta-blockers	• propranolol (Inderal) • metoprolol (Lopressor)	Decrease cardiac demand for oxygen by reducing heart rate, blood pressure, and force of contraction	• Inderal blocks both $beta_1$ and $beta_2$: caution in respiratory disease • Hold drug if pulse <60 or systolic BP <90, and notify RN/MD
Calcium channel blockers	• nifedipine (Procardia) • mibefradil dihydrochloride (Posicor) • diltiazem (Cardizem)	Decrease oxygen demand by decreasing the amount of calcium in the muscle cell and coronary vasodilation	• Monitor for hypotension, nausea, vomiting, and irregular pulse. Notify RN/MD
Antiplatelet agents	• aspirin (Ecotrin, Bayer, Bufferin)	Inhibit platelet aggregation, reduce inflammation	• Give with food if GI upset occurs • Monitor for bleeding

Data from Hodgson, B. B., & Kizior, R. J. (2001). *Saunders nursing drug handbook*. Philadelphia: W. B. Saunders; Ignatavicius, D. D., Workman, M. L. & Mishler, M. A. (1999). *Medical-surgical nursing across the health care continuum*. Philadelphia: W. B. Saunders.

Table 8–2

SURGICAL AND NONSURGICAL INTERVENTIONS FOR CORONARY ARTERY DISEASE

Intervention	Description	Nursing Implications
Coronary artery bypass graft (CABG)	Occluded coronary arteries are "bypassed" using the client's veins and/or arteries. Incision is made via median sternotomy approach	• Surgery requires the heart-lung bypass machine, sternal incision, mechanical ventilation, and ICU care up to 48 hours postoperatively • If saphenous vein used, assess additional leg incision • If internal mammary artery used, monitor for pulmonary complications • Discharge home in about 1 week; full recovery in 6–8 weeks
Minimally invasive direct coronary artery bypass (MIDCAB)	Surgery done via thorocotomy incision	• Shorter convalescence, as no bypass used • Relatively new procedure • Discharge home in 2–3 days
Percutaneous transluminal coronary angioplasty (PTCA)	Balloon-tipped catheter inserted into coronary artery, balloon inflated to compress occluding plaque against artery wall, balloon removed	• Performed in cardiac catheterization laboratory • May not provide a permanent solution for the client • Procedure may involve placement of a stent, a small metal mesh tube that remains in place to keep the artery patent

<table>
<tr><td>

Box 8-4 Common Causes of Congestive Heart Failure

- Myocardial infarction
- Coronary artery disease
- Hypertension
- Congenital heart disease
- Valvular disease
- Infection
- Alcoholism or other substance abuse
- Idiopathic causes

Adapted from Managing congestive heart failure: The role of ACE inhibitors (1998). *Clinical Reviews*, 9, 2–5. Available at http://www.medscape.com/CPG/Clin Reviews/ 1998/09.98s.mana/pnt-c0998smana.html

</td></tr>
</table>

restriction of salt, exercise, and weight control may be recommended. If drug therapy is prescribed, numerous medications can be used, alone or in combination. Medications can be effective in reducing the workload of the heart, thereby increasing cardiac output and **contractility** and sodium and water retention. Commonly used medications are listed in Table 8–3.

If heart failure is severe and surgical interventions are believed to be of value, possible

Box 8-5 Signs and Symptoms of Congestive Heart Failure

Signs

- Decreased urinary output
- Neck vein distention
- Crackles to auscultation
- Extra heart sounds
- Pulmonary edema
- Tachycardia
- Ankle edema

Symptoms

- Fatigue
- Dyspnea on exertion
- Night cough

Adapted from Managing congestive heart failure: The role of ACE inhibitors (1998). *Clinical Reviews*, 9, 2–5. Available at http://www.medscape.com/CPG/Clin Reviews/1998/09.98s.mana/pnt-c0998smana.html

operative repairs may include correction of a congenital defect, repair or replacement of damaged cardiac valves, or coronary artery bypass grafting to improve circulation to the myocardium. As a last resort, cardiac transplantation may be considered.

Hypertension —Silent Killer

Hypertension, or HTN (high blood pressure), is defined as a persistent systolic blood pressure reading greater than 140 mm Hg and a persistent diastolic blood pressure reading greater than 90 mm Hg. This disorder is common among older people, affecting more than half of all older adults. It affects even greater numbers of African-American older adults.

Hypertension is known as the "silent killer," because it often has few symptoms but can result in very serious consequences. Hypertension can place an individual at risk for cerebrovascular accident (CVA), cardiovascular disorders, and kidney disease owing to the constant elevation of blood pressure and the body's attempts to compensate.

Although growing older is a risk factor for HTN, other risk factors are associated with the disorder as well. As with many disorders, some of the risk factors (such as gender) are not modifiable; however many can be modified through changes in lifestyle habits. Risk factors for HTN are outlined in Box 8–6.

As has been stated earlier, some individuals may exhibit few signs or symptoms of HTN, especially in the early stages of the disorder. Others, however, have signs and/or symptoms that may occur regularly or intermittently. Many of these, such as headache, are associated with the high pressure of the blood flow. Other signs, such as palpitations or angina, are related to the stress the disorder imposes on other body systems. Still others, such as changes to the retina, may be entirely unnoticed by the older adult, but are detected upon examination by a physician or advanced practice nurse. Signs and symptoms of hypertension are outlined in Box 8–7.

As with other cardiac-related disorders, treatment of HTN begins with modification of risk factors that can be modified. Lifestyle changes that can improve the health of a client with HTN include smoking cessation, weight loss,

Table 8–3
DRUGS USED IN THE TREATMENT OF CONGESTIVE HEART FAILURE

Category	Examples	Mechanism of Action	Nursing Implications
Diuretics	• furosemide (Lasix) • hydrochlorothiazide (HCTZ) • spironolactone (Aldactone)	Reduce volume and pressure by increasing urine output	• Monitor serum potassium • Teach client to change positions gradually
Vasodilators	• hydralazine HCl (Apresoline) • isosorbide dinitrate (Isordil)	Decrease workload of the heart by primarily dilating either veins or arterioles	• Apresoline and Isordil often used together • Monitor orthostatic blood pressure (BP)
Angiotensin-converting enzyme (ACE) inhibitors	• captopril (Capoten) • enalapril (Vasotec)	Decrease cardiac workload by vasodilation; improve cardiac output	• Monitor pulse and BP • Teach client to change positions gradually
Inotropic agents	• digoxin (Lanoxin) • milrinone (Primacor)	Increase force of contractions	• Milrinone IV is for short-term use • Take apical pulse for 1 minute with Lanoxin; hold drug if pulse <60, and notify RN/MD
Beta-blockers	• carvedilol (Coreg)	Decrease cardiac demand for oxygen; reduce peripheral vascular resistance	• Use only in mild to moderate heart failure • Hold drug if pulse <60 or systolic BP <90, and notify RN/MD

Data from Cohn, J. N. (1998). Managing heart failure: Data from clinical trials and future directions. Online coverage from the American College of Cardiology, March 29–April 1, 1998. Available at http://www.medscape.com/Medscape/CNO/1998/ACC/04.01/acc0710.cohn/acc0710.cohn.html; Hodgson, B. B., & Kizior, R. J. (1999). *Saunders nursing drug handbook.* Philadelphia: W. B. Saunders; Managing congestive heart failure: The role of ACE inhibitors (1998). *Clinical Reviews, 9,* 2–5. Available at http://www.medscape.com/CPG/ClinReviews/1998/09.98s.mana/pnt-c0998smana.html Accessed 8/5/99; Whellan, D. J. (1998). Cardiac rehabilitation is associated with improved survival in CHF patients. Online coverage from American Heart Association 71st Scientific Sessions, November 8–11, 1998. Available at http://www.medscape.com/Medscape/CNO/1998/AHA/11.11/whel.41/whel.41.html

moderation of alcohol consumption, stress reduction, regular exercise, and moderation of caffeine consumption (Grauer, 1998). *Healthy People 2010* provides specific objectives related to HTN, some of which directly involve individual health-promoting behaviors (Box 8–8).

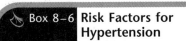 Health Promotion Tip

The most important lifestyle modifications for a client with hypertension are smoking cessation and weight loss.

Medical treatment of HTN involves the use of various categories of medications. More than 100 medications are available for the treatment of HTN; therefore, the most sensible way of learning about these medications is by studying the various categories of drugs to understand the

---

Box 8–6 Risk Factors for Hypertension

Nonmodifiable
• Advanced age
• Male gender
• African American race

Modifiable
• Obesity
• Smoking
• High-fat diet
• Caffeine intake
• High sodium intake
• Stress
• Sedentary lifestyle

Box 8–7 Signs and Symptoms of Hypertension

Signs

- Retinal hemorrhage
- Thickening of retinal arteries
- Patchy white areas on the retina
- Papilledema of the retina
- Epistaxis
- Vomiting
- Nocturia
- Hematuria

Symptoms

- Vertigo
- Lightheadedness
- Tinnitus
- Occipital headache upon arising
- Blurred vision
- Nausea
- Fatigue
- Angina
- Palpitations

Adapted from Ignatavicius, D. D., Workman, M. L., & Mishler, M. A. (1999). *Medical-surgical nursing across the health care continuum.* Philadelphia: W. B. Saunders, p. 375.

Box 8–8 Selected *Healthy People 2010* Hypertension Objectives

- Reduce the proportion of adults with high blood pressure.
- Increase the proportion of adults with high blood pressure whose blood pressure is under control.
- Increase the proportion of adults with high blood pressure who are taking action (e.g., losing weight, increasing physical activity, or reducing sodium intake) to help control their blood pressure.
- Increase the proportion of adults who have had their blood pressure measured within the preceding 2 years and can state whether their blood pressure was normal or high.

From U. S. Department of Health and Human Services. *Healthy People 2010: Understanding and Improving Health*, 2nd ed. Washington, D. C.: U. S. Government Printing Office, November 2000.

mechanism of action of each category. New drugs are always being developed for the treatment of this and other disorders.

Medications may be used alone or in combination with drugs from other categories. Clinicians have found that some clients respond better to smaller doses of two different drugs than to larger doses of only one drug. Drug categories and common examples of medications used for the treatment of HTN are outlined in Table 8–4.

Peripheral Arterial Disease

Peripheral arterial disease is a common disorder in the United States. The incidence of peripheral arterial disease increases steadily with age; it affects almost 20% of those older than 70 years of age (Michaels, 1999). Peripheral arterial disease is the most common form of peripheral vascular disease (PVD).

Peripheral arterial disease is similar to coronary artery disease; it too begins with atherosclerosis and narrowing of the blood vessel lumen. As the disease progresses, the client experiences symptoms of reduced blood flow to the affected body part, often the lower extremities. Risk factors for peripheral arterial disease are similar to those for coronary artery disease; however, diabetes mellitus plays a larger role in the risk of development of peripheral arterial disease. Risk factors for peripheral arterial disease, ranked in order of importance, are provided in Box 8–9.

The ranking of importance of risk factors is important to note and is associated with some very interesting statistics. For example, clients with diabetes mellitus are 3 to 4 times more likely to develop peripheral arterial disease than are those without diabetes mellitus. People who smoke have 2.5 to 3 times the risk of peripheral arterial disease when compared with nonsmokers; hypertension carries 1.5 to 2 times the risk (Michaels, 1999). To make matters worse, there is a strong additive effect when an individual has diabetes and hypertension, and is a smoker.

Health Promotion Tip

The most important lifestyle modification for a client with peripheral arterial disease is smoking cessation.

Table 8–4
DRUGS USED IN THE TREATMENT OF HYPERTENSION

Category	Examples	Mechanism of Action	Nursing Implications
Diuretics	• furosemide (Lasix) • spironolactone (Aldactone) • Indapamide (Lozol)	Help kidneys to excrete sodium and water; all except "potassium sparing" (Aldactone); help excrete potassium	• Monitor serum potassium • Teach client to change positions gradually
Beta-blockers	• atenolol (Tenormin) • metoprolol (Lopressor) • nadolol (Corgard)	Decrease cardiac output, sympathetic stimulation, and renin secretion	• Take apical pulse for 1 full minute • Hold drug if pulse <60 or systolic blood pressure (BP) <90, and notify RN/MD • Monitor for dyspnea in clients with pulmonary disorders
Angiotensin-converting enzyme (ACE) inhibitors	• captopril (Capoten) • enalapril (Vasotec)	Decrease blood pressure by reducing peripheral vascular resistance	• Monitor pulse and BP • Teach client to change positions gradually
Calcium channel blockers	• diltiazem (Cardizem) • mibefradil dihydrochloride (Posicor)	Decrease peripheral vascular resistance and dilate arterioles	• Hold drug if systolic BP <90, and notify RN/MD • Monitor for dizziness, headache
Alpha-blockers	• prazosin (Minipress)	Decrease peripheral vascular resistance and produce vasodilation	• Administer first dose at bedtime to avoid "first-dose syncope" • Monitor apical pulse (1 full minute) and BP before every dose
Alpha/beta-blockers	• labetalol HCl (Normodyne, Trandate)	Slow heart rate, decrease cardiac output, reduce blood pressure	• Monitor apical pulse for 1 full minute • Hold drug if pulse <60 or systolic BP <90, and notify RN/MD • Monitor for dyspnea in clients with pulmonary disorders

Data from Hodgson, B. B., & Kizior, R. J. (1999). *Saunders nursing drug handbook.* Philadelphia: W. B. Saunders; Ignatavicius, D. D., Workman, M. L., & Mishler, M. A. (1999). *Medical-surgical nursing across the health care continuum.* Philadelphia: W. B. Saunders, pp. 377–379; McCarthy, R. (1997). The pharmacologic treatment of hypertension: An update. *Drug Benefit Trends, 9*(9), 71–77.

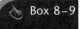

Box 8–9 │ Risk Factors for Peripheral Arterial Disease (in order of importance)

1. Diabetes mellitus
2. Smoking
3. Hypertension
4. Hyperlipidemia
5. Elevated homocysteine levels

Adapted from Michaels, A. D. (1999). Management of peripheral artery disease. Online coverage from the American College of Cardiology 48th Annual Scientific Session, March 7–10, 1999. Available at http://www.medscape.com/Medscape/CNO/1999/ACC/eng/03.08/02 02.mich/0202.mich.html

As was stated earlier, signs and symptoms of peripheral arterial disease are related to reduction of blood flow. Because oxygen delivery to skeletal muscles is reduced, skeletal muscle function becomes impaired and the muscles undergo atrophy. The most common symptom experienced by the client is the pain of **intermittent claudication.** This cramplike pain usually appears bilaterally in the calf muscles; it is associated with walking and relieved by rest. Intermittent claudication is a sign that the muscles are deprived of blood flow and therefore oxygen. The client may experience such pain after walking a certain distance, but he or she may find that the distance required to produce the intermittent claudication shortens as the disorder progresses. Other signs and symptoms of peripheral arterial disease are given in Box 8–10.

> **Box 8-10 Signs and Symptoms of Peripheral Arterial Disease**
>
> *Signs*
> - Muscle atrophy
> - Shiny, thin, dry skin
> - Hair loss on distal extremity
> - Thickened toenails
> - Pallor or cyanosis
> - Rubor in dependent position
> - Coolness to touch
> - Ulcerations
>
> *Symptoms*
> - Intermittent claudication
> - Pain at rest
> - Decreased or altered peripheral sensation

The first strategy for treating peripheral arterial disease is assisting the older adult in risk factor reduction. If the client smokes, smoking cessation is paramount. If the client has diabetes mellitus, the physician or advanced practice nurse must work closely with the client in management of the disorder. A referral to a Certified Diabetes Educator (CDE) may be provided. Other disorders, such as hypertension, are medically controlled to the greatest extent possible. Dietary modifications are advised in an attempt to decrease lipid and homocysteine levels. Other treatments for peripheral arterial disease, both medical and surgical, can be found in Table 8–5.

NURSING DIAGNOSES

As has been previously discussed, nursing diagnoses are derived from the assessment data and are unique to each individual client. The nursing diagnosis focuses on the client's response to the particular health problem that he or she is facing.

Common nursing diagnoses (written only as the problem portion of the *Problem, Etiology,* and *Signs and symptoms* [PES] nursing diagnosis statement) that apply to the older adult experiencing disorders covered in this chapter are listed in Table 8–6.

Not every nursing diagnosis identified in Table 8–6 is appropriate for every client with a given cardiovascular disorder. Likewise, there may be other nursing diagnoses that are suitable for your

client that have not been included. For example, not every client with coronary artery disease experiences fear about the disease. Carefully consider every nursing diagnosis as you individualize a plan of care for the older adult with disorders related to the heart and peripheral vascular system.

COLLABORATING ON THE PLAN OF CARE

After the nursing diagnoses are established, expected outcomes must be developed for your client. Set outcomes that are realistic, measurable, and tailored to the individual older adult.

Sample outcomes for a client with coronary artery disease are given in Table 8–7. These are samples only because the outcomes you set must be established with your individual client in mind. Similarly, sample outcomes for older adults with nursing diagnoses for the conditions of congestive heart failure, hypertension, and peripheral arterial disease are provided in Tables 8–8, 8–9, and 8–10, respectively.

IMPLEMENTING INTERVENTIONS FOR HEALTH PROMOTION

Interventions to Promote Safety

1. Perform careful assessments of pain in the older adult with coronary artery disease. Be alert for possible atypical signs and symptoms of cardiac pain, such as shoulder pain or nausea. Document and report immediately any suspicious symptoms. Unlike other forms of pain, which the client may be willing to tolerate to a certain level of discomfort, **your client should tolerate no cardiac pain**. Every episode of cardiac pain indicates that the heart is deprived of oxygen, which is a serious condition that must be corrected.
2. Educate the older adult with hypertension about the importance of taking his or her medications as prescribed. This aspect of health promotion is extremely important because few symptoms are associated with this disorder. A client may feel more or less the same whether or not antihypertensive medications have been taken, and therefore may see no immediate need to be consistent with therapy.

Table 8–5
MEDICAL AND SURGICAL TREATMENTS FOR PERIPHERAL ARTERIAL DISEASE

Treatment	Example	Benefits	Special Considerations
Exercise therapy	• 30- to 40-minute sessions, 3 to 4 times/week until moderate claudication, then rest (usually supervised)	• Increased exercise tolerance • Increased quality of life	• Treadmill test done before starting program
Hypolipidemic therapy	• simvastatin (Zocor)	• Decreases low-density lipoprotein cholesterol, triglycerides, and cholesterol • Improves claudication	• Administer in evening • Not used in client with liver disease
Antiplatelet therapy	• aspirin	• Decreases the incidence of arterial occlusion • Decreases the risk of cardiovascular events (myocardial infarction, cerebrovascular accident)	• Monitor for signs of bleeding
Revascularization therapy	• Peripheral bypass graft surgery (e.g., femoral-popliteal) • Peripheral angioplasty	• Restores circulation to affected extremity	• Surgical postoperative considerations apply • Requires diligent nursing assessment of circulation at frequent postoperative intervals

Data from Michaels, A. D. (1999). Management of peripheral artery disease. Online coverage from the American College of Cardiology 48th Annual Scientific Session, March 7–10, 1999. Available at http://www.medscape.com/Medscape/CNO/1999/ACC/eng/03.08/0202.mich/0202.mich.html

Table 8–6
NURSING DIAGNOSES RELATED TO THE HEART AND VASCULAR SYSTEM

	Coronary Artery Disease	Congestive Heart Failure	Hypertension	Peripheral Arterial Disease
Imbalanced nutrition: more than body requirements	X		X	X
Ineffective tissue perfusion	X	X	X	X
Fluid volume excess		X		
Decreased cardiac output	X	X	X	
Impaired gas exchange		X		
Risk for impaired skin integrity				X
Social isolation	X	X		X
Ineffective role performance	X	X	X	X
Sexual dysfunction	X		X	X
Impaired walking				X
Activity intolerance	X	X		X
Fatigue	X	X		X
Disturbed sleep pattern		X		X
Deficient knowledge	X	X	X	X
Pain	X		X	X
Anxiety	X	X	X	X
Fear	X	X	X	X

Table 8–7	
SAMPLE OUTCOMES FOR AN OLDER ADULT WITH CORONARY ARTERY DISEASE	
Nursing Diagnosis	**Sample Outcomes**
Pain	• Client will report all episodes of chest pain immediately • Client will experience pain relief within 30 minutes of onset • Vital signs will be within normal limits
Fear	• Client will verbalize concerns and fears about the disease process • Client will verbally identify strategies used in the past to successfully manage fear • Client will verbalize decreased fear
Knowledge deficit: cardiac medications	• Client will verbally describe the name, general action, and important adverse effects of every medication he or she takes • Client will correctly demonstrate measurement of his or her pulse and verbally identify which medications should be held if pulse is <60

Medication Safety Tip

A client who does not take his or her antihypertensive medications as directed is at risk of developing complications from hypertension, such as cerebrovascular accident.

3. Perform hourly neurovascular assessments of the lower extremities following revascularization therapy for peripheral arterial disease. Assess and document pulses, temperature, and capillary refill bilaterally. The initial assessment is performed by the RN; he or she marks the pulse sites with an "X" on the skin. If you are unable to palpate the pulse, notify the RN immediately; next, try using a

Table 8–8	
SAMPLE OUTCOMES FOR AN OLDER ADULT WITH CONGESTIVE HEART FAILURE	
Nursing Diagnosis	**Sample Outcomes**
Decreased cardiac output	• Vital signs will be within normal limits • Client's dyspnea will be improved as evidenced by client statement • Client will maintain perfusion to body organs as evidenced by: alert and oriented mental status, urine output ≥240 mL/shift, extremities warm to touch, and palpable peripheral pulses
Fluid volume excess	• Client's respiratory rate will be ≤24 • Client's dyspnea will be improved as evidenced by client statement • Lung sounds will be clear to auscultation • Client will demonstrate improvement of peripheral edema
Activity intolerance	• Client will gradually increase activity level each day • Client will resume previous level of activity without experiencing dyspnea

Table 8–9	
SAMPLE OUTCOMES FOR AN OLDER ADULT WITH HYPERTENSION	
Nursing Diagnosis	**Sample Outcomes**
Imbalanced nutrition: more than body requirements	• Client will reduce daily calorie intake to prescribed 2000-calorie American Diabetes Association diet • Client will exhibit gradual weight loss of 2 pounds per week
Anxiety	• Client will verbalize questions and concerns about disorder and treatment • Client will describe methods of stress reduction that have been effective in past situations • Client will acknowledge reduction in anxiety level • Client's vital signs will be within normal limits
Deficient knowledge: modifiable risk factors	• Client will verbally list the modifiable risk factors for hypertension • Client will explain the mechanism whereby elimination of each risk factor contributes to symptom improvement • Client will verbalize specific plan for risk factor reduction

Doppler. If you and the RN both are unable to locate the pulse via Doppler, the RN will notify the surgeon immediately.

Interventions to Promote Health Education

1. Educate the older adult about the benefits of regular physical activity. Physical activity has important positive effects on the musculoskeletal, cardiovascular, respiratory, and endocrine systems. Regular physical activity appears to reduce anxiety and depression, improve mood, and enhance one's ability to perform daily activities.

2. Educate people at risk about the atypical signs and symptoms of myocardial infarction. Emphasize the importance of seeking medical care promptly to optimize health outcomes.

Table 8–10	
SAMPLE OUTCOMES FOR AN OLDER ADULT WITH PERIPHERAL ARTERIAL DISEASE	
Nursing Diagnosis	**Sample Outcomes**
Ineffective tissue perfusion	• Client's feet will be warm bilaterally • Pedal pulses will be palpable bilaterally • Capillary refill time will be ≤3 seconds bilaterally • Client will be free of leg pain at rest
Pain	• Client will report a decrease in pain with ambulation • Client will follow exercise recommendations made by physician/advanced practice nurse
Activity intolerance	• Client will identify factors that reduce activity tolerance • Client will progress to the recommended activity level established by the physician/advanced practice nurse

3. Educate the client with CHF about the importance of exercise and weight control in managing the disorder.
4. Educate the client with a cardiovascular disorder about the medications he or she is taking. A client may be taking multiple medications, and it is very important that he or she understand the desired effects, any required monitoring (such as measuring the pulse before taking the medication), and adverse effects to report. Instruct the client to keep a current list of all medications he or she is taking, including name, dose, and scheduled time. This list should be kept with the client at all times, perhaps in a wallet or purse.

Interventions to Promote Lifestyle Modification

1. Assist the older adult with cardiac-related disorders in modifying lifestyle factors to improve outcomes related to the disorder. For example, stress reduction techniques may be helpful for individuals with hypertension or coronary artery disease. Regular exercise is beneficial for all people. Dietary modifications pertinent to the disorder may greatly improve client outcome.
2. Encourage the older adult who smokes to quit. Smoking precipitates or aggravates most of the disorders described in this chapter; smoking cessation can greatly improve the client's health outcome.

Interventions to Promote Mobility

1. Encourage physical activity according to the recommendations of the National Institutes of Health (NIH) Consensus Development Conference, "Physical Activity and Cardiovascular Health." When you are applying these recommendations to an older adult with one or more physical or medical limitations, you should consult with the client's physician or advanced practice nurse. In these instances, the intensity of the activity may need to be lowered slightly, but the frequency and timing can usually be increased. The current and former recommendations are compared in Table 8–11. One method of determining the appropriate intensity of physical activity is called the "talk test." While exercising, one should be able to carry on a conversation with some labored breathing, but should never huff and puff to the point of not being able to talk. On the other hand, if, while exercising, one is able to carry on extensive, unlimited discussions, perhaps the intensity of the activity should be increased.
2. Encourage the client with CHF to participate in regular activity, alternating with rest.
3. Encourage the older adult with peripheral arterial disease to follow the exercise prescription advised by his or her physician or advanced practice nurse. Reinforce previous teaching, for example, instruct the client to ambulate until a moderate level of claudication occurs.

Interventions to Promote Nutrition

1. Encourage the older adult with coronary artery disease or peripheral arterial disease to consume a balanced, nutritious diet low in fat and cholesterol with plenty of vitamins B_6, B_{12}, A, C, and E, folic acid, beta carotene, and

Table 8–11		
PHYSICAL ACTIVITY RECOMMENDATIONS FROM NIH CONSENSUS CONFERENCE		
	Old Recommendations	New Recommendations
Frequency	Three times per week	Most, or preferably all, days of the week
Intensity	60% to 85% of maximum heart rate	At a "moderate" intensity
Timing	At least 20 consecutive minutes	Cumulatively 30 minutes; can be divided throughout the day

Source: Jones, J. M. (1997). Promoting physical activity in the senior years. *Journal of Gerontological Nursing, 23*(7), 42.

flavonoids. Table 8–12 lists foods high in each of these nutrients.

2. Encourage the older adult with CHF to reduce salt intake. Often the client will be placed on a 2- or 4-gram sodium restriction diet. Educate the older adult about the various salt substitutes available on the market, with a cautionary word to discuss these with his or her physician or advanced practice nurse before using them. Many of these products contain potassium chloride, an excess of which may be contraindicated for some clients.

3. Encourage the older adult with severe CHF to restrict fluid intake, if recommended by the physician or advanced practice nurse. Be creative in devising alternative ways to keep his or her oral mucosa moist.

4. Encourage the client with hypertension to reduce excessive intake of sodium, fat, caffeine, and alcohol.

Nutrition Tip

Keeping diabetes as well controlled as possible discourages the development of cardiovascular disease.

Table 8–12		
FOODS HIGH IN SELECTED NUTRIENTS		
Nutrient	**Classification**	**Good Sources**
Beta carotene	Precursor to vitamin A	• Spinach • Broccoli • Carrots • Pumpkin • Winter squash
Vitamin A (Retinol)	Fat-soluble vitamin	• Liver • All beta carotene foods
Vitamin B_6 (Pyroxidine)	Water-soluble vitamin	• Liver and red meats • Whole grains • Potatoes • Green vegetables • Corn
Vitamin B_{12} (Cobalamin)	Water-soluble vitamin	• Milk products • Meats • Organ meats • Egg yolks
Vitamin C (Ascorbic acid)	Water-soluble vitamin	• Citrus fruits • Tomatoes • Strawberries • Cantaloupe • Green leafy vegetables
Vitamin E (Tocopherol)	Fat-soluble vitamin	• Vegetable oils • Fish • Whole grains • Green leafy vegetables
Folicin (Folic acid)	Water-soluble vitamin	• Yeast • Dark green leafy vegetables • Legumes • Whole grains
Flavonoids	Bioactive compound/ antioxidant/nutrient	• Apples • Onions • Garlic • Fruits/vegetables • Parsley • Red wine

Data from Peckenpaugh, N. J., & Poleman, C. M. (1999). *Nutrition essentials and diet therapy.* Philadelphia: W. B. Saunders, pp. 85–89; Healthy Foods for the Heart. *Women's Health Interactive.* Available at http://www.womens-health.com/health center/nutrition/nta1.html Accessed 11/15/00.

5. Encourage the older adult with diabetes mellitus to adhere to the prescribed diet.

Interventions to Promote Rest and Sleep

1. Encourage the client with coronary artery disease to stop all activity immediately and rest, if cardiac pain occurs. (See earlier discussion for safety measures.)
2. Encourage the client with CHF to rest between physical activities. Planned rest periods throughout the day improve venous return to the heart, cardiac output, and renal perfusion.
3. Encourage the older adult with peripheral arterial disease to rest when moderate claudication occurs with ambulation.

GATHERING DATA FOR EVALUATION

Your collaboration with the RN in the evaluation and modification phases of the nursing process is crucial. As a licensed practical nurse/licensed vocational nurse (LPN/LVN), your observations, data gathering, and insight into the process ultimately help to determine whether or not the plan of care is successful (Fig. 8–3).

Evaluation of the plan of care should be aimed directly at the outcomes. Many of the outcomes identified earlier in the chapter are straightforward and objective; therefore, when they are used, evaluation of progress can be completed easily. For example, one outcome identified for the older adult experiencing congestive heart failure reads, "Lung sounds will be clear to auscultation." This outcome can be evaluated at the bedside with your stethoscope. In the evaluation column you can write, "4/23: clear to auscultation" followed by your initials. But, what if the lung sounds are improved but not fully clear? You could then write the appropriate data, such as, "4/23: clear in upper fields; inspiratory crackles at bases," which, when compared with the client's baseline, would indicate an improvement.

Evaluation of other outcomes may also require referral to baseline. For example, "Client will show improvement of peripheral edema" requires knowledge of how severe the edema was to begin with. Most care plan forms have a section for the pertinent assessment data on which the nursing diagnoses were based. It is very important that this section be completed thoroughly; otherwise,

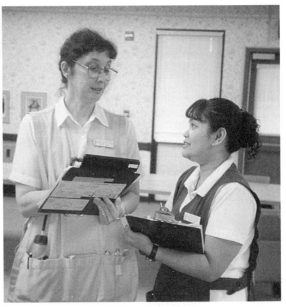

Figure 8–3. An RN and an LVN collaborating on the plan of care.

determination of whether or not an improvement has occurred is impossible.

In addition, your evaluation should take into consideration individual interventions employed. Consider the nursing diagnosis, "Anxiety," which was discussed in Chapter 7 but may also apply to many clients experiencing cardiac disorders. Remember that interventions effective in reducing one person's anxiety may not be effective for all anxious clients. Your written evaluation of which interventions were successful and which ones were ineffective will be very helpful to other nurses who are implementing the care plan.

Summary

- Normal aging does not change the size of the heart. Age-related changes of the heart will be observed during times of stress. The resting heart rate (HR), stroke volume (SV), and cardiac output (CO) are unchanged; however, the maximum HR decreases.
- Heart valves thicken and stiffen, and murmurs are more common with age. Some older adults have an irregular heartbeat.
- Blood vessels become less distensible and undergo atherosclerosis, especially in people

- who have high dietary cholesterol intake, who smoke, or who have diabetes mellitus. Systolic blood pressure (BP) may increase slightly.
- In the older adult, the temperature may run as low as 96.4°F. If any HR irregularities are detected, it is crucial that the apical pulse be taken for a full minute.
- Continue the cardiovascular assessment in a head-to-toe direction. Assess color of the head and face; auscultate heart sounds. Observe the chest and abdominal area for visible pulsations. Assess extremities for edema, bruising, hair distribution, pallor, cyanosis, thickened toenails, and thin, shiny skin. Compare temperature, pulses, and CRT bilaterally.
- Risk factors for CAD include obesity, HTN, smoking, and diet. Angina occurs when there is an imbalance between oxygen supply and demand. Oxygen depletion for a short time results in tissue ischemia. The client with unstable angina is at high risk for MI. Clients more likely to have an atypical presentation of MI include older adults, African Americans, women, and those with diabetes mellitus.
- Treatment for coronary artery disease includes reduction of risk factors. Other medical treatments include numerous drugs, as well as medical and surgical interventions.
- In CHF, the heart fails to pump blood adequately to meet the needs of the body. Common causes include CAD, HTN, and valve disease. Signs and symptoms include fatigue, dyspnea, and crackles upon auscultation. Treatment consists of medical interventions, medications, and sometimes surgery. Restriction of salt, exercise, and weight control may be recommended.
- HTN is a persistent systolic BP reading greater than 140 mm Hg and a diastolic BP reading greater than 90 mm Hg. It affects more than half of all older adults and places a client at risk for CVA, cardiovascular disorders, and kidney disease. Risk factors include advanced age, male gender, African American ethnicity, obesity, smoking, and a high-fat diet. When they occur, signs and symptoms of HTN include headache, palpitations, epistaxis, vomiting, and changes to the retina.
- Lifestyle changes that can improve the health of a client with HTN include smoking cessation, weight loss, moderation of alcohol consumption, stress reduction, regular exercise, and moderation of caffeine consumption. Medical treatment consists primarily of medications.
- Peripheral arterial disease is similar to coronary artery disease. As the disease progresses, the client experiences symptoms of reduced blood flow to the affected body part. Risk factors are similar to those for coronary artery disease, with diabetes mellitus playing a larger role. The most common symptom is the pain of intermittent claudication.
- The first strategy for treating peripheral arterial disease is assisting in risk factor reduction. This includes smoking cessation, dietary modification, and control of diabetes mellitus and HTN. Other treatments include exercise, medication, and vascular surgery.
- Nursing diagnoses are derived from the assessment data and are unique to the individual client. Outcomes that are set must be realistic, measurable, and tailored to the individual client.
- Interventions to promote safety include the following: perform pain assessments in the older adult with CAD; report symptoms immediately; educate the client to take medications as prescribed; and perform hourly neurovascular assessments following revascularization therapy for peripheral arterial disease.
- Interventions to promote health education include the following: educate the older adult about medications, diet, and exercise, and about the atypical signs and symptoms of MI.
- Interventions to promote lifestyle modification include the following: assist the older adult to modify lifestyle factors; encourage smoking cessation.
- Interventions to promote mobility include the encouragement of physical activity.
- Interventions to promote nutrition include the following: encourage a balanced, nutritious diet low in fat and cholesterol with vitamins B_6, B_{12}, A, C, and E, folic acid, beta carotene, and flavonoids; encourage the older adult with CHF to reduce salt intake and fluids; encourage the client with HTN to reduce excessive intake of sodium, fat, caffeine,

Ischemia — decreased supply of Oxygenated Blood
hypoxia — lack of O₂ @ cellular level

Couple-n Pe'n
Debies   Am or
PM

and alcohol; encourage the older adult with diabetes mellitus to adhere to the prescribed diet.

- Interventions to promote rest and sleep include the following: encourage the client with coronary artery disease to stop activity immediately and to rest upon the occurrence of cardiac pain; encourage the client with CHF to rest between activities; encourage the older adult with peripheral arterial disease to rest when claudication occurs.
- Evaluation should be aimed directly at the expected outcomes.

STUDY QUESTIONS

Multiple-Choice Review

1. You are performing an assessment on your older adult client with peripheral arterial disease. While palpating the feet, you notice that they are slightly cool bilaterally. You are unable to locate a pedal pulse on either foot. What action should you take?
   1. Nothing—this is a normal finding in older adults.
   2. Nothing—if the client has peripheral arterial disease, the physician probably knows there is no pulse.
   — 3. Document the absence of pulse and notify the RN immediately.
   4. Document the absence of pulse and take no further action.

2. The symptoms of coronary artery disease are a reflection of:
   — 1. Lack of oxygen to the myocardium
   2. Turbulent blood flow through the coronary arteries
   3. Decreased pumping ability of the heart
   4. Decreased sinoatrial cells

3. Atypical presentation of a myocardial infarction is more likely to occur in which of the following groups?
   1. Chinese Americans
   2. Men
   — 3. People with diabetes mellitus
   4. None of the above

4. The primary form of treatment for congestive heart failure is:
   — 1. Lifestyle modification and drug therapy

2. Surgical valve repair
3. Cardiac transplantation
4. Stress reduction

5. If you could convince your older adult client with peripheral arterial disease to eliminate *one* risk factor of the disease, which one would it be?
   1. High-cholesterol diet
   2. Hypertension
   3. High homocysteine levels
   — 4. Smoking

Critical Thinking

1. Under what situations would you expect to see evidence of age-related changes to the cardiovascular system in an older adult?

2. List each of the physical findings that you may find during your assessment of the older adult with peripheral arterial disease. What is the basis of each of these symptoms?

3. Why is hypertension called the silent killer, and what implication does this have for your client-teaching efforts?

4. Compare and contrast the similarities and differences in drug therapy for the four disorders discussed in this chapter.

Resources

Internet Resources

American Heart Association
http://www.americanheart.org
Centers for Disease Control and Prevention
- FASTATS on hypertension
  http://www.cdc.gov/nchswww/fastats.htm
- Physical activity and health: A report of the Surgeon General
  http://www.cdc.gov/nccdphp/sgr/summ.htm
Vascular Disease Foundation
http://www.vdf.org/main.htm
World Hypertension League
http://www.mco.edu/whl/know.html

Organizations

American Association of Cardiovascular and Pulmonary Rehabilitation
7611 Elmwood Avenue, Suite 201
Middletown, WI 53562

American Heart Association
7272 Greenville Avenue
Dallas, TX 75231

Selected References

Alexander, M., Grumbach, K., Remy, L., Rowell, R., & Massie, B. M. (1999). Congestive heart failure hospitalizations and survival in California: Patterns according to race/ethnicity. *American Heart Journal, 137*(5), 919–927.

Cohn, J. N. (1998). Managing heart failure: Data from clinical trials and future directions. Online coverage from the American College of Cardiology, March 29–April 1, 1998. Available at http://www.medscape.com/Medscape/CNO/1998/ACC/04.01/acc0710.cohn/acc0710.cohn.html

Confronting aging and disease: CVD and estrogen. *Women's Health Treatment Updates, 1999, Medscape.* Available at http://cardiology.medscape.com/Medscape/WomesHealth/TreatmentUpdate/1999/tu01/tu01–10.html Accessed 8/1/99.

Gaziano, J. M. (1998). When should heart disease prevention begin? *New England Journal of Medicine, 338*(23), 1690–1692.

Graham, I. M., Daly, L. E., Refsum, H. M., et al. (1997). Plasma homocysteine as a risk factor for vascular disease: The European Concerted Action Project. *Journal of the American Medical Association, 277*(22), 1775–1781.

Grauer, K. (1998). Management of hypertension: JNC-VI guidelines and beyond. Online coverage from the 50th Annual Meeting of the American Academy of Family Physicians Scientific Assembly, September 16–20, 1998. Available at http://www.medscape.com/Medscape/CNO/1998/AAFP/09.17/AAFP..../AAFP.17.556.Grau.htm Accessed 8/5/99.

Healthy Foods for the Heart. Women's Health Interactive Available at http://www.womens-health.com/health_center/nutrition/nt_a_1.html Accessed 11/15/00.

Healthy People 2010 website. Available at http://www.health.gov/healthypeople/Document/tableofcontents.htm Accessed 11/15/00.

Hodgson, B. B., & Kizior, R. J. (1999). *Saunders nursing drug handbook.* Philadelphia: W. B. Saunders.

Homocysteine: Discovering a new predictor for coronary artery disease. *Clinical Reviews, 8*(5), 203–206, 208–210, 1998. Available at http://www.medscape.com/CPG/ClinReviews/1998/v08.n05/c0805.04..../pnt-c0805.04.food.htm Accessed 8/4/99.

Homocysteine, fibrinogen, Lp(a), small dense LDL, oxidative stress, and *C pneumoniae* infection: How important are they? Online coverage from the American College of Cardiology 48th Annual Scientific Session, March 7–10, 1999.

Available at http://www.medscape.com/Medscape/CNO/1999/ACC/eng/03.10/0251.chan/0251.chan.htm Accessed 8/4/99.

Ignatavicius, D. D., Workman, M. L., & Mishler, M. A. (1999). *Medical-surgical nursing across the health care continuum.* Philadelphia: W. B. Saunders.

Jones, J. M. (1997). Promoting physical activity in the senior years. *Journal of Gerontological Nursing, 23*(7), 41–48.

Lee, H. (1997). Typical and atypical clinical signs and symptoms of myocardial infarction and delayed seeking of professional care among blacks. *American Journal of Critical Care, 6*(1), 7–13.

Managing congestive heart failure: The role of ACE inhibitors (1998). *Clinical Reviews, 9*, 2–5. Available at http://www.medscape.com/CPG/ClinReviews/1998/09.98s.mana/pnt-c0998smana.html Accessed 8/5/99.

Matteson, M. A., McConnell, E. S., & Linton, A. D. (1998). *Gerontological nursing: Concepts and practice.* Philadelphia: W. B. Saunders.

McCarthy, R. (1997). The pharmacologic treatment of hypertension: An update. *Drug Benefit Trends, 9*(9), 71–77.

Michaels, A. D. (1999). Management of peripheral artery disease. Online coverage from the American College of Cardiology 48th Annual Scientific Session, *March 7–10, 1999.* Available at http://www.medscape.com/Medscape/CNO/1999/ACC/eng/03.08/0202.mich/0202.mich.html

Papademetriou, V., Narayan, P., Rubins, H., Collins, D., & Robins, S. (1998). Influence of risk factors on peripheral and cerebrovascular disease in men with coronary artery disease, low high-density lipoprotein cholesterol levels, and desirable low-density lipoprotein cholesterol levels. *American Heart Journal, 136*(4), 734–740.

Peckenpaugh, N. J., & Poleman, C. M. (1999). *Nutrition essentials and diet therapy.* Philadelphia: W. B. Saunders.

Physical activity and health: A report of the Surgeon General. Available at http://www.cdc.gov/nccdphp/sgr/summ.htm Accessed 8/23/98.

Tyson, S. R. (1999). *Gerontological nursing care.* Philadelphia: W. B. Saunders.

Whellan, D. J. (1998). Cardiac rehabilitation is associated with improved survival in CHF patients. Online coverage from the American Heart Association 71st Scientific Sessions, November 8–11, 1998. Available at http://www.medscape.com/Medscape/CNO/1998/AHA/11.11/whel.41/whel.41.html

Promoting Oxygenation

OBJECTIVES

After completing this chapter, you will be able to:

- Discuss the normal changes of aging that affect the lung.
- Describe the sequence of assessment for the respiratory system.
- Compare the key clinical features of disorders commonly affecting the respiratory system of older adults.
- Identify atypical presentation of pneumonia in the older adult.
- Examine the nursing process in care planning for the older adult with disorders of chronic obstructive pulmonary disease and pneumonia.

CHAPTER OUTLINE

KEY TERMS

Accessory muscles
Alveoli
Anterior-posterior diameter
Aspiration
Atelectasis
Cilia
Circulation
Dyspnea

Ecchymoses
Exacerbation
Extrapulmonary
Extravasation
FEV_1
Hypoxemia
Hypoxia
Inhalation

Interstitial

Intrapulmonary

Kyphosis

Negative pressure

Nonproductive cough

Obstructive lung diseases

PaO_2

Productive cough

Pulse oximetry

Restrictive lung diseases

Sepsis

Tachycardia

Tachypnea

AGE-RELATED CHANGES OF THE RESPIRATORY SYSTEM

The respiratory system undergoes changes with age. Most of these changes may go unnoticed on a day-to-day basis; for example, no change may be evident as the older adult client gets out of bed, walks to the grocery store, prepares meals, and carries out ordinary daily activities. Instead, these changes become noticeable under circumstances in which the older adult is forced to call upon reserves—those times when extra energy is required, for example, to run to catch a plane, to run to answer the telephone, or to fight off an infection.

The changes that occur happen both inside the lung tissue (**intrapulmonary** changes) and outside of it (**extrapulmonary** changes). In the lung itself, a loss of elasticity develops. The lungs are like two small balloons, which would prefer to be deflated—and would be, if not for **negative pressure**, which keeps them inflated. Lung tissue is normally very elastic, but aging reduces this elasticity. One contributing factor is the replacement of smooth muscle fibers in the bronchioles with fibrous tissue. The cartilage in the walls of the trachea and in the bronchi undergoes progressive calcification. The net result of these changes is a reduced ability of the older adult to move air rapidly, which is measured by a parameter called **FEV$_1$**, or forced expiratory volume in 1 second. As the name implies, to take this measurement, the older adult is asked to take in a very deep breath, then is timed while exhaling the maximum amount of air possible in 1 second. This exhaled volume is then measured. Typically, FEV$_1$ is reduced in the older adult. Lung

volumes and capacities and changes with aging are listed in Table 9–1.

Extrapulmonary changes of the lung that occur with age include changes to the chest wall that impair the older adult's ability to take a very deep breath. For example, the chest wall may become stiffer as a result of calcification and osteoporosis. The thoracic cage shortens, and the **anterior-posterior diameter** increases. This leaves the older adult with more of a "barrel-shaped" chest than he or she had earlier. In addition, muscles associated with respiration weaken with age. As a result, the older adult has a greater residual volume of air remaining in the lung after expiration, and vital capacity is reduced (Fig. 9–1).

The **alveoli** enlarge and become thinner, which impairs gas exchange. A lower percentage of the oxygen in alveolar air is able to diffuse into the lung capillaries. The result of this impairment is that the partial pressure of arterial oxygen (**PaO$_2$**) is reduced with age by approximately 4 mm Hg per decade. Therefore, a 20-year-old who has a PaO$_2$ of approximately 90 mm Hg may, at age 70, have a PaO$_2$ closer to 75 mm Hg. Of course, 75 is still adequate for tissue oxygenation under normal circumstances; however, it is clear that the older adult is at a disadvantage when faced with additional oxygenation requirements.

Over the course of many years, the **cilia** become atrophied, which impairs their ability to cleanse and rid the respiratory tract of mucus. The strength of the cough is also reduced somewhat, which is related to the decreased strength of respiratory muscles described earlier. In addition, changes to the immune system with age make an older adult more susceptible to infection. All of

Table 9–1

LUNG VOLUMES AND CAPACITIES

Parameter	Symbol	Normal Value	Description	Remarks
Tidal volume	V_T	500 mL	Volume of breath inhaled and exhaled with a normal breath	Unchanged with aging; can be decreased in **restrictive lung disease**
Inspiratory reserve volume	IRV	3000 mL	Maximum amount of air that can be inspired after a normal inhalation	Reduced in **obstructive lung disease**
Expiratory reserve volume	ERV	1000 mL	Air remaining in the lungs after expiration that can be forcibly exhaled	Reduced in restrictive lung disease
Residual volume	RV	1500 mL	Amount of air remaining in the lungs after maximum exhalation	Increases with aging
Inspiratory capacity	IC	3500 mL	Maximum amount of air that can be inspired after a normal exhalation	Decreased with restrictive lung disease
Functional residual capacity	FRC	2500 mL	ERV plus RV	Increases with aging
Vital capacity	VC	4500 mL	Amount of air that can be expelled from the lungs after maximum inspiration	Reduced with aging
Total lung capacity	TLC	6000 mL	Amount of air in the lungs after maximum inspiration	Reduced with restrictive lung disease

Adapted from Tyson, S. R. (1999). *Gerontological nursing care.* Philadelphia: W. B. Saunders, p. 295.

these factors make it more difficult for an older adult to fight off respiratory infection.

Along with normal aging, certain lifestyle factors can further impair lung function in the older adult. It is well known that smoking accelerates the aging process in lung tissue in numerous ways

(Box 9–1). Obesity increases the work of breathing and makes it more difficult for the lower portions of the lung to be oxygenated because the large abdomen makes it difficult for the lungs to fully expand. Immobility can further impair lung function in the older adult.

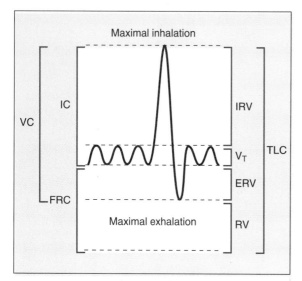

Figure 9–1. Lung volumes and capacities.

Health Promotion Tip

Quitting smoking, increasing activity, and reducing excess body weight can all lead to improved lung function in the older adult.

ASSESSMENT OF THE RESPIRATORY SYSTEM

Begin your assessment with the measurement of vital signs, paying special attention to the pulse and respiratory rate. If the older adult has an impairment of the respiratory system, the pulse and respiratory rate may be slightly to

Box 9–1 | Harmful Effects of Smoking on Lung Tissue

- Reduction in FEV_1 of 50 to 160 mL/yr
- Further inhibition of cilia
- Increased mucus production
- Bronchoconstriction
- Increased risk of complications from heart and lung disease (both active and passive exposure to smoke)

Data from Matteson, M. A., McConnell, E. S., & Linton, A. D. (1998). *Gerontological nursing: Concepts and practice.* Philadelphia: W. B. Saunders, pp. 264–265.

moderately elevated, as the body attempts to compensate. A client in respiratory distress will present with marked **tachypnea** and **tachycardia**, along with possible alterations in blood pressure. Observe and document the regularity or irregularity of both the pulse and the respiratory rate (Fig. 9–2).

After vital signs have been assessed, measure and document the **pulse oximetry** reading for your client, if available on your unit. Continue with a head-to-toe approach for the assessment. Assess the level of orientation of the older adult. If an older adult is having difficulty oxygenating the body because of a respiratory impairment, he or she may present with mild confusion or disorientation, as the brain is deficient in oxygen.

Beginning with the head, observe the color of the skin. Lack of tissue oxygen can appear as pallor or cyanosis. Cyanosis most commonly appears near the lips and nose. Some respiratory diseases leave the cheeks of a client with a ruddy appearance. Observe the neck muscles: hypertrophy may indicate lung disease, as the body must work harder to breathe and use the **accessory muscles** of respiration, including the sternocleidomastoid muscles in the neck region. Next, examine the chest area and upper back. It is normal with age for the thorax to take on a more rounded or "barrel-chest" appearance, although this finding is more pronounced with chronic lung disease. Observe for and document the presence of musculoskeletal abnormalities such as **kyphosis**, which can have an adverse effect on breathing, as the lungs are unable to fully expand.

Auscultate the lung fields with your stethoscope. Lung sounds are best heard from the back of the client, although the right middle lobe must be auscultated from the anterior or lateral aspect of the chest. Most assessment books advise beginning auscultation from the top of the lungs (apices) to the bottom (base); however, you may get better assessment data by doing the opposite with the older adult. Beginning assessment at the bases allows the older adult to generate his or her best respiratory effort to your instructions to "take a deep breath." After four or five deep breaths, the older adult is often beginning to fatigue, and each "deep breath" may be less deep than the first ones; if you begin at the apices, you may merely hear and chart "diminished bases," when in fact there could be abnormal lung

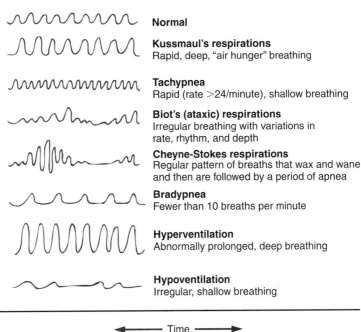

Figure 9–2. Breathing patterns. (From Monahan, F. D., & Neighbors, M. [1998]. *Medical-surgical nursing: Foundations for clinical practice* [2nd ed.]. Philadelphia: W. B. Saunders, p. 553.)

sounds present (Table 9–2). If the older adult becomes fatigued during lung auscultation, stop this portion of the assessment, continue with another part of the assessment, and then resume lung auscultation after a few minutes.

Assess the extremities of the older adult. A client receiving long-term steroid therapy for chronic lung disease may have multiple **ecchymoses** on his or her arms, due to increased capillary fragility. An older adult with chronic **hypoxia** may have fingernails with a clubbed appearance (Fig. 9–3).

The older adult with a long smoking history may have brownish discoloration of the fingers, teeth, and lips resulting from years of tobacco use.

During the examination, note the presence or absence of a cough. Ask the client if he or she experiences a frequent cough. If so, inquire as to whether it is a **productive** or **nonproductive** cough. If productive, ask about the characteristics of the sputum produced in terms of color and thickness. If the client demonstrates a cough for you, observe and document the color and consistency of the sputum. After the cough, auscultate the lung fields again if adventitious lung sounds were present upon initial auscultation. Sometimes a client may have inspiratory crackles that disappear

after coughing. This would be documented, "Inspiratory crackles, clearing after cough."

Ask the older adult if he or she has any history of respiratory disorders, such as asthma or bronchitis, or of another disorder that would affect the respiratory system. Inquire about the presence or absence of **dyspnea**. If the client complains of dyspnea, it is important to determine under what circumstances he or she experiences this discomfort. Some older adults experience dyspnea on exertion (DOE). If this is the case, try to determine approximately how much exertion is required to produce the dyspnea, and document this information. Older adults with severe respiratory disease may experience dyspnea even at rest. It is very important not to fatigue these individuals during the assessment.

Inquire about other types of pain related to the respiratory system, such as pleurisy. Ask if it is painful to take a deep breath. Assess for and document other types of pain that can have an effect on breathing. A client with abdominal pain from surgery may breathe shallowly in an attempt to reduce his or her pain. This information is important to relay, because nursing interventions to reduce this pain may make taking a deep breath easier for the client, thereby minimizing the likelihood that respiratory problems will develop.

Table 9–2
ADVENTITIOUS LUNG SOUNDS

Finding	Description	Cause
Fine crackles	Short, high-pitched sounds audible just prior to end-inspiration; sound is similar to rolling hair between fingers just behind the ear	Rapid equalization of gas pressure when collapsed alveoli or terminal bronchioles suddenly snap open; often audible with atelectasis
Coarse crackles	Series of short, low-pitched sounds during inspiration and/or expiration; sound is similar to blowing through a straw under water	Air passing through airway intermittently occluded by mucus, unstable bronchial wall, or fold of mucosa; often audible in clients with COPD
Rhonchi	Continuous rumbling, snoring, or rattling sounds, most prominent on expiration (may change after coughing or suctioning)	Obstruction of large airways with secretions; may be present in clients with chronic bronchitis or pneumonia if secretions are present
Wheezes	Continuous high-pitched squeaking sounds, usually on expiration, but may occur on inspiration as condition worsens	Rapid vibration of bronchial walls from bronchospasm; can be caused by airway obstruction
Stridor	Continuous musical sound of constant pitch	Partial obstruction of larynx or trachea
Absent breath sounds	No sounds audible over entire lung or area(s) of lung	Reduced or absent airflow, such as with main-stem bronchial obstruction, large atelectasis, lobectomy, or pneumonectomy
Pleural friction rub	Creaking or grating sound during inspiration and/or expiration associated with discomfort upon inspiration	Roughened, inflamed pleural surfaces rubbing together; may occur in clients with pneumonia

COPD, chronic obstructive pulmonary disease.
Adapted from Lewis, S. M., Heitkemper, M. M., & Dirksen, S. R. (2000). *Medical-surgical nursing: Assessment and management of clinical problems.* St. Louis: Mosby Inc., p. 570.

DISORDERS COMMON IN OLDER ADULTS

Chronic Obstructive Pulmonary Disease

Chronic obstructive pulmonary disease, commonly referred to as COPD, is a disease state characterized by the presence of chronic airflow obstruction caused by chronic bronchitis or emphysema. In the past, asthma was also classified under the umbrella of COPD; however, recently it has been categorized separately, owing to its distinguishing feature of lung inflammation.

COPD is a growing health problem in the United States: the number of individuals diagnosed

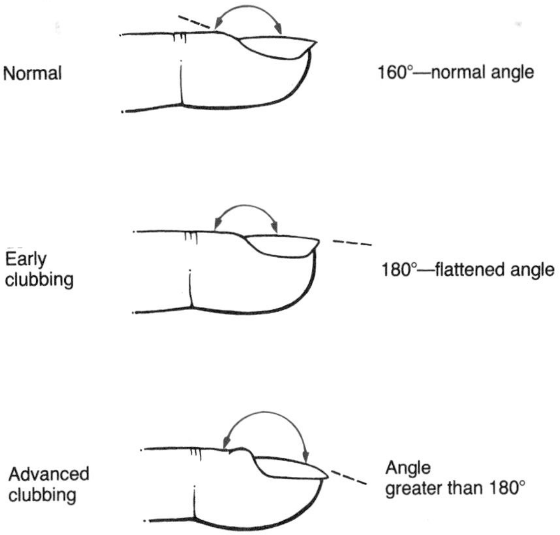

Figure 9–3. Clubbing of fingernails. (From Monahan, F. D., & Neighbors, M. [1998]. *Medical-surgical nursing: Foundations for clinical practice* [2nd ed.]. Philadelphia: W. B. Saunders, p. 535.)

with COPD has doubled over the past 25 years to over 15 million people affected. *Healthy People 2010* contains specific objectives related to COPD, listed in Box 9–2.

The number of women affected by COPD has increased steadily, as the number of women who smoke cigarettes continues to rise. Cigarette smoking is the primary cause of COPD, and patterns of incidence of the disease tend to reflect prior societal patterns of cigarette smoking. Other risk factors are listed in Box 9–3.

As was stated earlier, obstruction of airflow in the lungs is the primary problem characterizing COPD. The course of the illness is generally progressive, with symptoms worsening over time. The

---

Box 9–2 | *Healthy People 2010* COPD Objectives

- Reduce the proportion of adults whose activity is limited owing to chronic lung and breathing problems.
- Reduce deaths from chronic obstructive pulmonary disease (COPD) among adults.

From U. S. Department of Health and Human Services. *Healthy People 2010: Understanding and Improving Health*, 2nd ed. Washington, D. C.: U. S. Government Printing Office, November 2000.

Box 9–3 | Risk Factors for Chronic Obstructive Pulmonary Disease

- Cigarette smoking
- Cigar smoking
- Recurrent respiratory tract infection
- Aging
- Male sex
- Family history of COPD
- Air pollution
- Genetic deficiency of alpha$_1$-antitrypsin

Data from Berglund, D. J., Abbey, D. E., Lebowitz, M. D., et al. (1999). Respiratory symptoms and pulmonary function in an elderly nonsmoking population. *Chest, 115*(1), 49–59; Iribarren, C., Tekawa, S. S., & Friedman, G. D. (1999). Effect of cigar smoking on the risk of cardiovascular disease, chronic obstructive pulmonary disease, and cancer in men. *New England Journal of Medicine, 340*(23), 1773–1780; Lewis, S. M., Heitkemper, M. M., & Dirksen, S. R. (2000). *Medical-surgical nursing: Assessment and management of clinical problems.* St. Louis: Mosby.

airflow obstruction associated with emphysema is related to alveolar destruction by proteases and elastase. This destruction leads to collapse and narrowing of smaller airways, hyperinflation, trapping of air, and **atelectasis or airway closure.** Elastin and collagen, which are responsible for lung tissue elasticity, are destroyed in emphysema. The net result is that lung tissue takes on what can be thought of as a "floppy" characteristic: it is easy for air to get in, but more difficult for air to get *out*, as lung tissue collapses upon itself.

Imagine a healthy pair of lungs as a balloon. Air will go into the lungs under pressure (in our lungs, this is negative pressure), and air escapes the lungs passively. Now, imagine lungs with the disorder emphysema as a paper bag. When you blow air into a paper bag, it will enter quite easily, but waiting for it to leave the paper bag and return to the external environment is more difficult because the paper bag has no elastic properties. Although extreme, this analogy may help you remember that the primary disorder with

emphysema is difficulty in getting the air out of the lungs because of decreased elasticity.

Chronic bronchitis is characterized by excessive mucus production, due to hyperplasia of the mucus-producing glands in the trachea and bronchi. Cilia in the airways normally help the body adapt to increases in mucus production; however, in chronic bronchitis, there is a decrease in the number and effectiveness of cilia, which further compounds the problem. Mucus plugs may develop, which can lead to respiratory infection. Additionally, edema and bronchospasm further limit airflow in clients with chronic bronchitis. The pathophysiology of chronic bronchitis and emphysema is depicted in Figure 9–4.

Symptoms of a client with COPD can be related to either chronic bronchitis or emphysema, or both, as most clients have features of both disorders. The most notable sign of an older adult with chronic bronchitis is cough with mucus production. In the beginning stages, it can be described as a "smoker's cough," which reflects the

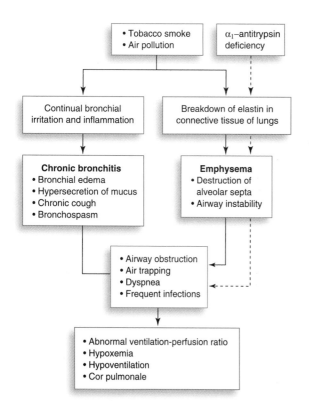

Figure 9–4. Pathophysiology of chronic bronchitis and emphysema. (From Lewis, S. M., Heitkemper, M. M., & Dirksen, S. R. [2000]. *Medical-surgical nursing: Assessment and management of clinical problems* [5th ed.]. St. Louis: Mosby, p. 684.)

fact that most clients with COPD have a significant smoking history. The cough is coarse and is most notable in the morning, or during cold, damp weather. The mucus produced increases in thickness and volume, and becomes more foul-smelling over time. Later symptoms of chronic bronchitis include dyspnea and cyanosis due to a reduced oxygen supply to the body.

🍴 Nutrition Tip _____

The client with chronic bronchitis is usually malnourished, even if overweight.

If the primary disorder of an older adult is emphysema, the earliest and most notable symptom is dyspnea. The dyspnea progresses in severity, first appearing with exertion and gradually worsening to the point that it occurs with rest. In the later stages of the illness, even the simple task of eating a meal can produce dyspnea. The client with emphysema will eventually experience cough with mucus production, but to much less degree than the client whose primary disorder is chronic bronchitis. Signs and symptoms of chronic bronchitis and emphysema, along with the pathophysiologic basis, are listed in Table 9–3. Also see Figure 9–5.

Treatment for COPD includes drug therapy, respiratory therapy, pulmonary rehabilitation, and close monitoring of nutritional status. Smoking cessation is of the utmost importance in helping to slow the disease process and preserve as much respiratory function as possible.

Numerous medications may be prescribed for the client with COPD. Initially, bronchodilator medications of various types are employed, often in inhalation form. Corticosteroids may be prescribed, to be taken either via inhaler or orally. Oral corticosteroids are controversial for long-term use, as adverse effects are numerous

	Table 9–3		
	COMPARISON OF SIGNS AND SYMPTOMS IN CHRONIC BRONCHITIS AND EMPHYSEMA		
Sign/Symptom	Chronic Bronchitis	Emphysema	Causes
Cough	• Early sign • Productive of thick mucus • "Hallmark" feature of disorder	• Later sign • Less significant feature of disorder • Non- or only slightly productive	Excess mucus production/ hypertrophy of mucus-secreting glands
Dyspnea	• Later sign	• Early sign • "Hallmark" feature of disorder	Hypoxemia
Weight loss	• May be present or absent	• Present	Unknown, but may be related to dyspnea associated with act of eating or hypermetabolism
Malnourishment	• Usually present	• Almost always present	Same as above
Clubbed fingernails	• Later sign	• Later sign	Chronic hypoxia
Skin color	• Reddish "ruddy" appearance	• Pallor or cyanosis	"Ruddy" appearance related to polycythemia; pallor/cyanosis related to hypoxia

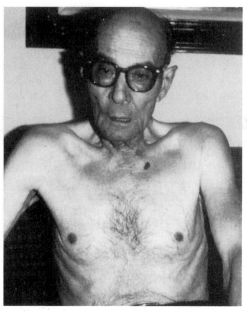

Figure 9–5. Older adult male with classic presentation of emphysema. Note the malnourished appearance, hypertrophy of accessory muscles of respiration, and slight kyphosis to ease the work of breathing. (From Kersten, L. D. [1989]. *Comprehensive respiratory nursing: A decision making approach.* Philadelphia: W. B. Saunders, p. 109.)

and can be quite severe. It is more common for oral corticosteroids to be used on a short-term basis during an acute **exacerbation** of the disease process. Table 9–4 lists medications commonly used for chronic obstructive pulmonary disease.

Respiratory therapy is another important component of COPD management. Components of respiratory therapy include oxygen therapy, chest physiotherapy, and use of breathing and/or coughing techniques. Oxygen therapy may be used under certain circumstances for the client with COPD, but very cautiously and only under a physician's order (Fig. 9–6). A physician may prescribe a very low amount of oxygen, for example, 2 L/minute, on a temporary basis for a client experiencing an acute exacerbation of the illness. It is critical that physician orders be followed precisely. Certain clients with COPD may experience suppression of respiratory drive because of build-up of carbon dioxide in the blood when oxygen is administered at high levels. In other

words, it is possible to make the client worse by administering too much oxygen. Oxygen therapy is sometimes used on a long-term basis for certain clients, including use at home. Whatever the circumstances, oxygen safety is a top nursing care priority.

Medication Safety Tip

Principles of oxygen safety:

- Administer oxygen according to specific physician orders.*
- Place "No smoking" signs in a highly visible area; reinforce to any staff or visitors in the vicinity the importance of not smoking.
- Monitor the client's vital signs on each shift; report these to the registered nurse (RN).
- Every 4 hours, monitor the client's respiratory rate, respiratory pattern, and level of orientation; report any changes to the RN.
- Instruct the client to **not** self-adjust the oxygen level.
- Pad any areas where the oxygen device irritates the client's skin.
- Provide frequent oral hygiene and skin care around the oxygen device.
- Avoid the use of electric razors, portable radios, open flames, wool blankets, or mineral oils in the vicinity of oxygen use.

*Although respiratory therapists are largely responsible for oxygen administration, you must verify that the oxygen is implemented as ordered.

Chest physiotherapy, sometimes abbreviated CPT, consists of percussion, vibration, and postural drainage. It may be used for the client with excessive bronchial secretions and difficulty clearing those secretions. The three components of CPT are outlined in Table 9–5.

An important part of caring for the older adult with COPD is the reinforcement of effective breathing and coughing techniques. Teach the client to breathe slowly, and to use the abdominal muscles to facilitate expiration. Many older adults find that exhalation through pursed lips (such as with blowing out a candle) provides a controlled method of slowing down the expiratory phase of the respiratory cycle. Remember, especially with emphysema, exhalation is often the most difficult

Table 9–4

COMMON MEDICATIONS USED IN THE TREATMENT OF CHRONIC OBSTRUCTIVE PULMONARY DISEASE

Category/Drug Action	Examples	Usual Route	Nursing Considerations
Beta-agonist (bronchodilating effect)	• albuterol • terbutaline	Inhalation	• Onset is within 5 minutes • Monitor for tachycardia • Hold medication/notify physician if pulse >120
Anticholinergic (bronchodilating effect)	• ipratropium • oxitropium	Inhalation	• Slower onset (within 15 minutes) • Instruct client to wait at least 1 minute between inhalations
Methylxanthine (bronchodilating effect)	• theophylline	Oral, intravenous	• Monitor for tachycardia or tremors
Corticosteroid (decrease airway inflammation)	• prednisone	Inhalation, oral	• Monitor for signs of infection, hyperglycemia • Other adverse effects include mood swings, insomnia, irritability, and increased appetite

Data from Hafner, J., & Ferro, T. J. (1998). Recent developments in the management of COPD. *Hospital Medicine, 34*(1), 29–38; Hodgson, B. B., & Kizior, R. J. (1999). *Saunders nursing drug handbook.* Philadelphia: W. B. Saunders.

phase. It is also important to teach effective coughing to promote the removal of bronchial secretions. Timing of coughing is just as important as technique; the most effective coughing may occur when the client is well rested, such as upon arising, or before meals, rather than afterward. Instructions for effective coughing can be found in Box 9–4.

Breathing and coughing techniques are also components of a larger program of pulmonary rehabilitation for clients with COPD. Pulmonary rehabilitation programs are expensive and may be difficult to access, but are growing in popularity as they can increase exercise capacity, reduce dyspnea, and improve quality of life for older adults with COPD. Components of an effective pulmonary rehabilitation program can be found in Box 9–5.

Another vital nursing intervention for the client with COPD is maintaining good nutritional status. This intervention can be difficult to implement, as food may by the last thing on the mind of people with difficulty breathing. Also, dyspnea makes it difficult to consume food and fluids in adequate amounts. However, proper nutrition is crucial in maintaining the respiratory muscle strength needed for breathing and achieving effective airway clearance.

Unless contraindicated, encourage the client with COPD to consume 2 to 3 L of fluid each day. Keeping well hydrated decreases the viscosity of respiratory secretions, making them easier to expectorate. Encourage the client to eat smaller, more frequent meals rather than 3 large meals each day to decrease abdominal bloating and reduce the fatigue associated with eating.

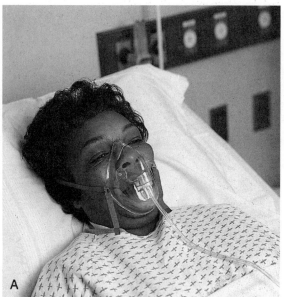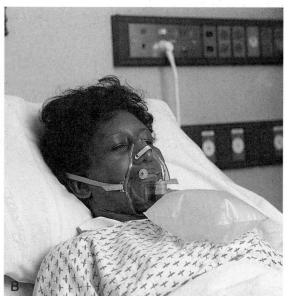

Figure 9–6. Oxygen therapy. *A,* Simple face mask. *B,* Plaster face mask with reservoir bag. (From Lewis, S. M., Heitkemper, M. M., & Dirksen, S. R. [2000]. *Medical-surgical nursing: Assessment and management of clinical problems.* St. Louis: Mosby, p. 695.)

| | Table 9–5 | |
| | CHEST PHYSIOTHERAPY | |
Mode	**Description**	**Nursing Implications**
Percussion	Rhythmic clapping of cupped hands over various segments of lungs to mobilize secretions	• Avoid sternum, spinal cord, kidneys, or tender/painful areas • Performing over hospital gown or T-shirt may improve comfort • Contraindications include hemoptysis, carcinoma, and bronchospasm
Vibration	Pressure and a shaking movement of the hand are applied to various segments of the lung to mobilize secretions	• Better tolerated than percussion in older adults • Commercial vibrators may also be used for the same purpose
Postural drainage	Use of gravity and various positions to facilitate drainage of secretions from bronchial airways to the trachea for expectoration	• Perform 1 hour before meals or 3 hours after meals • Positions are maintained for 5 to 15 minutes; 2 to 4 times per day • Older adults may need nursing assistance to assume positions • Some positions are contraindicated with chest trauma, head injury, heart disease, or unstable client conditions

Data from Lewis, S. M., Heitkemper, M. M., & Dirksen, S. R. (2000). *Medical-surgical nursing: Assessment and management of clinical problems.* St. Louis: Mosby Inc; O'Toole, M. T. (1997). *Encyclopedia and dictionary of medicine, nursing, and allied health.* Philadelphia: W. B. Saunders.

Nutrition Tip

Nutritional tips for the client with COPD:

- Rest for 30 minutes prior to each meal.
- Select highly nutritious foods: high-calorie, high-protein choices.
- Choose foods that are easy to prepare.
- Eat 5 to 6 small meals each day.
- Select nutritious between-meal beverages, such as Pulmocare.
- Assume a comfortable eating position: upright with elbows propped on the table top may decrease the work of breathing.
- Avoid exercise and treatments 1 hour before and 1 hour after eating.
- Avoid large meals and gas-forming foods.

Pneumonia

Pneumonia is inflammation of the lung tissue, usually related to an infectious process. The inflammatory process affects the **interstitial** lung tissue, leading to leaking, or **extravasation,** of fluid into the alveoli. As the body attempts to defend itself from the invading organism, white blood cells rush to the scene, causing thickening of the alveolar wall. These two processes result in **hypoxemia** because the alveolus is the location at which gas exchange must take place. Many of the symptoms of pneumonia are related to this impairment of gas exchange. As the infection takes hold, the body tries to fight it in the usual ways: increasing heat production and raising the metabolic rate. Other symptoms of pneumonia are related to this attempt by the body to fight the infection. Signs and symptoms of pneumonia are outlined in Box 9–6.

Unfortunately, the older adult may not present with the usual signs or symptoms of pneumonia, or the signs may be more subtle. He or she may simply have a slight decrease in appetite or weight, or may experience a falling episode or an acute exacerbation of another chronic illness. Often, tachycardia and tachypnea are the only signs of pneumonia in the older adult. Because of this, the illness often progresses to a very serious stage by the time it is discovered.

 Signs and Symptoms Tip

Atypical presentation of pneumonia:

- Decreased appetite
- Slight weight loss
- Episodes of falling
- Altered mental status
- Weakness
- Exacerbation of underlying illness: COPD, heart failure, diabetes mellitus

Source: Ely, E. W. (1997). Pneumonia in the elderly: Diagnostic and therapeutic challenges. *Infectious Medicine, 14*(8), 643–654.

Box 9–4 | Instructions for Effective Coughing

- Sit upright with feet placed firmly on the floor.
- Turn shoulders inward and bend head slightly downward, while hugging a pillow.
- Take two deep breaths, using your diaphragm: inhale through the nose and exhale through pursed lips.
- Bend forward slowly, while producing two or three strong coughs from the next exhalation.
- Repeat the procedure twice, then rest before undertaking additional coughing.

Adapted from Ignatavicius, D. D., Workman, M. L., & Mishler, M. A. (1999). *Medical-surgical nursing across the health care continuum.* Philadelphia: W. B. Saunders, p. 631.

Box 9–5 | Components of a Pulmonary Rehabilitation Program

- Breathing control techniques
- Chest physiotherapy
- Lower extremity exercise training
- Respiratory muscle training
- Upper extremity muscle group training
- Occupational therapy
- Respiratory therapy
- Education
- Psychosocial support
- Nutritional education

Data from Ambrosino, N., Foglio, K., & Bianchi, L. (1997). Pulmonary rehabilitation programs in COPD: Patient selection, therapeutic modalities, and outcome measures. Available at http://www.medscape.com/Medscape/RespiratoryCare/journal/1997/.../mrc3098 ambrosino.htm Accessed 8/25/99.

> **Box 9-6   Signs and Symptoms of Pneumonia**
>
> - Fever
> - Chills
> - Productive cough
> - Tachypnea, tachycardia, and hypotension
> - Muscular chest wall pain
> - Malaise
> - Dyspnea
> - Crackles or wheezes to auscultation
> - Dullness to percussion

There are many different ways to classify pneumonia: by organism, site of inflammation, or physical environment in which the patient contracted the illness, to name a few. Common classifications of pneumonia are outlined in Table 9-6.

Pneumonia is a serious threat to the health of the older adult. Most older adults who contract pneumonia require hospitalization and are hospitalized longer than their younger counterparts because of the presence of coexisting illnesses they may have. To make matters worse, the older adult with pneumonia often has an atypical presentation of the illness. This is why your astute nursing observations and assessments are crucial.

The older adult is especially vulnerable to pneumonia caused by *Streptococcus pneumoniae*. This type of pneumonia, referred to as pneumococcal pneumonia, has a much higher mortality rate among the older adult population: it is three to five times more likely to result in death for adults over age 65 than for their younger counterparts. The pneumococcal vaccine, also known as Pneumovax, is designed to provide protection against this organism.

> **Health Promotion Tip**
>
> It is important for nurses to educate older adult clients about the importance of being vaccinated against pneumococcal pneumonia.

Older adults are at risk for the development of pneumonia simply because of their age. With age comes a decline in immunity, a weakened cough reflex, and often the presence of other illnesses and treatments that can promote the development of pneumonia. Risk factors for community- and hospital-acquired pneumonia are listed in Table 9-7.

Organisms and other agents responsible for causing pneumonia reach the lung tissue in one of three ways: **aspiration, inhalation, or circulation.** The older adult at greatest risk for aspiration pneumonia has a decreased level of consciousness, an endotracheal or nasogastric tube, or a disorder of the esophagus. The fact that aging can weaken one's cough and gag reflex also helps to explain why older adults may be vulnerable to aspiration pneumonia. **Inhalation** of microorganisms suspended in water droplets is often the cause of viral pneumonia. The third way in which microorganisms can reach the lung is by way of **circulation.** This occurs when an infection in another part of the body spreads to, or "seeds," the lung tissue. An example of this is a client who develops pneumonia as a result of **sepsis.** This very serious mode of transmission is, fortunately, the most infrequent type.

Table 9-6
CLASSIFICATIONS OF PNEUMONIA

Classification	Examples	Description
Anatomic location	• Lobar • Bronchial	Lobar affects a segment or entire lobe of the lung and is more serious. Bronchial is more prevalent, affects a smaller area.
Location acquired	• Community acquired • Hospital acquired	Community-acquired pneumonias are often viral. Hospital-acquired pneumonia has a mortality rate of 30%.
Causative agent	• Bacterial • Viral • Aspiration	Bacterial often caused by *Streptococcus pneumoniae* or *Haemophilus influenzae.* Viral usually caused by type A virus.

Data from McKay, C. (1999). Best practices: Reducing nosocomial pneumonia. *A Supplement to RN,* February 1999; Monahan, F. D., & Neighbors, M. (1998). *Medical-surgical nursing: Foundations for clinical practice.* Philadelphia: W. B. Saunders.

Table 9–7
RISK FACTORS ASSOCIATED WITH PNEUMONIA

Community Acquired	Hospital Acquired
• Age 65 or older	• Age 65 or older
• Chronic illness	• Chronic lung or cardiac
• Recent exposure to	disease
infectious organisms	• Immobility
• Malnutrition	• Abdominal or thoracic
• Tobacco or	surgery
alcohol abuse	• Endotracheal,
• No history of having	tracheostomy, or
received the	nasogastric tube
pneumococcal	• Mechanical ventilation
vaccine	• Weak cough or gag
• No history of	reflex
influenza vaccine	• Medications that
the previous year	increase gastric pH
• Immunosuppressed	• Antibiotics
state	• Immunocompromised
	state
	• Malnutrition
	• Altered level of
	consciousness

Data from Cassiere, H. A. (1998). Severe pneumonia in the elderly: Risks, treatment, and prevention. *Medscape Respiratory Care, 2*(2), 1998; Ignatavicius, D. D., Workman, M. L., & Mishler, M. A. (1999). *Medical-surgical nursing across the health care continuum.* Philadelphia: W. B. Saunders, p. 669; Monahan, F. D., & Neighbors, M. (1998). *Medical-surgical nursing: Foundations for clinical practice.* Philadelphia: W. B. Saunders, p. 642.

Treatment of pneumonia varies according to the causative agent. In bacterial pneumonia, the physician or advanced practice nurse prescribes antibiotic therapy (oral or intravenous) appropriate to the organism being treated. Some common antibiotic therapies used in the treatment of pneumonia are listed in Table 9–8.

Medication Safety Tip

Antibiotics may interact with other medications that the older adult client is taking, and may cause a serious allergic reaction. It is important that the nurse observe the client who is taking new medication for any unusual signs and symptoms, and report them immediately.

Depending on the severity of the illness and the types of therapies ordered, treatment of the older adult with pneumonia may take place in the hospital setting. Bedrest is important to help the body combat the infection and to prevent unnecessary strain on the heart and lungs. Administration of fluids, either orally or intravenously, is important in promoting circulation and keeping sputum thin enough to be expectorated. The physician or advanced practice nurse may order oxygen therapy and/or chest physiotherapy to

Table 9–8
COMMON ANTIBIOTIC THERAPIES FOR TREATMENT OF PNEUMONIA

Antibiotic	Considerations
Erythromycin	• Effective against *Streptococcus pneumoniae* • Generally the #1 choice because of low cost and wide organism coverage • If client is severely ill, may be combined with a cephalosporin
Amoxicillin	• Good choice in uncomplicated mild infections • Organisms may develop resistance
Trimethoprim-sulfamethoxazole (TMP-SMX)	• Often used against *Haemophilus influenzae, Staphylococcus aureus,* or *Legionella* species • Inexpensive • Watch for drug interactions with warfarin, oral hypoglycemic agents, phenytoin
Cefuroxime, ceftriaxone, or cefotaxime	• Effective against a wide variety of organisms • Often used in clients with COPD
Doxycycline	• Used for mild, uncomplicated infections • Inexpensive
Ampicillin	• Often used parenterally for gram-positive cocci, gram-negative rods, or anaerobic organisms

COPD, chronic obstructive pulmonary disease.
Data from Ely, E. W. (1997). Pneumonia in the elderly: Diagnostic and therapeutic challenges. *Infectious Medicine, 14*(8), 643–654.

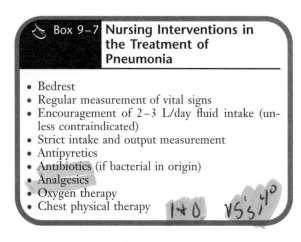

Box 9–7 **Nursing Interventions in the Treatment of Pneumonia**

- Bedrest
- Regular measurement of vital signs
- Encouragement of 2–3 L/day fluid intake (unless contraindicated)
- Strict intake and output measurement
- Antipyretics
- Antibiotics (if bacterial in origin)
- Analgesics
- Oxygen therapy
- Chest physical therapy

help promote optimal gas exchange in the older adult with pneumonia. Common nursing interventions for the client with pneumonia can be found in Box 9–7.

NURSING DIAGNOSES

As you are aware, nursing diagnoses are derived from the assessment data and are unique to each older adult. The focus of the nursing diagnosis is the client's response to the particular health problem that he or she faces.

Common nursing diagnoses (written only as the "problem" portion of the *Problem, Etiology,* and *Signs* and symptoms [PES] in the nursing diagnosis statement) that apply to the older adult experiencing disorders covered in this chapter are listed in Table 9–9.

Not every nursing diagnosis identified in Table 9–9 will be appropriate for every client with a given respiratory disorder. Likewise, there may be other nursing diagnoses suitable for your older adult client that cannot be found in the table. For example, not every client with pneumonia will experience pain. Carefully consider every nursing diagnosis to individualize a plan of care for your older adult client with a disorder related to the respiratory system.

COLLABORATING ON THE PLAN OF CARE

After the nursing diagnoses are established, you must develop outcomes for your client. Set outcomes that are realistic, measurable, and tailored to the individual older adult.

Based on the nursing diagnoses discussed in the previous section, sample outcomes for a client with chronic obstructive pulmonary disease can be found in Table 9–10. These are samples only because the outcomes you set must be established with your individual client in mind.

Similarly, sample outcomes for older adults with nursing diagnoses for pneumonia can be found in Table 9–11.

IMPLEMENTING INTERVENTIONS FOR HEALTH PROMOTION

Interventions to Promote Safety

1. Perform careful assessments of the older adult with actual or potential respiratory impairment. Be alert for possible atypical signs and symptoms of pneumonia, such as decreased appetite or altered mental status. Remember that the first sign of hypoxia in the older adult is often confusion and/or restlessness. Report and document any suspicious symptoms immediately.

2. Frequently assess vital signs of the client with pneumonia or respiratory difficulty. Immediately report and document any variations from the client's baseline.

Table 9–9		
NURSING DIAGNOSES RELATED TO OXYGENATION		
	COPD	Pneumonia
Imbalanced nutrition: less than body requirements	X	
Risk for infection	X	X
Risk for imbalanced body temperature		X
Risk for constipation	X	X
Ineffective tissue perfusion: cardiopulmonary	X	X
Risk for imbalanced fluid volume	X	X
Impaired gas exchange	X	X
Risk for activity intolerance	X	X
Fatigue	X	X
Disturbed sleep pattern	X	X
Deficient knowledge	X	X
Pain		X
Anxiety	X	

COPD, chronic obstructive pulmonary disease.

Table 9–10

SAMPLE OUTCOMES FOR AN OLDER ADULT WITH CHRONIC OBSTRUCTIVE PULMONARY DISEASE

Nursing Diagnosis	Sample Outcomes
Imbalanced nutrition: less than body requirements	• Client will consume 1500 kcal per day • Client will experience no respiratory difficulty during eating • Client's weight will increase by 2 pounds within a month
Impaired gas exchange	• Client's vital signs will remain within normal limits • Client will remain alert and oriented to person, place, time, and situation
Risk for activity intolerance	• Client will actively participate in activities of daily living • Client will participate in a supervised, planned exercise program • Client will state the rationale for alternating activity with rest periods

Table 9–11

SAMPLE OUTCOMES FOR AN OLDER ADULT WITH PNEUMONIA

Nursing Diagnosis	Sample Outcomes
Ineffective tissue perfusion: cardiopulmonary	• Client's temperature, pulse, and respiratory rate will be within normal range within 6 hours of beginning antibiotic therapy • Client will have decreased dyspnea within 2 days
Pain	• Client will be free from pain during coughing episodes
Deficient knowledge: pneumonia and its treatment	• Client will state the importance of following measures to prevent transmission of organisms • Client will explain the basic mechanism of action of each medication he or she is taking and major adverse effects to watch for • Client will explain the importance of taking medications for the entire duration prescribed

3. Encourage your older adult clients with COPD to receive annual immunization against influenza to avoid infectious complications.

4. Encourage the older adult to discuss the pneumococcal vaccine with his or her physician or advanced practice nurse. Inform the older adult that this is often a one-time injection, although it may be repeated after 6 years if decreased antibody titer is present.

5. Instruct clients who work or reside in an environment of respiratory irritants to wear personal protective equipment (PPE) such as masks.

6. Teach clients to avoid crowded public areas during the flu season.

7. Educate the client to avoid close contact with persons who have respiratory infection to decrease the chance of contracting it.

8. Teach older adults who must use oxygen at home about safety precautions that must be taken at home and when traveling (Fig. 9–7).

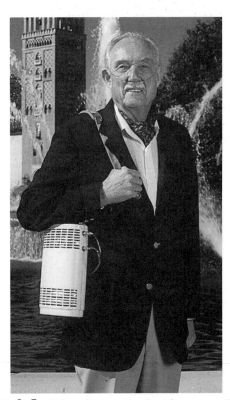

Figure 9–7. Older client using liquid oxygen. (From Lewis, S. M., Heitkemper, M. M., & Dirksen, S. R. [2000]. *Medical-surgical nursing: Assessment and management of clinical problems* [5th ed.]. St. Louis: Mosby, p. 698.)

9. Instruct the client to discuss any over-the-counter medications or herbal therapies with his or her physician or advanced practice nurse before consuming them. Many medications may interact with other medications being taken or may interfere with the client's respiratory drive.

Interventions to Promote Health Education

1. Teach the older adult to avoid substances that irritate the respiratory system, such as household cleaners, aerosol sprays, and known allergens.
2. Reinforce instructions to take medications as directed by the physician or advanced practice nurse. If antibiotic therapy is prescribed, the older adult should take the full course of medications—even if the symptoms have gone away.
3. Instruct the older adult to watch for early signs or symptoms of respiratory infection and to report them immediately. Early recognition and treatment of respiratory infection are crucial in maintaining optimal respiratory functioning for the older adult.
4. Teach the client with chronic obstructive pulmonary disease to report any change in sputum characteristics to his or her physician or advanced practice nurse.
5. Reinforce client teaching regarding the correct technique for metered-dose inhaler (MDI) usage (Box 9–8).
6. Reinforce proper breathing and coughing techniques for clients with COPD or pneumonia.
7. Include the client's family in your teaching.

Interventions to Promote Lifestyle Modification

1. Explain the negative health effects of smoking, such as an exaggeration of age-related decline in FEV_1 and overall respiratory function decline.
2. Encourage the client who does smoke to begin a smoking cessation program. Adjuncts to a smoking cessation program may include nicotine replacement (gum, transdermal, or intranasal methods) and the use of bupropion,

an antidepressant. Other important components of a smoking cessation program involve assisting the older adult with coping skills and providing psychological support. A respiratory support group may provide needed social support to the individual who is trying to quit smoking. Often lifelong smoking cessation is achieved after multiple (often between three and ten) relapses.

Interventions to Promote Mobility

1. Encourage the older adult to engage in a program of physical activity that incorporates cardiopulmonary endurance and diaphragmatic breathing.
2. Educate the older adult with COPD about proper breathing techniques that may ease breathing difficulties and enhance mobility (Fig. 9–8).
3. Encourage the bedridden older adult with pneumonia to turn, perform deep-breathing exercises, and cough every 2 to 4 hours.
4. Instruct the client regarding the use of the incentive spirometer (IS).

Interventions to Promote Nutrition

1. Explain to obese clients that reduction of excess body weight helps to promote optimal respiratory function.
2. Encourage the client with a respiratory disorder to consume a nutritious diet to decrease the risk of respiratory infection.
3. Encourage the older adult to maintain adequate hydration to keep respiratory secretions thin enough to expectorate. In general, a good target is intake of 2 to 3 liters of nonalcoholic, noncaffeinated beverages daily, unless contraindicated.
4. Maintain accurate intake and output records for the client with pneumonia.
5. Educate the older adult that the consumption of small, frequent meals rather than large meals decreases dyspnea and improves oxygenation by decreasing the need for oxygen during digestion.
6. Instruct the client with pneumonia that a minimum of 1500 calories per day is required for optimal tissue healing.

Box 9–8 How to Use an Inhaler Correctly*

Without a Spacer (Preferred Technique)

1. Before each use, remove the cap and shake the inhaler according to the instructions in the package insert.
2. Tilt your head back slightly and breathe out fully.
3. Open your mouth and place the mouthpiece 1 to 2 inches away.
4. As you begin to breathe in deeply through your mouth, press down firmly on the canister of the inhaler to release one dose of medication.
5. Continue to breathe in slowly and deeply (usually over 3 to 5 seconds).
6. Hold your breath for at least 10 seconds to allow the medication to reach deep into the lungs, then breathe out slowly.
7. Wait at least 1 minute between puffs.
8. Replace the cap on the inhaler.
9. At least once a day, remove the canister and clean the plastic case and cap of the inhaler by thoroughly rinsing in warm, running tap water.

Without a Spacer (Alternative Method)

1. Follow steps 1 and 2 above.
2. Place the mouthpiece in your mouth, over your tongue, and seal your lips tightly around it.

3. Follow steps 4 to 9 above.

With a Spacer

1. Before each use, remove the caps from the inhaler and the spacer.
2. Insert the mouthpiece of the inhaler into the nonmouthpiece end of the spacer.
3. Shake the whole unit vigorously 3 or 4 times.
4. Place the mouthpiece in your mouth, over your tongue, and seal your lips tightly around it.
5. Press down firmly on the canister of the inhaler to release one dose of medication into the spacer.
6. Breathe in slowly and deeply. If the spacer makes a whistling sound, you are breathing in too rapidly.
7. Remove the mouthpiece from your mouth and, keeping your lips closed, hold your breath for at least 10 seconds, then breathe out slowly.
8. Wait at least 1 minute between puffs.
9. Replace the caps on the inhaler and the spacer.
10. At least once a day, clean the plastic case and cap of the inhaler by thoroughly rinsing in warm, running tap water; at least once a week, clean the spacer in the same manner.

---

* Avoid spraying in the direction of the eyes.

From Ignatavicius, D. D., Workman, M. L., & Mishler, M. A. (1999). *Medical-surgical nursing across the health care continuum* (3rd ed.). Philadelphia: W. B. Saunders, p. 628.

Interventions to Promote Rest and Sleep

1. Instruct the client with a respiratory illness to alternate activity with rest periods to conserve energy and prevent fatigue.
2. Encourage the older adult to use relaxation techniques that have been helpful in the past. Explain the beneficial effects of relaxation and deep-breathing exercises on promoting respiratory function.
3. Educate the older adult with pneumonia that analgesics can be helpful toward achieving the relaxation needed to obtain sleep.

GATHERING DATA FOR EVALUATION

As was stated earlier in this text, your collaboration with the registered nurse (RN) in the evaluation and modification phases of the nursing process is crucial. Your observations and the data gathered from client interactions will ultimately help guide the care planning process toward successful nursing interventions.

Evaluation of the plan of care must be aimed directly at the outcomes. Many of the outcomes identified earlier in this chapter are very objective; therefore, it is easy to evaluate progress

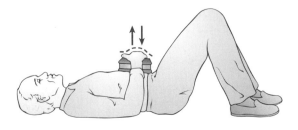

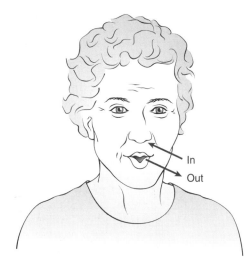

In
Out

Figure 9–8. Breathing exercises. (From Ignatavicius, D. D., Workman, M. L., & Mishler, M. A. [1999]. *Medical-surgical nursing across the healthcare continuum* [3rd ed.]. Philadelphia: W. B. Saunders, p. 630.)

toward attaining them. For example, one outcome identified for the nursing diagnosis, Impaired Gas Exchange, reads, "Client will remain alert and oriented to person, place, time, and situation." You can evaluate this outcome at the bedside through careful observation and questioning. In the evaluation column you can write, "2/22: Client alert and oriented X4," followed by your initials. If the client was partially correct in answering your orientation questions, you could note his or her actual statements and allow the reader to evaluate the responses. For example, you could write, "2/22: Client oriented to person, place, and situation, but states the month is January."

Evaluation of outcomes may also require referral to the client's baseline. One outcome written for the nursing diagnosis, Ineffective Tissue Perfusion: Cardiopulmonary, states, "Client will have decreased dyspnea within 2 days." Evaluation of this outcome requires knowledge of how severe the dyspnea was on initial assessment. It is very important that the "pertinent assessment data" section of the care plan be completed thoroughly to enable the health care professional to determine if client improvement has occurred.

Your evaluation should take into consideration individual interventions employed. Consider the nursing diagnosis, "Imbalanced Nutrition: Less than Body Requirements." It would be helpful to document on the care plan food preferences and dislikes. Or, perhaps while you were assisting your client with a meal, you discovered some environmental modification, such as soft music, that seemed to stimulate his or her appetite. This would be valuable information to communicate to other nurses—via the care plan—that could help your client meet the outcome of consuming 1500 calories per day. Nursing care plans are much more than "busy work." They are useful tools for sharing information with one another so that health care providers are not constantly "reinventing the wheel." By using them as they were designed, caregivers can meet the needs of older adult clients much more efficiently.

Summary

- Age-related changes in the respiratory system include loss of <u>lung elasticity</u>, weakening of respiratory muscles, thinner alveoli, atrophied cilia, weakened cough, and a declining immune system. Certain lifestyle factors, such as smoking and obesity, can further impair lung function.
- Begin your assessment with measurement of vital signs and pulse oximetry. Continue with a head-to-toe approach. Monitor for signs of hypoxia, and note the appearance of musculoskeletal variations such as "barrel chest" and kyphosis.
- Auscultate the lung fields, beginning at the bases. Assess the extremities for ecchymoses, discoloration, and "clubbed" fingernails. Document signs and symptoms such as cough, sputum, dyspnea, and pain.

PPC—personal protective equipment

- COPD is characterized by airflow obstruction caused by chronic bronchitis or emphysema. Cigarette smoking is the primary cause of COPD. Emphysema is characterized by alveolar destruction; lung tissue develops a "floppy" characteristic because of the destruction of elastin and collagen. Chronic bronchitis is characterized by excessive mucus production. Symptoms of a client with COPD can be related to either chronic bronchitis or emphysema, or both. Treatment includes drug therapy, respiratory therapy, pulmonary rehabilitation, and close monitoring of nutritional status.
- Pneumonia is inflammation of the lung tissue, usually related to infection. The older adult with pneumonia may have an atypical presentation. Pneumococcal pneumonia has a higher mortality rate in the older adult population than among younger people. Pneumovax is designed to give protection against this type of pneumonia.
- Older adults are at risk for development of pneumonia because of physical changes associated with their age: decreased immunity, weakened cough reflex, and other illnesses or treatments. Organisms responsible for causing pneumonia reach the lung tissue by aspiration, inhalation, or circulation. The inflammatory process affects the interstitial lung tissue, leading to extravasation of fluid and hypoxemia. The older adult may have an atypical presentation. Treatment depends on the causative agent, and may include antibiotic therapy, bedrest, fluids, and oxygen and/or chest physiotherapy.
- Nursing diagnoses must be unique to the individual client. Once the nursing diagnosis is established, outcomes must be set. They must be realistic, measurable, and tailored to the individual client.
- Interventions to promote safety include the following: perform careful assessment; encourage older adults with COPD to discuss with their physician immunizations against influenza and pneumococcal pneumonia; instruct clients to wear PPE; teach clients to avoid crowds during the flu season and to avoid close contact with persons who have respiratory infection; teach older adults about

oxygen safety; and instruct the client to discuss use of any over-the-counter products or herbs with the physician.
- Interventions to promote health education include the following: teach the older adult to avoid respiratory irritants; reinforce medication instructions; instruct the older adult to watch for early signs or symptoms of respiratory infection or a change in sputum characteristics; and reinforce teaching regarding the MDI, as well as breathing and coughing techniques.
- Interventions to promote lifestyle modification include encouraging the client who smokes to begin a smoking cessation program.
- Interventions to promote mobility include the following: encourage the older adult to engage in physical activity; teach proper breathing techniques; encourage turning, coughing, and deep-breathing exercises for bedridden older adults.
- Interventions to promote nutrition include the following: explain that reduction of excess body weight helps to promote respiratory function; encourage a nutritious diet and adequate hydration; maintain accurate intake and output records; encourage the consumption of small, frequent meals; and instruct the client with pneumonia to consume 1500 calories per day for tissue healing.
- Interventions to promote rest and sleep include the following: encourage relaxation techniques; instruct the client to alternate activity with rest periods; and educate that analgesics can be helpful for promoting relaxation.
- Evaluation should be aimed directly at the outcomes, and should take into consideration the effectiveness of individual interventions.

STUDY QUESTIONS

Multiple-Choice Review

1. Which of the following statements *best* describes age-related changes of the lung?
    1. Residual volume becomes decreased with age.
    2. Smooth muscle is replaced by fibrous connective tissue.

3. Lung tissue becomes more elastic with normal aging.
4. FEV$_1$ increases with age.

2. The primary problem in emphysema is:
   1. Decreased elasticity of lung tissue.
   2. Excess mucus production.
   3. Increased elasticity of lung tissue.
   4. Proliferation of elastin and collagen in the lung tissue.

3. Select the statement that *best* describes the safe use of oxygen therapy for the older adult with COPD:
   1. Oxygen should be used liberally to prevent hypoxia.
   2. Oxygen should be used very cautiously and only under a physician's order.
   3. Clients should be taught to self-adjust the oxygen level.
   4. Mineral oil should be applied to the nares to prevent skin breakdown.

4. The organism to which older adults are especially vulnerable, owing to increased mortality rates from pneumonia caused by this organism, is:
   1. *Staphylococcus aureus.*
   2. *Streptococcus pneumoniae.*
   3. *Pneumocystis carinii.*
   4. *Haemophilus influenzae.*

5. Which of the following is the best example of an *atypical* presentation of pneumonia?
   1. Cough, fever, and pleuritic chest pain
   2. Cough, dyspnea, and crackles
   3. Fever and tachypnea
   4. Fall and decreased appetite

Critical Thinking

1. Describe the effects of smoking, obesity, and immobility on normal aging of the lung.

2. Why should a client with COPD receive low-flow oxygen?

3. Explain why rates of COPD are increasing among women.

4. How would you respond to your client who states, "I've smoked for 50 years and I've never been sick a day in my life. Why should I quit now?"

5. Identify factors that place an older adult at risk for aspiration pneumonia.

Resources

Internet Resources

American Lung Association
www.lungusa.org

National Emphysema Foundation
www.emphysemafoundation.org

National Heart, Lung, and Blood Institute
www.nhlbi.nih.gov

Organizations

American Association of Cardiovascular and Pulmonary Rehabilitation
7611 Elmwood Avenue, Suite 201
Middletown, WI 53562

American Lung Association
1740 Broadway
New York, NY 10019-4373
(212) 245-8000

National Interagency Council on Smoking and Health
Room 1005
291 Broadway
New York, NY 10007

Selected References

Ambrosino, N., Foglio, K., & Bianchi, L. (1997). Pulmonary rehabilitation programs in COPD: Patient selection, therapeutic modalities, and outcome measures. Available at http://www.medscape.com/Medscape/RespiratoryCare/journal/1997/.../mrc3098ambrosino.htm Accessed 8/25/99.

Berglund, D. J., Abbey, D. E., Lebowitz, M. D., et al. (1999). Respiratory symptoms and pulmonary function in an elderly nonsmoking population. *Chest, 115*(1), 49–59.

Cassiere, H. A. (1998). Severe pneumonia in the elderly: Risks, treatment, and prevention. *Medscape Respiratory Care, 2*(2), 1998. Available at http://www.medscape.com/Medscape/RespiratoryCare/1998/v02.n02/mrc4601.cass/mrc4601.cass.html

Early identification and active intervention essential in the long-term management of stable COPD. Available at http://www.medscape.com/adis/DTP/1998/v12.n11/dtp1211.02/pnt-dtp1211.02.html Accessed 8/25/99.

Ely, E. W. (1997). Pneumonia in the elderly: Diagnostic and therapeutic challenges. *Infectious Medicine, 14*(8), 643–654.

Hafner, J., & Ferro, T. J. (1998). Recent developments in the management of COPD. *Hospital Medicine, 34*(1), 29–38.

Healthy People 2010. Available at http://www.health.gov/healthypeople/Document/tableofcontents.htm Accessed 11/15/00.

Hodgson, B. B., & Kizior, R. J. (1999). *Saunders nursing drug handbook.* Philadelphia: W. B. Saunders.

Ignatavicius, D. D., Workman, M. L., & Mishler, M. A. (1999). *Medical-surgical nursing across the health care continuum.* Philadelphia: W. B. Saunders.

Iribarren, C., Tekawa, S. S., & Friedman, G. D. (1999). Effect of cigar smoking on the risk of cardiovascular disease, chronic obstructive pulmonary disease, and cancer in men. *New England Journal of Medicine, 340*(23), 1773–1780.

Lewis, S. M., Heitkemper, M. M., & Dirksen, S. R. (2000). *Medical-surgical nursing: Assessment and management of clinical problems.* St. Louis: Mosby.

Matteson, M. A., McConnell, E. S., & Linton, A. D. (1998). *Gerontological nursing: Concepts and practice.* Philadelphia: W. B. Saunders.

McKay, C. (1999). Best practices: Reducing nosocomial pneumonia. *Supplement to RN,* February 1999.

Monahan, F. D., & Neighbors, M. (1998). *Medical-surgical nursing: Foundations for clinical practice.* Philadelphia: W. B. Saunders.

O'Toole, M. T. (1997). *Encyclopedia and dictionary of medicine, nursing, and allied health.* Philadelphia: W. B. Saunders.

Tyson, S. R. (1999). *Gerontological nursing care.* Philadelphia: W. B. Saunders.

Promoting Sensory/Perceptual Functioning

OBJECTIVES

After completing this chapter, you will be able to:

- Discuss the normal changes of aging that affect sensory/perceptual functioning.
- Describe assessment of sensory organs and expected variations in the older adult.
- Compare the key clinical features of disorders commonly affecting sensory/perceptual functioning of older adults.
- Examine the nursing process in care planning for the older adult with disorders of presbycusis, cerumen impaction, presbyopia, cataracts, glaucoma, and macular degeneration.

CHAPTER OUTLINE

KEY TERMS

Aphakia

Arcus senilis

Central vision

Cerumen

Cochlea

Conductive hearing loss

Hyperopia

Macular degeneration

Myopia

Neovascularization

Otosclerosis

Presbycusis

Presbyopia

Sensorineural hearing loss

Tinnitus

AGE-RELATED CHANGES OF THE SENSE ORGANS

We rely on accurate functioning of our sense organs to correctly perceive our environment, avoid danger, and enjoy many of life's sensory pleasures. With age, some of our sensory abilities decrease, although in a gradual manner, and quality of life need not be affected greatly. Nurses must be able to recognize normal sensory changes of aging to be able to help the older adult compensate for deficits that develop and avoid injury.

Some normal age-related changes involve the external structure of the eye. Some of these changes, such as graying of eyebrows and wrinkled skin around the eyes, are easy to recognize and are commonly thought of as signs of aging (Fig. 10–1). Because of decreased fat tissue around the eyes, they may appear more sunken. The older adult may be at greater risk for injury from a foreign object in the eye owing to decreased tear secretion and fragile conjunctiva.

The internal structure of the eye also undergoes change with aging. Most of these changes are not visible to the eye of the observer, with the exception of loss of iris pigment leading to the appearance of light blue/gray eyes and decreased pupil size. The body compensates for other changes associated with aging. For example, although there is less secretion of aqueous humor in the eye, there is also decreased outflow of fluid from the anterior and posterior chambers; therefore, most older adults do not develop glaucoma from this age-related change. Still

other age-related changes have very important nursing implications for client education. For example, because the older adult has difficulty discriminating between blues and greens, the client with diabetes mellitus should not rely on urine testing for daily monitoring, as discrimination between blues and greens is required. Common age-related changes to the internal structure of the eye are summarized in Box 10–1.

In addition to the structural changes, functional changes develop that affect everyday living for the older adult. Common functional changes

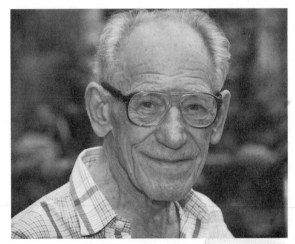

Figure 10–1. Wrinkles are a visible age-related sign of aging. (From Leahy, J. M. & Kiziloy E. [1998]. *Fundamentals of nursing practice*. Philadelphia: W. B. Saunders, p. 352.)

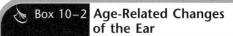

Box 10–1 Age-Related Changes: Internal Eye Structure

- Corneal reflex: diminished or absent
- Aqueous humor secretion: decreased
- Ciliary muscle: shortened
- Lens: yellowed, opaque, with decreased elasticity
- Color discrimination: greater difficulty discriminating between shorter wavelengths of light (violet, blue, and green)
- Iris: loss of pigment
- Pupil: smaller, less reactive to light
- Vitreous humor: begins to liquefy and collapse
- Retina: degeneration

Data from Matteson, M. A., McConnell, E. S., & Linton, A. D. (1998). *Gerontological nursing: Concepts and practice.* Philadelphia: W. B. Saunders.

Box 10–2 Age-Related Changes of the Ear

External Ear

- Increased wrinkling of the skin
- Increased size due to continued growth of cartilage
- Longer, more coarse hairs
- Decreased number and activity of cerumen glands

Middle Ear

- Thickening of tympanic membrane
- Degeneration of ossicles

Inner Ear

- Degeneration of vestibular structures
- Atrophy and neuron loss in cochlea

Data from Matteson, M. A., McConnell, E. S., & Linton, A. D. (1998). *Gerontological nursing: Concepts and practice.* Philadelphia: W. B. Saunders.

---

in vision and implications for nursing care are outlined in Table 10–1.

The process of aging also affects the ear and one's ability to hear. As with the eye, changes are more visible on the external part of the ear than in the middle and inner ear. The most significant effects of age-related changes of the ear include the propensity toward earwax impactions, altered equilibrium, and hearing loss, usually of higher frequencies. Some degree of hearing loss is almost inevitable with advancing age, although institutionalized older adults experience greater hearing deficits than do those living in the community. Age-related changes to the ear are summarized in Box 10–2.

Because the senses of taste and smell are so closely related, age-related effects are described together here. The older adult may experience either a distorted or a diminished sense of taste because of atrophy and a decreased number of taste

---

Table 10–1
FUNCTIONAL CHANGES IN VISION

Category	Age-Related Change	Nursing Implication
Visual acuity	Decreased	• Encourage regular eye examinations
Tolerance of glare	Decreased	• Use soft lighting and nonshiny floor in environment • Encourage limited night driving if especially problematic
Adaptation to dark and light	Decreased	• Allow extra time to make transitions from dark to light and vice versa before moving about • Encourage only limited night driving if oncoming headlights are problematic • Encourage use of red night light (stimulates the cones,* allowing the older adult to see better in the dark)
Peripheral vision	Decreased	• Encourage the older adult to be aware of this change and compensate for it (turn head regularly, etc.)
Depth perception	Distorted	• Encourage caution when descending stairs or driving

*Cone, photoreceptor in the eye that detects color.
Data from Matteson, M. A., McConnell, E. S., & Linton, A. D. (1998). *Gerontological nursing: Concepts and practice.* Philadelphia: W. B. Saunders.

buds. Usually, any age-related impairment of the sense of taste is minor; greater impairments may occur as the result of medications or disease processes.

Nutrition Tip

Assist older adults in identifying foods that appeal to their senses of taste and smell. Choosing foods with a variety of aromas, colors, and textures may help compensate for the diminished sensory appeal of foods.

Aging appears to affect the sense of smell to a greater degree than it affects taste. The mechanism responsible for this is unknown, although researchers postulate that it may be related to degenerative changes in the upper airway or neurologic systems. The sense of smell, like taste, is affected to a much greater degree by various medications and diseases. Other factors that might be to blame include airborne toxins and smoking. Common diseases and medications that diminish the senses of taste and smell are listed in Box 10–3.

The effect of aging on the senses of touch, vibration, and pain is unclear. Some researchers report a decline in these sensations, although further study is needed before we can clearly identify patterns of normal aging of these sensory modalities. In addition, pain is a complex phenomenon, and people vary greatly in their tendency to report pain. There may be a higher pain threshold for the older adult, or the experience of pain may be altered with aging. It is important to consider that pain sensation might be altered with aging: a client experiencing only slight pain will probably not seek medical attention. As a nurse, you must always observe not only for verbal complaints of pain, but also for physical signs, such as tachycardia, tachypnea, guarding of body areas, and stiff movements.

Signs and Symptoms Tip

Atypical presentation of many disease states may be related to decreased pain perception with aging.

ASSESSMENT OF SENSORY/PERCEPTUAL FUNCTIONING

Bedside assessment of sensory organs begins with inspection. Observe the client's eyes for color and clarity. The eyes of a client with cataracts have an opaque appearance. **Arcus senilis,** thought to be due to accumulation of lipids, may be visible on the periphery of the cornea. Observe the eyes for redness, excess tearing, or discharge. Inspect the pupils: are they round and equal? Check the pupil response to light: shine a penlight on the pupil and observe for constriction. When performing this procedure, it is important to make certain that the room is darkened; place the palm of your hand over the bridge of the client's nose to illuminate only the eye being assessed.

If the *p*upils are *e*qual and *r*ound and *r*eact to *l*ight, this may be charted using the acronym

Box 10–3 Diseases and Medications that Diminish the Senses of Taste and Smell

Disease Processes

- Nervous system disorders: Alzheimer's disease, epilepsy, head trauma, Parkinson's disease, and tumors
- Nutritional impairments
- Endocrine disorders: diabetes mellitus, hypothyroidism
- Viral infections
- Local inflammatory processes: bronchial asthma, sinusitis

Medications

- Anti-inflammatory medications
- Antihypertensives
- Cardiac medications
- Lipid-lowering agents
- Antihistamines
- Bronchodilators
- Chemotherapy
- Anticonvulsants
- Vasodilators

Data from Alspach, G. (1998). Chemosensory impairments: Nothing to sniff at. *Critical Care Nurse, 18*(2), 16–18.

PERRL. Perform a gross visual examination by asking the client to read a large sign or to identify an object across the room. Alternatively, you can ask the client to read a large print document held at arm's length. Document and report any unusual findings to the registered nurse (RN).

Next, inspect the ears of the client. Observe the size, shape, and symmetry of the ears. Inspect for any excess accumulation of **cerumen**. A gross assessment of hearing can be done at the bedside by whispering a question into the client's ear. Document and report unusual findings.

Taste and smell can be grossly evaluated at mealtime. Select an aromatic item from the client's tray, such as coffee, and ask the older adult to close his or her eyes and identify the source of the aroma. Select a different item from the tray, such as a dessert item, and provide the client with a taste of the food, again with eyes closed. Ask the client to identify whether the item was sweet, salty, sour, or bitter. Document your findings.

To assess touch, ask the client to close his or her eyes while you lightly touch the forehead with a wisp of cotton. Ask which part of the face is being touched. You may also touch the forearms, hands, and fingertips. Vibration can be assessed with a tuning fork, if one is available. This author does not recommend inflicting pain on the older adult for purposes of assessment; however, it is very important to ask about its presence and to assess for nonverbal signs of pain, such as those described earlier.

As was described in earlier chapters of this book, *Healthy People 2010* contains goals and objectives that relate to the health of individuals. Selected *Healthy People 2010* objectives that address vision and hearing can be found in Box 10–4.

DISORDERS COMMON IN OLDER ADULTS

Presbycusis

Presbycusis is a progressive loss of hearing associated with aging. This hearing loss is bilateral, and predominantly affects the ability to hear sounds at high frequencies. Speech discrimination may be affected, and the ability to hear when background noise is present becomes more difficult. Presbycusis is a form of **sensorineural hearing loss**. The differences between the two major

---

Box 10–4 **Selected *Healthy People 2010* Vision and Hearing Objectives**

- Increase the proportion of persons who have a dilated eye examination at appropriate intervals.
- Reduce visual impairment due to glaucoma.
- Reduce visual impairment due to cataract.
- Increase the use of appropriate personal protective eyewear in recreational activities and hazardous situations around the home.
- Increase vision rehabilitation.
- Increase access by persons who have hearing impairments to hearing rehabilitation services and adaptive devices, including hearing aids, cochlear implants, or tactile or other assistive or augmentative devices.
- Increase the proportion of persons who have had a hearing examination on schedule.
- Increase the number of persons who are referred by their primary care physician for hearing evaluation and treatment.
- Increase the use of appropriate ear protection devices, equipment, and practices.
- Reduce adult hearing loss in the noise-exposed public.

From U. S. Department of Health and Human Services. *Healthy People 2010: Understanding and Improving Health*, 2nd Edition. Washington, D. C.: U. S. Government Printing Office, November 2000.

---

categories of hearing loss, sensorineural and **conductive hearing loss**, are outlined in Box 10–5.

Tinnitus may accompany hearing loss. Tinnitus affects approximately 11% of people with presbycusis (Podoshin, Ben-David, & Teszler, 1997) and can be especially troublesome. Generally, one thinks of tinnitus as ringing in the ears, but that description is actually a bit oversimplified. Tinnitus can consist of a variety of sounds, such as ringing, buzzing, hissing, or a sound similar to that of a generator humming. It can affect one or both ears, and may affect each ear differently. It can be uncomfortably loud at times, especially if the client speaks loudly or shouts. The chronic nature of it can be particularly distressing, especially if the individual wishes to enjoy a quiet activity, such as reading. Imagine how much more difficult it would be for you to focus on your reading right now with one more thing—tinnitus—to contend with!

Box 10–5 Differences Between Sensorineural and Conductive Hearing Loss

Sensorineural Hearing Loss

- Inner ear disorder
- Results from damage to the cochlea or cochlear portion of the eighth cranial nerve
- Transmission of the auditory signal to the brain is interrupted
- Numerous causes include ototoxicity, presbycusis, Meniere's disease, birth trauma, exposure to excessive noise, multiple sclerosis, autoimmune disease, and congenital abnormalities

Conductive Hearing Loss

- Middle or external ear disorder
- Results from obstruction or reduction in the passage of sound to the cochlea
- Causes include infection, congenital deformity, tumor, trauma, **otosclerosis,** and cerumen impaction
- Often treatable

Data from Murphy, M. P., & Gates, G. A. (1997). Hearing loss: Does gender play a role? *Medscape Women's Health*, 2(10).

Controversy exists as to whether there is a gender difference in susceptibility to age-related hearing loss. Older women generally do have superior hearing in the high tones, although it is hypothesized that this may be due to less exposure to hazardous noise levels, rather than a gender difference per se. Because of changes in work and social environments, it remains to be seen whether these gender differences in hearing will continue over the coming years.

Various treatment strategies have been developed to help the older adult maintain effective communication. Newer digital hearing aids make use of computer chip technology, and can be programmed similarly to a stereo to amplify or diminish only the specific sounds with which the client needs assistance. Because these devices are new, the price may be expensive for an older adult on a fixed income; however, as with all new technology, the price is expected to decrease over time. Descriptions of treatments available to individuals with hearing loss are outlined in Table 10–2.

Current research in the field focuses on hair cell regeneration. This involves the regeneration and replacement of damaged hair cells in the inner ear, and is believed to be the ultimate cure for sensorineural hearing loss.

Cerumen Impaction

Cerumen impaction is an occurrence for which many older adults are at risk because of age-related changes to the cerumen glands. Remember that these glands decrease in number and

The primary risk factor for presbycusis is advanced age, owing to the changes that occur to the middle and inner ear. Other factors contribute, such as a lifetime of recreational and occupational noise exposure. Cardiovascular disease has been linked to hearing loss, resulting from altered perfusion of the **cochlea.**

Table 10–2	
TREATMENTS FOR HEARING LOSS	
Example	**Description/Examples**
Speech reading	• The integration of lip movement, body gestures, facial expressions, situation cues, and other factors
Personal listening devices	• Telephone amplifiers • Infrared television listening systems • Closed-caption television adapters • Light systems that flash when activated by television, alarm clock, doorbell, or smoke detector
Amplification	• Four types of hearing aids: body, behind the ear, in the ear, and in the ear canal • Newer devices are programmable and use remote control units
Cochlear implants	• Provide electrical stimulation to the auditory nerve, bypassing damaged hair cells • Include a microphone, a processor located outside the body, and a surgically implanted electrode

Data from Murphy, M. P., & Gates, G. A. (1997). Hearing loss: Does gender play a role? *Medscape Women's Health, 2*(10).

activity as one ages, thus producing a thicker substance. An additional risk factor is the use of hearing aids, as the presence of a foreign body in the ear canal affects the body's ability to remove cerumen. Approximately one third of older adults living in the community experience cerumen impaction, and the incidence is believed to be much higher in institutional settings (Stone, 1999).

Impaction of cerumen in the ear canal leads to a conductive hearing loss. Cerumen in the ear canal blocks the transmission of sound to the tympanic membrane, middle ear, and inner ear. This can often go unnoticed, as the cerumen builds up over time. You may mistake cerumen impaction for confusion or a lack of cooperation by the client, when, in reality, the client cannot clearly hear your instructions. It is important to detect cerumen impaction, as it is easily treated.

Signs of cerumen impaction include the obvious one of the individual asking you to repeat information; less obvious signs include confusion or paranoia. Examination of the ear canal with an otoscope by the registered or advanced practice nurse will reveal the build-up of cerumen, and possibly redness, swelling, or discharge. Symptoms that the client may experience include dizziness, pain, pruritus, and a feeling of fullness or pressure in the ear.

Treatment for removal of cerumen includes lavage or irrigation and curette. Licensed personnel may perform gentle lavage using body temperature water or another solution (such as a weak hydrogen peroxide solution) ordered by the physician or advanced practice nurse, if permitted by institutional policy. Only the physician or advanced practice nurse should perform curette. Neither procedure should be performed if a perforated tympanic membrane is suspected.

Presbyopia

Presbyopia is the inability of the eyes to accommodate to close and detailed work. It is a normal age-related change of the eye that occurs because of changes in the ligaments, muscles, and nerves of the eyes. Presbyopia begins in the fourth decade of life, although it appears earlier in individuals with **hyperopia** and those living in warm climates, and later in individuals with **myopia**.

Presbyopia generally does not present great danger to the older adult, but rather is an inconvenience. Reading material or detailed work, such as needlepoint, must be held at arm's length for the best view.

Treatment for presbyopia primarily consists of corrective lenses or contact lenses. Most individuals with presbyopia will require an increase in the strength of their reading glasses every 2 to 3 years between the ages of 45 and 65.

Cataracts

A cataract is an opacity or clouding of the normally clear crystalline lens of the eye. Cataracts are a very common occurrence in the older adult, affecting approximately 70% of adults over the age of 75 (Lewis, Heitkemper, & Dirksen, 2000). The occurrence of cataracts is one of the most common causes of preventable blindness in the older adult. They can occur in one or both eyes.

With cataract formation, the client experiences a gradual loss of vision. The most common symptom is that of seeing halos around objects as light is diffused around them. Other visual symptoms experienced by the client include blurring, decreased perception of light, abnormal color perception, and sensitivity to glare.

Cataract development in the older adult appears to be related to age-related alterations in metabolic processes within the lens of the eye. These age-related changes lead to an accumulation of water and an alteration in lens fiber structure, and result in decreased transparency. Factors in addition to age, outlined in Box 10–6, can lead to the development of cataracts.

> **Box 10–6   Risk Factors for Cataract Development**
>
> - Advanced age
> - Physical trauma
> - Ultraviolet light
> - X-ray radiation
> - Medications such as corticosteroids
> - Congenital factors such as maternal rubella
> - Ocular inflammation
>
> ---
>
> Data from Lewis, S. M., Heitkemper, M. M., & Dirksen, S. R. (2000). *Medical-surgical nursing: Assessment and management of clinical problems.* St. Louis: Mosby.

Cataract development can be worsened when the older adult has diabetes, hypertension, or kidney disease. Both oral and inhaled corticosteroid use have been associated with increased incidence of cataracts; however, intranasal steroid use does not seem to increase the likelihood of cataract development.

Health Promotion Tip

There are no proven measures to prevent the development of cataracts; however, the following interventions *may* help:

- Wear sunglasses in bright sunlight.
- Avoid unnecessary radiation.
- Avoid exposure to toxins.
- Maintain good nutrition for antioxidant vitamin intake.
- Appropriately manage medical conditions such as diabetes and hypertension.

Treatment of cataracts is primarily surgical. Several years ago, older adults were forced to allow cataracts to ripen and did not receive the surgical procedure until nearly blind. More modern thinking has led to earlier intervention, however, and surgery is usually performed once the decrease in visual acuity affects one's daily life. During the surgical procedure, the damaged lens is removed from the eye and replaced with an artificial lens. Success rates with this type of procedure are very good, and it can lead to a dramatic improvement in the quality of life for the older adult.

Glaucoma

Glaucoma is a chronic, progressive disorder that leads to blindness if left untreated. It is one of the leading preventable causes of blindness and has been described as a thief in the night because often the symptoms are absent or so subtle that the client is unaware of the disorder until vision has been lost.

Health Promotion Tip

Encourage all older adults to undergo glaucoma screening annually.

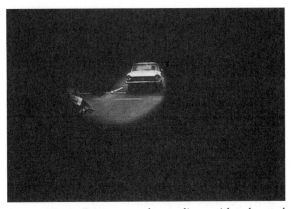

Figure 10–2. Image seen by a client with advanced glaucoma. Note small center island of vision. (From American Foundation for the Blind, 15 West 16th Street, New York, NY 10011, with permission.)

In glaucoma, intraocular pressure (IOP) of the eye is increased, which leads to damage of the optic nerve and irreversible blindness. Most clients with glaucoma experience a very gradual loss of vision, but no pain (Fig. 10–2). There are two types of glaucoma: open-angle glaucoma and angle-closure glaucoma. Open-angle glaucoma is the chronic, insidious type, whereas angle-closure glaucoma is the result of a sudden obstruction of the angle of the anterior chamber, leading to an acute increase in IOP. Because this increased IOP occurs rapidly, the client with angle-closure glaucoma will have symptoms of eye pain, headache, nausea, vomiting, and blurred vision. Open-angle glaucoma is far more common, accounting for 80% of all cases.

Age is the most important predictor for glaucoma, although there are other important risk factors, such as family history and race. Risk factors for glaucoma are outlined in Box 10–7.

Early treatment of glaucoma is extremely important in arresting progression of the disorder. If detected early, loss of vision may be prevented or slowed. The aim of treatment is threefold: to prevent vision loss, to prevent further damage to optic nerve fibers, and to reduce intraocular pressure. To assess severity of the disorder and evaluate response to treatment, the ophthalmologist performs examination of the eye, examination of the optic nerve, and visual field assessment. In addition, IOP measurements are taken.

Box 10–7 Risk Factors for Glaucoma

- Advanced age
- Races: African American, Chinese
- Family history of glaucoma
- Female gender
- Elevated intraocular pressure
- Associated conditions: diabetes mellitus, thyroid disease, myopia, hypertension, and cardiovascular disease

---

Adapted from Ebersole, P., & Hess, P. (1998). *Toward healthy aging.* St. Louis: Mosby-Year Book, p. 447.

Treatments employed for glaucoma usually begin with medications aimed at decreasing the IOP. These medications are given in the form of eyedrops. Drugs from various classifications, which either enhance outflow or reduce production of aqueous humor, are used to treat glaucoma. Table 10–3 lists categories and common examples of medications used in glaucoma treatment.

If medications are unsuccessful in lowering IOP, laser treatment may be used. This procedure is called *argon laser trabeculoplasty* and is usually

---

Table 10–3
CATEGORIES AND COMMON EXAMPLES OF MEDICATIONS USED IN GLAUCOMA TREATMENT

Category	Examples
Beta-blockers	• timolol (Timoptic)
	• levobunolol (Betagan)
	• betaxolol (Betoptic)
	• carteolol (Ocupress)
Prostaglandin analogs	• latanoprost (Xalatan)
Adrenergic agonists	• epinephrine (Glaucon)
	• dipivefrin (Propine)
	• apraclonidine (Iopidine)
	• brimonidine (Alphagan)
Carbonic anhydrase inhibitors	• dorzolamide (Trusopt)
	• acetazolamide (Diamox)
	• methazolamide (Neptazane)
	• dichlorphenamide (Daranide)
Cholinergic agonists	• pilocarpine (Isopto Carpine)
	• echothiophate (Phospholine Iodide)
	• physostigmine (Eserine)

Data from Hodgson, B. B., & Kizior, R. J. (1999). *Saunders nursing drug handbook.* Philadelphia: W. B. Saunders.

---

done in an ophthalmologist's office. Using a slit-lamp mounted laser, a series of small laser burns are created in the trabecular meshwork. This pulls the drainage channels open, allowing outflow of aqueous humor, thus lowering IOP. This procedure effectively lowers IOP at first in most clients, but may need to be repeated and usually loses its effectiveness over time.

Intraocular surgery is another treatment that may be employed if both medications and laser treatment are no longer successful in maintaining IOP at an acceptable level. Different types of surgery either create alternate pathways for the drainage of aqueous humor or destroy structures responsible for its production.

Age-Related Macular Degeneration

Age-related **macular degeneration**, or AMD, is the leading cause of blindness in older adults. It affects both the retina and the layers beneath the retina, and leads to the loss of **central vision**.

Although the disorder affects more than 40% of people over age 70, most individuals have the early form of the disorder, and it does not worsen to advanced disease and blindness. When advanced AMD strikes, one of two processes is usually to blame: choroidal **neovascularization** (wet AMD) or geographic atrophy (dry AMD). Early AMD is compared with these two late forms in Table 10–4.

With the loss of central vision, the older adult experiences greater difficulty seeing fine details. Certain tasks become more difficult, such as reading, writing, sewing, or recognizing faces. Objects may appear bent, crooked, or distorted. The client may also complain of seeing a fixed gray spot just off the center of vision, similar to just having had a flash photograph taken (Fig. 10–3).

Peripheral vision remains intact with macular degeneration, however, allowing the client to ambulate easily and remain independent in most activities. To the casual bystander, the older adult with macular degeneration may appear to have normal vision. This can create problems in social situations, in which the inability to recognize faces can be perceived as rudeness.

Unfortunately, there is no medical, surgical, or laser treatment available to the client with

| Table 10–4 | | | |
| AGE-RELATED MACULAR DEGENERATION | | | |
	Early AMD	Choroidal Neovascularization ("Wet" AMD)	Geographic Atrophy ("Dry" AMD)
Pathophysiology	Yellow-white deposits beneath retina Altered pigment Atrophy of retinal pigment epithelium	Abnormal new blood vessels growing under retina, which leak, bleed, and ultimately scar	Areas of change in color and thickness on a background of relatively normal-appearing retina
Onset of central visual loss	Mild, gradual decrease	Acute decrease	Gradual decrease
Visual acuity	Good	Initially may range from mildly reduced to legal blindness	Initially may range from mildly reduced to legal blindness
Blind spots	Yes	No	No
Reading	Not or minimally affected	Reduced reading rate, need large-print materials	Reduced reading rate, may need large-print materials, depending on location of blind spot
Face recognition	Not affected	Difficult	Difficult
Other symptoms	Mild difficulty in dim lighting	Distortion, waviness of lines near center	Severe difficulty in dim lighting
Prognosis	Most do not develop advanced AMD	Most develop legal blindness within 2 years	May develop legal blindness over a number of years

AMD, age-related macular degeneration.
Adapted from Weksler, M. E. (1998). Age-related macular degeneration: How science is improving clinical care (an interview with Janet S. Sunness, MD). *Geriatrics, 53*(2), 71.

geographic atrophy. The treatment options are only slightly better for one with choroidal neovascularization. He or she may be a candidate for laser therapy. In this instance, laser therapy is used to seal the blood vessels, thus stopping leaking and bleeding and further neovascularization. Whether or not the client is a candidate for this procedure depends on a variety of factors; although the procedure does not improve vision, it may reduce the amount of distortion present.

NURSING DIAGNOSES

Nursing diagnoses for the client with a sensory or perceptual impairment are derived from the assessment data and are unique to each older adult. The focus of the nursing diagnosis, as always, is the client's response to the particular health problem.

Common nursing diagnoses (written only as the "problem" portion of the *Problem, Etiology,* and *Signs* and symptoms [PES] in the nursing

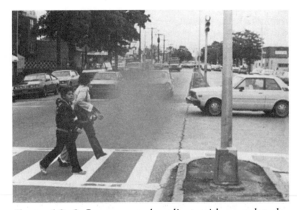

Figure 10–3. Image seen by client with macular degeneration. (From American Foundation for the Blind, 15 West 16th Street, New York, NY 10011, with permission.)

Table 10–5
NURSING DIAGNOSES RELATED TO SENSORY/PERCEPTUAL FUNCTIONING

	Presbycusis	Cerumen Impaction	Presbyopia	Cataracts	Glaucoma	Macular Degeneration
Risk for injury	X	X		X	X	X
Impaired social interaction	X	X		X	X	X
Social isolation	X			X	X	X
Impaired verbal communication	X	X				
Disturbed sensory perception	X	X	X	X	X	X
Deficient knowledge	X	X	X	X	X	X
Anticipatory grieving						X
Anxiety	X	X	X	X	X	X
Pain				X	X	

diagnosis statement) that apply to the older adult experiencing sensory/perceptual disorders are listed in Table 10–5.

Not every nursing diagnosis identified in Table 10–5 will be appropriate for every client with a given sensory/perceptual disorder. Likewise, there may be other nursing diagnoses suitable for your older adult client that cannot be found in the table. For example, if the client with glaucoma has been diagnosed early and has minimal or no vision loss, social isolation may not be an issue. The client with a small cerumen impaction will probably have just a few nursing diagnoses. Carefully consider every nursing diagnosis to individualize a plan of care for your older adult client with any type of sensory/perceptual disorder.

COLLABORATING ON THE PLAN OF CARE

After the nursing diagnoses are established, you must develop outcomes for your client. Set outcomes that are realistic, measurable, and tailored to the individual older adult.

Based on the nursing diagnoses discussed in the previous section, sample outcomes for a client with presbycusis can be found in Table 10–6.

These are samples only; the outcomes that you set must be established with your individual client in mind.

Similarly, sample outcomes for older adults with nursing diagnoses for cerumen impaction can be found in Table 10–7.

Sample outcomes for clients with visual disorders of presbyopia, cataracts, glaucoma, and age-related macular degeneration can be found in Tables 10–8, 10–9, 10–10, and 10–11, respectively.

Table 10–6
SAMPLE OUTCOMES FOR AN OLDER ADULT WITH PRESBYCUSIS

Nursing Diagnosis	Sample Outcomes
Social isolation	• Client will state methods for compensating in social situations for the loss of high-frequency hearing • Client will participate in social activities within his or her level of comfort
Disturbed sensory perception	• Client will function within his/her environment with the use of optical devices
Anxiety	• Client will verbalize concerns about presbycusis • Client will identify methods of reducing anxiety that have worked in the past

Table 10–7
SAMPLE OUTCOMES FOR AN OLDER ADULT WITH CERUMEN IMPACTION

Nursing Diagnosis	Sample Outcomes
Risk for injury	• Client will describe a safe method for removing cerumen from the ear • Client will describe rationale for not using cotton swab to clean ear canal • Client will remain free from injury
Deficient knowledge	• Client will state the physiologic reason why older adults are prone to cerumen impaction • Client will state the rationale for weekly cleaning of the ears and hearing aid
Impaired verbal communication	• Client will communicate effectively with others

IMPLEMENTING INTERVENTIONS FOR HEALTH PROMOTION

Interventions to Promote Safety

1. Educate the older adult about the effect of aging on the senses of smell and taste and how to avoid danger in his or her environment. For example, the older adult living alone may not

Table 10–8
SAMPLE OUTCOMES FOR AN OLDER ADULT WITH PRESBYOPIA

Nursing Diagnosis	Sample Outcomes
Sensory/perceptual alteration: visual	• Client will function within his or her environment using optical devices • Client will avoid injury
Deficient knowledge	• Client will describe, in lay terms, the age-related changes to vision that occur • Client will verbalize the importance of obtaining the correct prescription for visual correction
Anxiety	• Client will verbalize his or her concerns about the aging process • Client will accept visual changes

Table 10–9
SAMPLE OUTCOMES FOR AN OLDER ADULT WITH CATARACTS

Nursing Diagnosis	Sample Outcomes
Risk for injury	• Client will implement safety measures to compensate for the alterations in visual acuity • Client's eye heals without postoperative evidence of trauma • Client will refrain from rubbing eye postoperatively
Deficient knowledge	• Client will demonstrate correct application of eye shield • Client will state name, purpose, and schedule of medications • Client will state signs and symptoms of complications that must be reported • Client will describe activity restrictions and the rationale for such
Anxiety	• Client will verbalize his or her concerns about surgery • Client will verbalize a decrease in anxiety level

Table 10–10
SAMPLE OUTCOMES FOR AN OLDER ADULT WITH GLAUCOMA

Nursing Diagnosis	Sample Outcomes
Risk for injury	• Client will describe how to use existing vision to promote safety • Client will avoid injury
Deficient knowledge	• Client will verbalize the importance of the treatment regimen • Client will state name, purpose, and schedule of medications • Client will develop a schedule for administration of eye medications
Pain	• Client will identify both pharmacologic and nonpharmacologic pain management measures that are available • Client will verbalize a decrease in pain level

Table 10–11 SAMPLE OUTCOMES FOR AN OLDER ADULT WITH MACULAR DEGENERATION	
Nursing Diagnosis	**Sample Outcomes**
Risk for injury	• Client will describe how to use existing vision to promote safety • Client will describe changes he or she can make to the home environment to maximize remaining vision • Client will avoid injury
Social isolation	• Client will identify and use support systems • Client will interact with others on a daily basis • Client will verbalize feeling of decreased social isolation
Anxiety	• Client will identify measures that have helped decrease anxiety in the past • Client will verbalize anxieties and fears • Client will report a decreased anxiety level

identify a gas leak as quickly as a younger adult might; therefore, it is very important to keep household appliances in good working order and regularly inspected. In addition, the older adult may have difficulty identifying foods that have begun to spoil; therefore, it is important to buy smaller portions of perishable foods and discard by the dates recommended on the packaging.

2. Recommend to the older client screening for hearing loss on an annual basis.
3. Encourage the older adult with hearing loss to have safety features installed into his or her home. For example, flashing light systems can be installed that are activated by smoke detectors.
4. Teach the older adult with macular degeneration how to partially compensate for the loss of central vision by using his or her peripheral vision. If the client looks above the object to be viewed, he or she can often see it better because the "blind spot" of the eye is now above the object, and the peripheral vision will take over.
5. Explain the importance of adequate, nonglare lighting to all older adults, especially those with any type of visual impairment.

6. Educate the older adult with diabetes that blood glucose measurement with a digital numeric readout ("fingerstick") is safer than urine testing for at-home monitoring. The urine test requires subtle discrimination between blue and green colors, which may be difficult for the aging eye.
7. Encourage the client with any visual deficit to plan effective safety measures in his or her environment. This includes such changes as removing small items from frequently traveled pathways and eliminating throw rugs.

Interventions to Promote Health Education

1. Educate the older adult about the importance of regular examination of the ear canals for cerumen. This should be included as a regular part of any routine screening examination, and should be performed more frequently for individuals who wear hearing aids (Fig. 10–4).
2. Teach the family of the older adult with macular degeneration about the role of central versus peripheral vision.
3. Educate older adults to undergo screening for glaucoma annually, or more frequently if risk

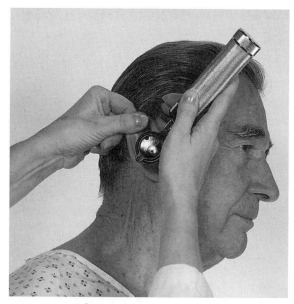

Figure 10–4. Otoscopic examination. (From Jarvis, C. [2000]. *Physical examination and health assessment* [3rd ed.]. Philadelphia: W. B. Saunders, p. 355.)

factors are present. This simple test, using a hand-held device, blasts a "puff of air" onto the client's cornea, and can be done quickly. If pressures appear to be elevated, more precise tonometry can be performed.

4. Review medication actions, dosages, and potential adverse effects with the older adult. The client with prescribed eyedrops may not consider these "real" medications because they are not taken orally. It is important to point out, however, that many of these medications may cause systemic adverse effects and could interact with other medications the client is taking.

Interventions to Promote Lifestyle Modification

1. Encourage the older adult with visual difficulties to select large-print materials or a magnifying glass.
2. Assist the older adult with hearing impairment in finding items to modify the environment to promote independence. For example, lights to signal a ringing telephone or doorbell may be helpful.
3. Inform the client who has undergone cataract removal to avoid contact sports. The absence of the body's crystalline lens, a condition known as **aphakia**, places the client at increased risk for retinal detachment. A sudden blow to the head in a susceptible individual can lead to detachment of the retina.

Interventions to Promote Mobility

1. Encourage the client with a visual impairment to keep the floor environment free from clutter, such as dog dishes, throw rugs, and extension cords.
2. Encourage the client with a visual impairment to avoid using furniture to assist balance. Following cataract surgery, depth perception is altered, and objects may not be where they appear to be.

Interventions to Promote Nutrition

1. Inform the older adult that his or her senses of taste and smell may be diminished as a process of aging.

2. Assess carefully for weight loss or signs of malnutrition as a result of diminished sensation.

Interventions to Promote Rest and Sleep

1. Assist the client with tinnitus to explore methods to promote relaxation and sleep. Some individuals have reported success by using "white noise" or a low-volume radio. Others have tried biofeedback with successful results.
2. Assist the client with pain management, including both pharmacologic and nonpharmacologic methods. Pain management is an important aspect of postoperative care for clients who have had eye surgery. Pain management may also be needed for some clients with glaucoma who experience eye pain with increased intraocular pressure. Instruct the client to notify the physician about any pain that is not relieved by acetaminophen.
3. Instruct the postoperative client to sleep with the head of the bed up slightly to promote comfort and reduce edema.
4. Suggest refrigeration of eyedrop medications for the postoperative cataract surgery client. Refrigeration will provide a cool, comfortable sensation when the medication is applied and will help reduce the sensation of pruritus that accompanies the healing process.

GATHERING DATA FOR EVALUATION

Your collaboration with the RN in the evaluation and modification of the plan of care for the older adult with a sensory/perceptual alteration is crucial. Your observations and data gathering regarding the older adult's sensory functioning will provide valuable information to facilitate the choice of successful nursing interventions.

As was pointed out in earlier chapters, evaluation of the care plan must be aimed directly at the outcomes. Many of the outcomes identified earlier in the chapter are very objective; therefore, it is easy to evaluate progress toward attaining them. For example, one outcome identified for the nursing diagnosis, Knowledge Deficit, reads, "Client will state the rationale for weekly cleaning of ears and hearing aid." This outcome can be evaluated at the bedside through your questioning of the client. In the evaluation column, you can write, "11/6: Client able to state rationale for weekly cleaning," followed by your initials. If the client was partially correct in answering your orientation questions, you could note his or her actual statements and allow the reader to evaluate the responses.

Evaluation of outcomes may also require referral to the client's baseline. For example, one expected outcome written for the nursing diagnosis, Pain, states, "Client will verbalize a decrease in pain level." Although the client's statement will serve as the primary source of information, you may wish to refer to your baseline nursing information to validate this information.

In addition, your evaluation should take into consideration individual interventions employed. Consider the nursing diagnosis, Pain. It will be helpful to document on the care plan which medications were most effective for pain relief. Or, perhaps while you were assisting your client with activities of daily living, you discovered an effective nonpharmacologic intervention that provided pain relief. This would be valuable information to communicate to other nurses—via the care plan—that could help your client meet the outcome of pain reduction.

Summary

- Age-related changes to the eye include graying of eyebrows, wrinkled skin, sunken-appearing eyes, decreased tear secretion, and fragile conjunctiva. Eyes appear more blue/gray with decreased pupil size. Functional changes include decreases in: depth perception, adaptation to dark and light, tolerance to glare, visual acuity, and peripheral vision.
- Age-related changes of the ear include the risk for earwax impaction, altered equilibrium, and hearing loss, usually of higher frequencies.
- The senses of taste and smell are affected more by medications, diseases, and nutritional deficiencies than by aging.
- Assessment begins with inspection. Observe the client's eyes for color, clarity, redness, discharge, and PERRL. Inspect the ears, noting size, shape, symmetry, and excess cerumen. Perform a gross assessment of vision and hearing. Evaluate taste and smell at mealtime; assess light touch.

- Presbycusis is a progressive, bilateral, sensorineural hearing loss, characterized by high-frequency hearing loss and sometimes tinnitus. The primary risk factor is age. Treatment strategies include the use of hearing aids and personal listening devices.
- Cerumen impaction leads to a conductive hearing loss. Signs include evidence of hearing deficit, confusion, or paranoia. The ear canal shows build-up of cerumen, redness, swelling, or discharge. Treatments include lavage or irrigation and curette.
- Presbyopia is the inability of the eyes to accommodate to close work. It is a normal age-related change; treatment consists primarily of corrective or contact lenses.
- A cataract is a clouding of the lens of one or both eyes, and is very common with age. The client experiences gradual vision loss, sees halos around objects, and develops blurring and sensitivity to glare. Ultraviolet light and medications are risk factors. Treatment is primarily surgical, involving replacement of the lens with an artificial lens.
- Glaucoma is a progressive disorder involving an increase in IOP, damage to the optic nerve, and blindness if untreated. Open-angle glaucoma is chronic, insidious, and more common. Angle-closure glaucoma occurs when a sudden obstruction of the angle leads to an acute increase in IOP, characterized by eye pain, headache, nausea, vomiting, and blurred vision. Age, family history, and race are risk factors. Early treatment is crucial, and begins with eyedrops. Laser treatment or intraocular surgery may be performed.
- AMD is the leading cause of blindness in older adults, involving the loss of central vision. Most individuals have the "early" form of the disorder, and it does not worsen to blindness. With the loss of central vision, the older adult experiences greater difficulty seeing fine details; however, peripheral vision remains intact. There are no medical, surgical, or laser treatments available for the client with geographic atrophy; however, the client with choroidal neovascularization may be a candidate for laser therapy.
- Nursing diagnoses are unique to the individual client. Once the nursing diagnosis is

established, outcomes must be set. It is important that they be realistic, measurable, and tailored to the individual client.

- Interventions to promote safety include the following: educate about the effect of aging on smell and taste and how to avoid danger; recommend annual screening for hearing loss; encourage the older adult with hearing loss to have safety features installed into the home; teach the older adult with macular degeneration how to use peripheral vision; teach the importance of adequate, nonglare lighting; and encourage the client with a visual deficit to plan and implement safety measures in the environment.

- Interventions to promote health education include the following: educate the older adult about regular examination of the ear canals for cerumen; teach the family of the older adult with macular degeneration about central versus peripheral vision; encourage annual screening for glaucoma; and review medication actions, dosages, and adverse effects.

- Interventions to promote lifestyle modification include the following: encourage selection of large-print materials or a magnifying glass; assist the older adult with hearing impairment in finding items to modify the environment; and inform the client who has undergone cataract surgery to avoid contact sports.

- Interventions to promote mobility include the following: encourage the client with a visual impairment to keep the floor environment free from clutter and to avoid using furniture to assist balance.

- Interventions to promote nutrition include the following: inform the older adult that taste and smell may be diminished owing to aging; assess carefully for weight loss or signs of malnutrition.

- Interventions to promote rest and sleep include the following: assist the client with tinnitus to find methods to promote relaxation; assist with pain management; instruct the postoperative client to sleep with the head of the bed up slightly; suggest refrigeration of eyedrop medications post cataract surgery.

- Evaluation should be aimed directly at the outcomes, and should take into consideration the effectiveness of individual interventions.

STUDY QUESTIONS

Multiple-Choice Review

1. Which of the following findings would accurately represent a normal change of aging?
   1. Increased fat tissue around the eye
   2. Increased tear secretion
   3. Increased pupil size
   4. Increased fragility of conjunctiva

2. Which of the following statements is true regarding hearing loss in one's older years?
   1. Some degree of hearing loss is common as one ages.
   2. Older adults living in the community experience a greater degree of hearing loss than do those living in extended-care facilities.
   3. Hearing loss with age usually affects sounds of lower frequencies.
   4. Thinning of the tympanic membrane is the major cause of hearing loss in older adults.

3. Which of the following assessment findings in the older adult should immediately be reported to the registered nurse?
   1. Increased size of the ear pinna
   2. Purulent discharge from the client's left eye
   3. Lack of visible cerumen in the ear canal
   4. Inability to differentiate sweet from salty taste

4. Which of the following accurately describes presbycusis?
   1. Hearing loss involving sounds of higher frequencies
   2. Hearing loss involving sounds of lower frequencies
   3. Visual deficit involving difficulty seeing objects close up
   4. Visual deficit involving difficulty seeing objects at a distance

5. Which of the following accurately describes the expected outcome of treatment for a client with glaucoma?
   1. Reduction of IOP
   2. Prevention of vision loss
   3. Prevention of further damage to optic nerve fibers
   4. All of the above

Critical Thinking

1. The wife of a client with macular degeneration dropped a safety pin on the floor. The client pointed out where the pin had fallen, to which the wife asked, "If you can't see well, how can you see the pin?" Explain the probable answer given the client.

2. Considering age-related changes to the eye regarding tolerance to light and glare, what are some nursing interventions that could be implemented to increase safety in the hospital setting? While driving a car at night?

3. The husband of your client who just received new hearing aids states, "It will be so much easier now that we don't have to clean her ears out every day." What would your response be?

4. You are caring for an older adult who was recently diagnosed with age-related macular degeneration. Describe appropriate nursing interventions for the nursing diagnosis Anticipatory Grieving.

Resources

Internet Resources

American Academy of Ophthalmology
http://www.eyenet.org

National Eye Institute
http://www.nei.nih.gov

Macular Degeneration Foundation
http://www.eyesight.org

Talking Books: National Library Service for the Blind and Visually Handicapped
Library of Congress
http://lcweb.loc.gov/nls./nls.html

Organizations

American Foundation for the Blind
11 Penn Plaza, Suite 300
New York, NY 10001
(212) 502-7600

Prevent Blindness America
(800) 331-2020

National Association for the Deaf
814 Thayer Avenue
Silver Spring, MD 20910-4500
(301) 587-1788

Selected References

Alspach, G. (1998). Chemosensory impairments: Nothing to sniff at. *Critical Care Nurse, 18*(2), 16–18.

Derby, L., & Maier, W. C. (2000). Risk of cataract among users of intranasal corticosteroids. *Journal of Allergy and Clinical Immunology, 105*(5), 912–916.

Ebersole, P., & Hess, P. (1998). *Toward healthy aging.* St. Louis: Mosby-Year Book.

Garbe, E., Suissa, S., & LeLorier, J. (1998). Association of inhaled corticosteroid use with cataract extraction in elderly patients. *Journal of the American Medical Association, 280*(6), 539–543.

Glanton, E. (1998). New device may aid hearing—at a price. *Sacramento Bee,* October 7, 1998.

Glaucoma Guidelines: A Way to Improve Care? *Drug & Therapeutic Perspective, 15*(1), 8–10, 2000. Available at http://www.medscape.com/adis/DTP/2000/v15.n01/dtp1501.03/pnt-dtp1501.03.html Accessed 5/24/00.

Healthy People 2010. Available at http://www.health.gov/healthypeople/Document/tableofcontents.htm Accessed 11/15/00.

Hodgson, B. B., & Kizior, R. J. (1999). *Saunders nursing drug handbook.* Philadelphia: W. B. Saunders.

Ignatavicius, D. D., Workman, M. L., & Mishler, M. A. (1999). *Medical-surgical nursing across the health care continuum.* Philadelphia: W. B. Saunders.

Lewis, S. M., Heitkemper, M. M., & Dirksen, S. R. (2000). *Medical-surgical nursing: Assessment and management of clinical problems.* St. Louis: Mosby.

Matteson, M. A., McConnell, E. S., & Linton, A. D. (1998). *Gerontological nursing: Concepts and practice.* Philadelphia: W. B. Saunders.

Monahan, F. D., & Neighbors, M. (1998). *Medical-surgical nursing: Foundations for clinical practice.* Philadelphia: W. B. Saunders.

Murphy, M. P., & Gates, G. A. (1997). Hearing loss: Does gender play a role? *Medscape Women's Health,* 2(10). Available at http://www.medscape.com/WomensH...v02.n10/wh3101.murphy/wh3101.murphy.html

Podoshin, L., Ben-David, J., & Teszler, C. B. (1997). Pediatric and geriatric tinnitus. *Internal Tinnitus Journal, 3*(2), 101–103.

Stone, C. M. (1999). Preventing cerumen impaction in nursing facility residents. *Journal of Gerontological Nursing, 25*(5), 43–45.

Weksler, M. E. (1998). Age-related macular degeneration: How science is improving clinical care (an interview with Janet S. Sunness, MD). *Geriatrics, 53*(2), 70–80.

Promoting Cognitive Abilities

Dysarthria

Embolism

Homeostasis

Infarction

Ischemia

Level of consciousness

Long-term memory

Necrosis

Neurofibrillary tangles

Orientation

Pallidotomy

Paresis

Plantar flexion

Plaques

Prodromal

Short-term memory

Thalamotomy

Thrombolytic agents

Thrombosis

AGE-RELATED CHANGES OF THE BRAIN AND NERVOUS SYSTEM

In Chapter 1 we discussed several myths about aging. Two of the myths mentioned were that older adults are senile, and that "you can't teach an old dog new tricks." We will now disprove these myths and describe the changes to the brain and central nervous system that actually do occur with age.

The brain undergoes structural changes with age, which can translate into minor differences that you will observe in your data collection. There is a loss of neurons, both in the brain and in the spinal cord, especially after the age of 70. The brain atrophies, showing a decrease in both size and weight. The good news is that there has never been a strong correlation demonstrated between atrophy of the brain and one's intelligence. As with other areas of the body, the brain must be stimulated and challenged to maximize mental acuity. The old adage, "use it or lose it," applies to mental processes. Activities that stimulate and challenge the brain, such as solving crossword puzzles, are considered health-promoting activities.

With age, the synthesis and metabolism of neurotransmitters are reduced, leading to nerve impulses being conducted more slowly in the central nervous system. The older adult demonstrates slower movements, a delayed response time, and slower reflexes than the younger adult. When using complex machinery or driving, the older adult may sacrifice speed for more precise movements. The older adult may take longer to make important decisions.

Movement of large muscle groups is generally easier for the older adult than is fine movement. Some older adults may experience a tremulousness that is not associated with any sort of disease process. This is referred to as **benign senile**

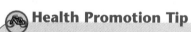
Health Promotion Tip

Activities to promote mental acuity:

- Solving crossword puzzles
- Completing jigsaw puzzles
- Playing musical instruments
- Learning foreign languages
- Reading
- Driving
- Cooking new recipes
- Sewing and/or needlepoint
- Knitting
- Dancing
- Exercising
- Learning how to use computers
- Internet "surfing"
- Playing games
- Debating
- Art/painting
- Writing: letters to the editor, articles for publication
- Swimming
- Building a family tree
- Tracking down long-lost friends
- Campaigning in elections

tremor, and is an intermittent tremor that becomes more pronounced with emotional stress and fatigue.

Regarding memory and aging, memories from the past tend to be well preserved in the older adult. This memory, called **long-term memory**, refers to memories that are stored for future retrieval, and involves memories from days to weeks old. Long-term memory is the result of a permanent neuronal change in the brain whereby information is stored on a protein. **Short-term memory** involves information presented seconds to minutes ago and no permanent neuronal change occurs in the brain. Short-term memory is not as well preserved in the older adult. For example, although the older adult may be able to provide accounts from long ago that include detailed information, he or she may be unable to recall last evening's meal quite as easily. Age-associated memory impairment, first described in Chapter 4, is a term that refers to these changes in memory that may occur with age. It is important to take into consideration age-related changes in short-term memory when implementing health care teaching with the older adult.

Although the myth about not being able to teach an old dog new tricks is certainly *not* true, learning complex information may take more time for the older adult. There are important nursing interventions, however, that you can employ that will assist the older adult to compensate for this alteration in learning (Box 11–1).

Lifelong patterns of intelligence and personality remain stable with age. If someone loved to learn and explore intellectual pursuits as a young adult, this trait will usually continue into older adulthood. If one had a rather pleasant disposition as a young adult, chances are that he or she will remain pleasant. On the other hand, if a young adult is rigid and grumpy, he or she will probably continue to exhibit those tendencies as an older adult.

Functioning of the **autonomic nervous system** (ANS) is less efficient with age. Because of this, maintenance of body **homeostasis** is more difficult, leading to a more prolonged and difficult recovery from stressors such as heat, cold, or intensive exercise. Related to this, the older adult takes longer to recover from major surgeries and illnesses, and is more vulnerable to

---

Box 11–1 Strategies to Compensate for Age-Related Alterations in Learning

- Eliminate environmental distractions.
- Provide information in a variety of ways: print, video, return demonstration.
- Ensure that the older adult has eyeglasses or hearing aids, if appropriate.
- Present new concepts one at a time.
- Use a slightly slower pace of presentation.
- Repeat important information.
- Summarize.
- Relate the information to familiar concepts.
- Add color, texture, and meaning to the information when possible.
- Use mnemonics to introduce lists of information.

---

hypothermia and hyperthermia, as was discussed in Chapter 3. Another effect of the decline in ANS functioning is the tendency for the older adult to experience orthostatic hypotension. Dehydration and certain medications, discussed in Chapter 6, make one even more susceptible to orthostatic hypotension.

Although mild forgetfulness can be common owing to age-related changes in recent memory, dementia is *never* considered normal aging of the brain. Any serious deficits in thinking and cognition must be investigated. There are numerous treatable causes of **confusion**.

Signs and Symptoms Tip

Confusion may be a sign of numerous treatable illnesses and conditions:

- Pneumonia
- Urinary tract infection
- Medication toxicity
- Dehydration
- Fever
- Sleep deprivation
- Hypoxia
- Relocation
- Hospitalization
- Anesthesia
- Emotional strain
- Depression

The list of medications potentially responsible for causing confusion in the older adult is huge. Because drug effects last longer in the older adult, it is important to explore any new onset of confusion. Consider any new medications being taken not only over the past few days, but also over the past few weeks, even if the medications have since been discontinued.

⌨ Medication Safety Tip

Certain medications are notorious for causing confusion in the older adult. Some of the more common culprits include:

- Alcohol
- Analgesics
- Anticholinergics
- Antidepressants
- Antipsychotics
- Antiparkinson agents
- Beta-blocking agents
- Cimetidine
- Digitalis
- Diuretics
- Hypnotics
- Muscle relaxants
- Sedatives
- Benzodiazepines
- Antibiotics

Data from Ebersole, P., & Hess, P. (1998). *Toward healthy aging*. St. Louis: Mosby-Year Book, p. 361.

ASSESSMENT OF THE NERVOUS SYSTEM

The first step in assessment of the mental acuity of an older adult is to create an environment that will be comfortable and will encourage the best possible performance, especially regarding reflexes and recall. Attempt to remove any physical discomforts that may be present, such as pain, thirst, or anxiety. Make certain that the room temperature and lighting are at comfortable levels. Before you begin data collection, inform the older adult about what to expect from your assessment. Include in this preparation the explanation that some of the questions you will be asking may seem silly or simple, but that providing honest answers is important. Approach this type of

assessment with the same sense of routine that you would use to approach the measurement of vital signs.

Fatigue will have a negative effect on an older adult's performance of cognitive tasks. A complete examination of the nervous system and mental acuity may need to be broken into several short time periods in order to decrease fatigue and obtain a more accurate assessment of the older adult's capabilities. The older adult should be well rested when the examination is begun.

It is important to consider that certain physical obstacles may make it difficult to assess mental acuity and may affect assessment findings. These include aphasia, language barriers, and extreme hearing loss. Any of these conditions may give the impression of a mental deficit that simply is not there. It is important to note the presence of these or of any other conditions that may cause an inaccurate assessment.

Begin your data collection as always in a head-to-toe manner. An important first step, starting at the head, is to observe and document the client's **level of consciousness**, or LOC. One's LOC can range from full consciousness to deep coma. Although it is beyond your scope of practice to diagnose coma, it is important that you be familiar with commonly used medical terms that describe varying levels of consciousness. These terms are defined in Table 11–1.

A tool, such as the Glasgow Coma Scale (GCS), can be used to further address level of consciousness (Table 11–2). Any tool that you decide to use in your data collection should enhance your other observations, not replace them.

Note that the Glasgow Coma Scale addresses three major areas: eye opening, motor response, and verbal response. The client is evaluated in each of the three areas and is given a score for each area. The three scores are then added up, giving the client a total score somewhere between 3 and 15.

Level of **orientation** is different from level of consciousness. Level of orientation refers to one's awareness of his or her surroundings in terms of person, place, time, and situation. When someone is aware of who is around them, where they are, and what the date is, it is commonly written as "oriented X4." It is important not to *assume* someone is oriented simply because they are

Table 11-1
TERMS DESCRIBING LEVEL OF CONSCIOUSNESS

Term	Description
Full consciousness	• Awake, alert, appropriate in conversation • Oriented to person, place, and time
Confusion	• Short attention span • Poor memory • Difficulty following commands
Delirium	• Restlessness, agitation, occasional combativeness • Disoriented to time and place • Hallucinations possible
Obtundation	• Falls asleep when not stimulated but easily aroused and will engage in simple conversation • Synonyms: lethargy, somnolence, drowsiness
Stupor	• Very drowsy, appears unresponsive • Will show limited response to vigorous stimulation
Semicomatose	• Unresponsive to verbal stimulus • May moan or stir to painful stimulus • Corneal, pupil, gag, tendon reflexes (brain-stem reflexes) are intact
Comatose	• Unresponsive to verbal and painful stimuli • Brain-stem reflexes are intact
Deeply comatose	• Completely unarousable and unresponsive to all stimuli • Brain-stem reflexes are absent

Adapted from Monahan, F. D. & Neighbors, M. (1998). *Medical-surgical nursing: Foundations for clinical practice.* Philadelphia: W. B. Saunders, p. 726.

Mental Status (MMSE)

Table 11-2
GLASGOW COMA SCALE

Variable	Response	Score No.
Eye opening	Open spontaneously	4
	Open to verbal commands	3
	Open to pain	2
	No response	1
Motor response	Obeys verbal command to painful stimulus	6
	Localizes pain	5
	Flexion withdrawal	4
	Flexion abnormal	3
	Extension	2
	No response	1
Verbal response	Oriented and converses	5
	Disoriented and converses	4
	Inappropriate words	3
	Incomprehensible sounds	2
	No response	1
Highest possible score		15

Adapted from Monahan, F. D., & Neighbors, M. (1998). *Medical-surgical nursing: Foundations for clinical practice* (2nd ed.). Philadelphia: W. B. Saunders, p. 727.

acting appropriately—you truly need to ask the questions to determine that someone is oriented X4. To illustrate this point, consider the following true anecdote:

A new intensive care unit (ICU) nurse was caring for an older adult one rainy winter day in northern California. The older gentleman was on a ventilator and was unable to speak because of the endotracheal tube. During her assessment, the nurse asked the client to perform a variety of tasks: squeeze her hand, smile, roll over, wiggle toes, and so on. The client was very alert and appeared very interested in the program he was watching on television between nursing interventions. The new nurse charted the following: "Client alert and oriented X4." One hour later, it was determined that the gentleman was breathing effectively enough to have the endotracheal tube removed. After extubation, he looked over at his nurse and commented, "Boy, it's hot here in Korea!" He further proceeded to inform her of the trail of ants he was watching crawl all over the television and fall onto the floor beneath (there were no ants).

This anecdote clearly emphasizes the importance of not assuming someone is oriented X4 unless you've questioned them. How then, should the nurse have charted her assessment? She could have written that the client was alert, that he followed simple commands, that he was watching television, or other objective observations. To conclude that he was oriented X4, however, was an assumption that proved to be false.

Next, assess mental status of the older adult. The Mini Mental State Examination (MMSE) is an easy-to-use, widely accepted, and commonly available instrument that can be used for this purpose. It consists of eleven questions that measure five areas of cognitive functioning: orientation, registration, attention and calculation, recall, and language. The maximum score is 30, and a score of below 24 generally indicates dementia. The examination takes between 5 and 10 minutes to administer. The MMSE can be found in Appendix A.

Assessment of cranial nerves is the next step in a comprehensive neurologic examination that may be performed by the registered nurse (RN), the advanced practice nurse, or the physician. Although a full evaluation of cranial nerves is beyond the scope of this text, you should assess and document the pupils as described in Chapter 10.

After you have assessed LOC, level of orientation, and mental status, check for movement and strength in all extremities. Before beginning this, observe for any movement or tremulousness at rest. Beginning with the arms, ask the client to squeeze with both hands simultaneously, making certain the client's dominant hand squeezes your dominant hand. Note the strength of the hand grasp. Observe for any unequal strength on one side. Next, ask the client to push with his or her arms against your resistance. Record your findings and communicate any unusual findings to the RN.

Repeat your assessment for strength and movement in the lower extremities. Ask the client to wiggle toes, to flex the feet in both directions (**dorsiflexion** and **plantar flexion**), and then to push his or her legs against your resistance. Again, record your findings and communicate any unusual findings to the RN.

Next, observe the older adult standing and walking. Note his or her gait, balance, and coordination. Observe for any asymmetrical movement or weakness. Assess the older adult's coordination in the following way: hold up your index finger and direct the older adult to touch your fingertip with his or her index finger, then to touch his or her nose. Ask the older adult to repeat the motion as you move your finger to different areas. Observe for accuracy and smooth, even movement.

To complete the nervous system assessment of the older adult, assess sensory/perceptual functioning. Assessment of this area of function is outlined in detail in Chapter 10.

DISORDERS COMMON IN OLDER ADULTS

Cerebrovascular Accident

Cerebrovascular accident, or CVA, commonly known as *stroke*, is the third leading cause of death among Americans, affecting over 730,000 people each year. Older adults are especially at risk for stroke: the incidence more than doubles for each decade of life after age 55. The incidence of stroke is higher for men than for women; however, because there are far more female than male older adults, the mortality rate from stroke is greater for women. African Americans have two to three times the risk of CVA as their white counterparts.

Over the past 15 years, the rates of death from CVA have been declining, yet great physical challenges remain for individuals who have experienced stroke. It is one of the most common reasons for placement in a long-term care facility, second only to dementia. Rehabilitation from CVA can be painful, lengthy, and frustrating, and economic hardship can make the road to recovery even more difficult. Several advances have been made in recent years regarding management of clients with CVA that, if implemented early, can greatly reduce the disability associated with this disorder.

As was mentioned earlier, advanced age is a risk factor for CVA. Other risk factors include hypertension, cardiovascular disease, atherosclerosis, obesity, stress, smoking, high blood cholesterol, clotting disorders, and diabetes mellitus. Hypertension and diabetes mellitus are important risk factors because they accelerate the atherosclerotic process. In fact, most medical experts identify management of hypertension as the number one way to reduce one's risk of stroke.

🏍 Health Promotion Tip

Measures to reduce one's risk of CVA include:

- Maintain careful control of hypertension.
- Maintain careful control of diabetes.
- Avoid smoking.
- Eat a healthy diet low in sodium, fat, and cholesterol.
- Decrease alcohol consumption.
- Take medications as ordered by your physician.
- Have regular medical checkups.
- Maintain a healthy body weight.
- Exercise regularly.
- Be alert to the signs and symptoms of CVA.

CVA develops from an interruption of blood flow to the brain, due to one of three processes: **thrombosis**, **embolism**, or hemorrhage. Strokes due to thrombosis or embolism are by far the most common, accounting for about 85% of all strokes. The three types of strokes are compared in Figure 11–1.

When blood flow to the brain is interrupted, **ischemia** and **necrosis** of brain tissue occur, or cerebral **infarction**. This pathology is similar to what occurs in a myocardial infarction, and some of the newer treatments for stroke are the same medications used for treatment of a myocardial infarction, namely **thrombolytic agents**.

With the disruption of blood flow, the brain is unable to acquire the necessary nutrients—oxygen and glucose—that it requires for proper functioning. Several problems result, including accumulation of toxic substances, release of free radicals, breakdown of the blood-brain barrier, and the inflammatory response, which promotes further injury to brain cells. If treatment is not implemented promptly, potentially viable brain tissue becomes irreparably damaged.

Signs and symptoms of CVA can vary greatly depending on the location, type, and severity of the ischemia, and can range from headache and blurred vision to coma and death. The symptoms of each of the three types of stroke are outlined in Table 11–3.

🏍 Health Promotion Tip

Teach older adults and their families the warning signs of CVA and the importance of prompt treatment.

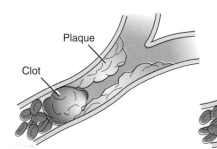

A. THROMBOTIC STROKE
Cerebral thrombosis is a narrowing of the artery by fatty deposits called plaque. Plaque can cause a clot to form, which blocks the passage of blood through the artery.

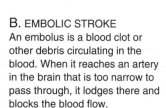

B. EMBOLIC STROKE
An embolus is a blood clot or other debris circulating in the blood. When it reaches an artery in the brain that is too narrow to pass through, it lodges there and blocks the blood flow.

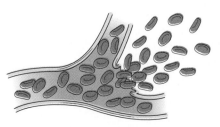

C. HEMORRHAGIC STROKE
A burst blood vessel may allow blood to seep into and damage brain tissues until clotting shuts off the link.

Figure 11–1. Three types of stroke. (From Lewis, S. M., Heitkemper, M. M., & Dirksen, S. R. [2000]. *Medical-surgical nursing: Assessment and management of clinical problems* [5th ed.]. St. Louis: Mosby, p. 1647.)

Table 11–3
CEREBROVASCULAR ACCIDENT: SIGNS AND SYMPTOMS

Classification	Signs and Symptoms
Thrombotic stroke	**Prodromal** episodes (30%–50%) are warning signs that occur hours to months before CVA, lasting 5 to 30 minutes, and may include: • **paresis** • **aphasia** • paralysis • confusion • visual disturbances • **diplopia** • numbness • visual impairment • headache • **dysarthria**
Embolic stroke	• Rapid onset • Usually no prodromal signs and symptoms • Headache and signs of neurologic deficit appear, depending on location
Hemorrhagic stroke	• Onset: minutes to days • Usually no prodromal signs and symptoms • May occur during activity • Signs and symptoms vary depending on severity and location, and include severe headache, vomiting, paresis, dysarthria, and coma

CVA, cerebrovascular accident.
Data from Lewis, S. M., Heitkemper, M. M., & Dirksen, S. R. (2000). *Medical-surgical nursing: Assessment and management of clinical problems.* St. Louis: Mosby Inc.

In addition, signs and symptoms of CVA depend on whether the right or left brain hemisphere is affected. Figure 11–2 depicts some of the differences you might see among your clients with stroke.

In the past, treatment of a stroke was not considered to be an urgent matter, except for the need to provide supportive care and to wait for the CVA to evolve, as there were no treatments believed to be effective in changing the outcome. In recent years, however, the medications given to clients experiencing a myocardial ⁓ (heart attack) have been shown to ⁓ r clients experiencing CVA from ⁓ embolism, if administered in a ⁓ r. When these medications, known ⁓ rs," are administered within 3 hours ⁓ of symptoms, valuable brain tissue

can be saved and the lengthy rehabilitation normally associated with stroke can be greatly shortened. Specialists in the field of neurology recognize that the public must be made aware of the urgency for fast treatment; they are beginning to refer to a stroke as a brain attack that requires emergency medical treatment, and they are teaching clients to telephone 911 for emergency medical help.

Before medications are administered, assist the emergency team with stabilizing the client who is experiencing a CVA. Attend to the ABCs of emergency care (airway, breathing, and circulation) first. Monitor vital signs closely, with special attention to blood pressure and respiration. Depending on the location of the CVA, the client's respiratory status may be compromised and support may be needed. The physician will order treatment for extreme hypertension but will usually allow the client to be slightly hypertensive as this helps maintain perfusion of the ischemic area. Other orders to expect may include placement of an intravenous line and possibly intravenous heparin administration to minimize further clot formation.

After the client is stabilized, the physician will usually order a computed tomography (CT) scan to determine if he or she is a candidate for thrombolytic therapy. The most common form of thrombolytic therapy is a medication called recombinant tissue plasminogen activator (rTPA). Although it can be extremely beneficial in limiting brain injury from CVA, it can also be deadly, causing brain hemorrhage if administered under the wrong circumstances. For this reason, important exclusion criteria exist specifying clients who should not be given this medication (Box 11–2).

From a nursing standpoint, it is important to anticipate any necessary invasive lines that will be needed, such as intravenous lines, nasogastric tubes, and Foley catheters, and to obtain orders for their placement *prior to* the start of rTPA therapy. Invasive devices not already in place, bloodwork, and injections must be avoided during the first hours after therapy owing to the increased risk of bleeding.

Other treatments for the client who experiences a CVA include close monitoring, including cardiac monitoring, and frequent measurement of vital signs. The client will remain on bedrest until neurologically stable, then mobilization

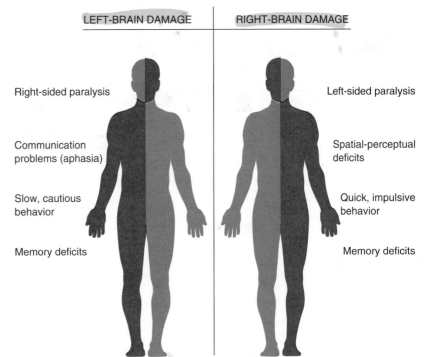

Figure 11–2. Right-sided versus left-sided cerebrovascular accident. (From Monahan, F. D., & Neighbors, M. [1998]. *Medical-surgical nursing: Foundations for clinical practice* [2nd ed.]. Philadelphia: W. B. Saunders, p. 807.)

LEFT-BRAIN DAMAGE

Right-sided paralysis

Communication problems (aphasia)

Slow, cautious behavior

Memory deficits

RIGHT-BRAIN DAMAGE

Left-sided paralysis

Spatial-perceptual deficits

Quick, impulsive behavior

Memory deficits

and rehabilitation will begin. Initiating range-of-motion exercises immediately, however, will reduce physical disability afterward.

Parkinson's Disease

Parkinson's disease is a disorder of the central nervous system that affects one's ability to move about normally (Fig. 11–3). It strikes men and women equally, affecting approximately 1.5% of the older adult population. Signs and symptoms of Parkinson's disease usually appear between the ages of 50 and 70. The cause of Parkinson's disease is unclear and there is no known cure for the disorder.

Because the exact cause of Parkinson's disease is unknown, identifying risk factors for the disorder is difficult. Some possible causes that have been identified by researchers include viruses, genetic predisposition, and premature aging. Newer research has identified environmental factors as a possible cause of Parkinson's disease, such as exposure to herbicides and pesticides, and diet. A surprising relationship that has been found in recent research, however, is that cigarette

---

Box 11–2 Exclusion Criteria for Treatment with rTPA

- Stroke longer than 3 hours from onset
- Neurologic deficit too large or too small
- Nonstroke cause of symptoms
- Presence of hemorrhage
- Prolonged blood coagulation laboratory values
- Low platelet count
- Blood pressure over 185 mm Hg systolic or 110 mm Hg diastolic
- CT findings suggestive of a large infarction
- History of recent stroke, myocardial infarction, or head injury
- History of recent surgery or hemorrhage
- Seizure at onset of symptoms

Data from Leira, E. C., & Adams, H. P. (1999). Management of acute ischemic stroke. *Clinics in Geriatric Medicine, 15*(4), 701–720.

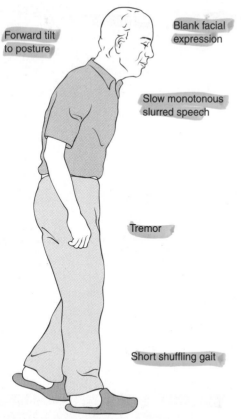

Forward tilt to posture

Blank facial expression

Slow monotonous slurred speech

Tremor

Short shuffling gait

Figure 11–3. Characteristic appearance of a client with Parkinson's disease.

are 50% less likely to develop Parkinson's disease than are nonsmokers (Fratiglioni & Wang, 2000). This is *not*, however, a rationale for starting to smoke.

The part of the brain affected by Parkinson's disease is the substantia nigra, which is responsible for the production of the neurotransmitter dopamine. Dopamine allows people to move about with fluid movements because balance is maintained between inhibitory and excitatory impulses. With a shortage of dopamine as in Parkinson's disease, movements become more jerky and difficult to control. The four classic signs of Parkinson's disease are tremor, rigidity, **bradykinesia,** and postural instability. These four signs are described in Box 11–3.

Other difficulties associated with Parkinson's disease are sleep disorders and pain. The most common sleep disorders are frequent awakening and early awakening. Many Parkinson's disease clients who experience sleep disorders also suffer from depression. Pain occurs in approximately 40% of clients with Parkinson's disease, and in some it is more bothersome than the primary motor symptoms of the disorder. The pain is often related to the rigidity of skeletal muscles kept in constant contraction. Another form of pain experienced by nearly one quarter of clients with Parkinson's disease is burning mouth. The reason for this symptom is unclear.

Box 11–3 Signs of Parkinson's Disease

Tremor

- Often the first sign   *tremors absent @ sleep*
- Mild initially
- More prominent at rest
- Areas involved: hands, tongue, lips, jaw, diaphragm
- "Pillrolling" motion of thumb and forefinger

Rigidity

- _____ to passive motion when extremities are _____ their range of motion
- _____ ty": muscles moving in a series of
- _____ lings of soreness due to sustained _____ on

Bradykinesia

- Slowed ordinary movements, such as walking or dressing
- Slowed semiautomatic gestures, such as crossing the legs or scratching
- Slowed spontaneous facial movements, resulting in a masklike stare ("masklike facies")

Postural instability

- Difficulty maintaining balance
- Leaning forward to maintain center of gravity
- May experience frequent falls

Sleep disorders
PAIN

...wis, S. M., Heitkemper, M. M., & Dirksen, S. R. (2000). *Medical-surgical nursing: Assessment and manage-...lems.* St. Louis: Mosby; Ebersole, P., & Hess, P. (1998). *Toward healthy aging.* St. Louis: Mosby-Year Book.

Table 11–4
DRUGS USED IN THE TREATMENT OF PARKINSON'S DISEASE

Category	Mechanism of Action	Examples
Dopamine agonists	Increase the release or supply of dopamine in the brain	• levodopa (L-dopa) • levodopa/carbidopa (Sinemet) • ropinirole (Requip) • pramipexole (Mirapex) • tolcapone (Tasmar)
Anticholinergics	Antagonize or block the effect of overactive cholinergic neurons	• trihexyphenidyl (Artane) • benztropine (Cogentin) • dicyclomine (Bentyl)
Antihistamines	Decrease the severity of tremors	• diphenhydramine (Benadryl) • promethazine (Phenergan)

Data from Hodgson, B. B., & Kizior, R. J. (1999). *Saunders nursing drug handbook.* Philadelphia: W. B. Saunders.

As was stated earlier, there is no known medical cure for Parkinson's disease. Drug therapy is aimed at controlling the symptoms of the disorder. Levodopa/carbidopa (Sinemet) is often the first drug to be employed. This medication is a dopaminergic agent that is able to cross the blood-brain barrier and help increase the supply of dopamine to the brain. Tolcapone (Tasmar) is a newer drug that enhances the effectiveness of Sinemet and allows the client to obtain symptom control at a lower dosage. These and other drugs commonly used to treat Parkinson's disease can be found in Table 11–4.

In recent years, neurosurgeons have begun performing surgical procedures, such as **thalamotomy** and **pallidotomy**, for select clients with Parkinson's disease. These procedures can help with decreasing the severity of the tremor, rigidity, and bradykinesia, but do not represent a cure for Parkinson's disease, and signs may reappear after treatment. These treatments are outlined in Table 11–5.

Dementia

Dementia is an all-encompassing term that refers to loss of short-term and long-term memory, as well as other cognitive deficits that occur gradually and worsen over time. As dementia progresses, the older adult loses the ability to perform self-care activities, to recognize familiar surroundings, and to recognize familiar faces, including those of loved ones. It is perhaps the cruelest disorder facing the families of older adult

Table 11–5
SURGICAL TREATMENTS FOR PARKINSON'S DISEASE

Category	Example	Comments
Ablative techniques (destructive)	• Thalamotomy • Pallidotomy	• Lesion is made in the thalamus or globus pallidus • Pallidotomy more commonly performed • Improve tremor, rigidity, pain, and bradykinesia, but may worsen speech
Augmentative techniques (stimulating)	• Deep brain stimulation	• Current trend • Similar symptom relief to ablative techniques, but achieved in a nondestructive manner
Restorative techniques	• Tissue transplantation • Gene therapy	• Experimental • Ethical considerations of human fetal tissue transplantation • Porcine (pig) fetal cells now being tried

Data from Favre, J., Burchiel, K. J., & Hammerstad, J. (2000). Outcome of unilateral and bilateral pallidotomy for Parkinson's disease: Patient assessment. *Neurosurgery, 46*(2), 344–355; Follett, K. A. (2000). The surgical treatment of Parkinson's disease. *Annual Review of Medicine, 51,* 135–147; Honey, C. R., Stoessl, A. J., Tsui, J. K., Schulzer, M., & Calne, D. B. (1999). Unilateral pallidotomy for reduction of parkinsonian pain. *Journal of Neurosurgery, 91*(2), 198–201; Mazzoni, P. (2000). Movement disorders: New and clarified options for treatment. Proceedings from the 52nd Annual Meeting of the American Academy of Neurology. Available at http://www.medscape.com/medscape/cno/2000/AAN/Story.cfm?stort—id=1213 Accessed 8/17/00.

Box 11-4 **Causes of Dementia**

- Alzheimer's disease — *most common*
- Vascular disease
- Pick's disease
- Diffuse Lewy body disease
- Normal-pressure hydrocephalus
- Creutzfeldt-Jakob disease
- Brain tumors
- Nutritional deficiencies

Data from Epstein, D. K., & Connor, J. R. (1999). Dementia in the elderly: An overview. *Generations, 23*(3), 9–16.

clients because gradually it becomes similar to living with a stranger.

Dementia is a significant problem throughout the world. More than 7 million people in North America and Europe have been diagnosed with dementia. An even larger number—as many as 11 million people—suffer from dementia in developing nations.

There are numerous types of dementia, but by far the most common one is Alzheimer's disease, which accounts for more than half of all cases of dementia. For this reason, Alzheimer's disease is discussed here in detail. The second most common cause of dementia is vascular disease, specifically cerebrovascular disease, which causes between 10% and 20% of cases. The reason behind this type of dementia is that in cerebrovascular disease,

the brain is deprived of blood flow and neurons deteriorate owing to lack of oxygen. Box 11–4 lists common causes of dementia.

Occasionally, an older adult shows signs of confusion and **disorientation** of a temporary nature, a condition called **delirium**. Delirium can be related to a number of factors, such as medication adverse effects, infection, hypoxia, or electrolyte imbalance. It would be a big mistake to assume that the older adult with delirium has dementia because delirium, unlike dementia, is reversible. Delirium and dementia are compared and contrasted in Table 11–6.

Alzheimer's Disease

Alzheimer's disease is thought to be the fourth or fifth leading cause of death in the United States. It is difficult to be sure, however, because people usually do not die of Alzheimer's disease, per se, but rather from complications associated with the disorder, such as pneumonia, infection, or accidents.

The major risk factor for Alzheimer's disease is aging. The prevalence of the disorder at age 65 is 1%, but it increases with age to somewhere between 20% and 50% after age 85. The exact cause of Alzheimer's disease is unknown. It is not considered to be a hereditary disorder in all cases; however, a subset of cases of Alzheimer's disease have been shown to have a genetic link, which is carried in certain types of proteins. Many factors have been investigated as influences on whether or not an individual will

Delirium is reversible & treatable

Table 11–6		
DELIRIUM VERSUS DEMENTIA		
	Delirium	**Dementia**
Onset	Sudden, acute (hours to days)	Gradual, insidious (months to years)
Reversibility	Reversible if cause is identified in a timely manner	Not reversible
Level of alertness	Reduced	Usually not reduced until end stages
Attention	Reduced ability to focus, sustain, or shift attention	Not impaired
Fluctuation	Usually worse at night	Stable throughout the day
Perceptual distortions (hallucinations, illusions)	Often present	Usually absent
Physical illness	Usually present	Usually absent

Data from Milisen, K., Foreman, M. D., Godderis, J., Abraham, I. L., & Broos, P. L. O. (1998). Delirium in the hospitalized elderly: Nursing assessment and management. *Nursing Clinics of North America, 33*(3), 417–436; Matteson, M. A., McConnell, E. S., & Linton, A. D. (1998). *Gerontological nursing: Concepts and practice.* Philadelphia: W. B. Saunders.

develop Alzheimer's disease. These include history of head injury, autoimmune disorders, viral causes, and low scores on tests of verbal ability and abstract reasoning. *Environmental*

The primary brain structural abnormalities that occur in Alzheimer's disease are the proliferation of **neurofibrillary tangles** and **plaques**, and the loss of neurons. The neurofibrillary tangles are bundles of proteins (neurofibrils) found in the cytoplasm of abnormal neurons. The plaques, sometimes referred to as senile plaques, are composed of a core of beta-amyloid. The plaques develop slowly and mature over time, interrupting normal neuron functioning. Exactly how these abnormal structures develop, in what sequence they develop, and what can be done to stop the abnormal development, are all important research questions that continue to be investigated.

Signs and symptoms of Alzheimer's disease depend on the stage of the disorder. Initially, the signs are very subtle and are often missed, even by loved ones. There may be a slight change in personality, such as apathy toward things normally of interest. Mild forgetfulness occurs,

although the individual can usually compensate for this with notes and lists. As the disorder progresses, more severe deficits become apparent, such as getting lost in familiar places, forgetting important things, and neglecting personal hygiene. In the final stage of Alzheimer's disease, the client becomes totally dependent on others for providing all aspects of personal care and is bedridden. The client with Alzheimer's disease usually dies as a result of a complication, often aspiration pneumonia. The three stages of Alzheimer's disease are described in detail in Table 11–7.

There is no known treatment to prevent or cure Alzheimer's disease, although certain medications may be administered to slow the progression of symptoms of the disorder. These drugs are from the classification of medications called **cholinesterase inhibitors**, which slow the breakdown of acetylcholine at the synapse, thus improving the transmission of nerve impulses. The first drug approved for this use is called tacrine (Cognex), but this medication can cause liver dysfunction and gastrointestinal upset in the client. Two newer drugs that physicians prefer are

Table 11–7	
STAGES OF ALZHEIMER'S DISEASE	
Early stage (2–4 years)	• Mild forgetfulness • Declining interest in people, environment, and current affairs • Uncertainty and hesitancy in initiating actions • Poor work performance
Middle stage (2–12 years)	• Progressive memory loss • Hesitates in response to questions; shows signs of aphasia • Difficulty following simple instructions • Difficulty with mathematics • Irritability • Evasive, anxious, physically active • Wanders • Loses important papers and possessions • Becomes lost in familiar surroundings • Lets instrumental activities of daily living slip: paying bills, disposing of garbage, taking medication • Neglects personal hygiene • Loses social graces
Late stage (1 year or less)	• Marked weight loss • Unable to communicate • Unable to recognize family • Incontinent of urine and feces • May have seizures • Bedridden

Adapted from Monahan, F. D., & Neighbors, M. (1998). *Medical-surgical nursing: Foundations for clinical practice.* Philadelphia: W. B. Saunders, p. 791.

most common

new drug (Reminyl)

Table 11–8

DRUGS AND THERAPIES UNDER INVESTIGATION FOR ALZHEIMER'S DISEASE

Drug/Therapy	Action
Calcium channel blockers	May promote nerve cell survival
Physostigmine	May inhibit acetylcholine breakdown
Besipirdine HCl	Mimics the action of acetylcholine
Melatonin	Helps insomnia
Vitamin E and selegiline	Antioxidants, may slow the course of Alzheimer's disease
NSAIDs	May lower the risk of developing Alzheimer's disease

NSAIDs, nonsteroidal anti-inflammatory drugs.
Adapted from Schweiger, J. L., & Huey, R. A. (1999). Alzheimer's disease: Your role in the caregiving equation. *Nursing99, 29*(6), 38.

donepezil (Aricept) and rivastigmine (Exelon) because they are safer and better tolerated by the older adult, with no need for monitoring of liver function. The most common adverse effect of both Aricept and Exelon is nausea; other adverse effects for which to watch include diarrhea, vomiting, dizziness, and fatigue. Pain and headache may be reported with Exelon. In addition to cholinesterase inhibitors, other drugs may be prescribed for clients with Alzheimer's disease to treat symptoms such as constipation, sleep disorder, or anxiety. New treatments for Alzheimer's disease are always being investigated. Some drugs and therapies recently investigated for Alzheimer's disease are presented in Table 11–8.

Table 11–9

NURSING DIAGNOSES RELATED TO COGNITIVE ABILITY

	Cerebrovascular Accident	Parkinson's Disease	Alzheimer's Disease
Imbalanced nutrition: more than body requirements	X		
Imbalanced nutrition: less than body requirements		X	X
Risk for imbalanced body temperature	X	X	X
Reflex urinary incontinence	X	X	X
Constipation	X	X	X
Ineffective tissue perfusion: cerebral	X		
Ineffective airway clearance	X		X
Risk for injury	X	X	X
Risk for trauma			X
Risk for aspiration	X	X	X
Risk for impaired skin integrity	X		X
Impaired verbal communication	X		X
Impaired social interaction			X
Risk for loneliness	X	X	X
Ineffective role performance	X	X	X
Interrupted family processes	X	X	X
Caregiver role strain	X	X	X
Impaired physical mobility	X	X	X
Impaired walking	X	X	X
Activity intolerance	X	X	
Fatigue	X	X	
Disturbed sleep pattern	X	X	X
Impaired home maintenance	X	X	X
Self-care deficit	X	X	X
Impaired swallowing	X	X	X
Disturbed body image	X	X	
Disturbed sensory perception	X	X	
Unilateral neglect	X		
Deficient knowledge	X	X	X
Chronic confusion			X
Impaired memory			X
Pain	X	X	
Anticipatory grieving		X	X
Anxiety	X	X	X
Situational low self-esteem	X	X	

NURSING DIAGNOSES

Nursing diagnoses for the client with an acute or chronic neurologic disorder are derived from the assessment data and are unique to each older adult. The focus of the nursing diagnosis is the client's response to the particular health problem.

Common nursing diagnoses (written only as the "problem" portion of the *Problem, Etiology,* and *Signs* and symptoms [PES] in the nursing diagnosis statement) that apply to the older adult experiencing neurologic disorders are listed in Table 11–9.

Not every nursing diagnosis identified in Table 11–9 will be appropriate for every client with a given neurologic disorder. For example, a client with Alzheimer's disease in the early stages will have fewer nursing diagnoses of a physical nature and more of a feeling or knowing nature, such as Anxiety and Altered Thought Processes. In the advanced stages of the disorder, however, the client will have more nursing diagnoses related to moving and exchanging, such as Impaired Swallowing or Incontinence. Additionally, there may be other nursing diagnoses that are suitable for your older adult client that cannot be found in the table. Carefully consider every nursing diagnosis to individualize a plan of care for your older adult client with any type of acute or chronic neurologic disorder.

Table 11–10
SAMPLE OUTCOMES FOR AN OLDER ADULT WITH CEREBROVASCULAR ACCIDENT

Nursing Diagnosis	Sample Outcomes
Ineffective airway clearance	• Client will expectorate secretions • Client will experience no respiratory distress • Client's airway will remain patent
Unilateral neglect	• Client will bring objects into his or her field of vision • Client will experience no physical injury on paralyzed side
Situational low self-esteem	• Client will verbalize concerns and feelings • Client will assist in setting realistic rehabilitation goals • Client will participate in daily rehabilitation activities

Table 11–11
SAMPLE OUTCOMES FOR AN OLDER ADULT WITH PARKINSON'S DISEASE

Nursing Diagnosis	Sample Outcomes
Disturbed body image	• Client will appear clean and well groomed at all times • Client will verbalize satisfaction with personal appearance
Constipation	• Client will maintain regular bowel evacuation • Client will avoid complications of constipation
Deficient diversional activity	• Client will identify activities in which he or she is able to participate • Client will participate in one diversional activity each day • Client will verbalize satisfaction with leisure time use

COLLABORATING ON THE PLAN OF CARE

After the nursing diagnoses are established, you must assist the RN in developing outcomes for the client with a neurologic disorder. Set outcomes that are realistic, measurable, and tailored to the individual older adult.

Based on the discussion of nursing diagnoses in the previous section, sample outcomes for a client with cerebrovascular accident can be found in Table 11–10. These are samples only; the outcomes you set must be established with your individual client in mind.

Similarly, sample outcomes for older adults with disorders of Parkinson's disease and Alzheimer's disease can be found in Tables 11–11 and 11–12, respectively.

IMPLEMENTING INTERVENTIONS FOR HEALTH PROMOTION

Interventions to Promote Safety

1. Closely monitor LOC and vital signs of the client with an acute neurologic disorder, paying close attention to respiratory status. Call for help immediately if an acute change in vital signs or LOC occurs.
2. Never offer oral food or fluids to a client with an acute neurologic disorder until swallowing has been tested.

Table 11–12
SAMPLE OUTCOMES FOR AN OLDER ADULT WITH ALZHEIMER'S DISEASE

Nursing Diagnosis	Sample Outcomes
Anxiety	• Client will identify a decrease in anxiety • Client will verbalize a sense of control over the situation
Caregiver role strain	• Caregiver will identify resources that are available • Caregiver will seek out appropriate resources • Client will have physical care needs met
Risk for injury	• Client will experience no injury

3. Turn the client on bedrest every 2 hours to help prevent complications of immobility. Encourage deep breathing with each turn.
4. Teach the client with Parkinson's disease techniques that will help with safe ambulation. For example, it may be helpful to instruct the client that, when experiencing "freezing" of movements while walking, he or she should step over an imaginary line or rock slightly from side to side to initiate leg movements.

Interventions to Promote Health Education

1. Help identify individuals at risk for CVA. Refer to Appendix A for a screening tool developed by neuroscience nurses to evaluate a client's risk for stroke.
2. Educate the public about the need for emergency medical attention if signs and symptoms of CVA are present.
3. Offer support for the family of an older adult with an acute or chronic neurologic disorder. Rehabilitation may be lengthy and frustrating for both client and family members.
4. Assist in the development of a teaching plan regarding the disease process for older adults with neurologic challenges. Remember that clients with neurologic deficits may have special learning needs. See Box 11–5 for suggestions.
5. Educate families and caregivers in methods of facilitating communication with the client with Alzheimer's disease. Strategies are presented in Box 11–6.

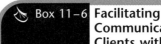

Box 11–5 Teaching Tips: Client with a Neurologic Disorder

• Tailor information to the individual based on his or her intellectual or physical challenges.
• Eliminate barriers to learning: make certain the client has eyeglasses, and hearing aids are in place.
• Provide information in the manner that makes the client most comfortable: discussion, video, demonstration.
• Present one concept at a time.
• Do not rush.
• Provide written instructions.
• Repeat information several times.
• Include family or significant other in teaching sessions.

Box 11–6 Facilitating Communication with Clients with Alzheimer's Disease

• Attract the client's attention.
• Maintain eye contact.
• Use gestures, pictures, and facial expression to convey more meaning.
• Repeat key words and phrases.
• Allow adequate time for comprehension.
• Keep sentences simple and direct.
• Provide "either/or" choices in questions.
• Supply missing words for the speaker.
• Avoid the use of pronouns.
• Paraphrase what the client has said, and ask if this is what was meant.
• Validate the client's emotional state rather than orienting the client to the fact or the "here and now" of the situation.
• Use memory books of life events to keep client stimulated.
• If the client is unable to stay still, continue the communication while walking.

Adapted from Hendryx-Bedalov, P. M. (2000). Alzheimer's dementia: Coping with communication decline. *Journal of Gerontological Nursing, 26*(8), 23.

Interventions to Promote Lifestyle Modification

1. Encourage the client at risk for CVA to modify factors that place him or her at increased risk.
2. Assist the client who has experienced a CVA in identifying areas at home that may require modification. Ideas to consider include removing throw rugs or other obstacles that may cause a fall, rearranging furniture for easier mobility, and reorganizing necessary items to promote self-care.
3. Identify with the client ways to arrange his or her environment to facilitate optimal self-care.
4. Encourage the client with a chronic neurologic disorder to perform activities of daily living within his or her ability, to prolong independence.
5. Assist the older adult with age-associated memory impairment in devising strategies to help compensate for memory lapses. Helpful strategies are presented in Box 11–7.

Interventions to Promote Mobility

1. Begin rehabilitation techniques and mobilization for the client with CVA as soon as he or she is neurologically stable. Early mobilization helps prevent venous stasis, contractures, and pressure ulcers. An explanation of the many facets of stroke rehabilitation can be found in Table 11–13.
2. Perform range-of-motion exercises with the client who has experienced a CVA or who has Parkinson's disease. Take care not to overstretch

Table 11–13	
COMPONENTS OF CVA REHABILITATION	
Discipline	**Areas of Expertise**
Physical therapy	Assist with regaining motor skills
Speech therapy	Help with language and articulation
Speech pathology	Assess ability to swallow
Occupational therapy	Assist clients to manage ADLs
Psychologists, counselors	Assist the client and family in dealing with feelings about new situations
Social workers	Make arrangements for client to return home or to another facility
Case manager	Coordinates management of the available resources

ADLs, activities of daily living; CVA, cerebrovascular accident.

the shoulder joint on the affected side of the client with CVA.
3. Elevate the arm of the client who has experienced a CVA to prevent edema.
4. Consider the possibility of pain in a cognitively impaired older adult. He or she may experience pain related to a musculoskeletal problem, such as arthritis, and be unable to effectively communicate this to you. In such a case, pain medication may encourage mobility.

Interventions to Promote Nutrition

1. Assist the client with an acute neurologic disorder in maintaining good nutrition. For the client with decreased LOC or dysphagia, a feeding tube may be required.
2. Weigh the client initially to obtain a baseline measurement, then weekly to assess adequacy of nutrition.

Box 11–7 Strategies to Help the Older Adult Compensate for Memory Lapses

- Use written reminders to perform important activities (such as activities of daily living) and place in strategic locations.
- Use verbal reminders, for example, offering water to drink.
- Recruit family and friends to help remind the older adult of activities and events.
- Use alarms or other audible reminders, such as setting an alarm clock, to remind the older adult to attend a group activity.

Health Promotion Tip

Encourage regular exercise according to the client's ability to stimulate appetite and keep the muscles in good condition.

3. Closely monitor the client with a neurologic disorder at mealtime and provide assistance with feeding as needed.

4. When providing assistance at mealtime, use an individualized approach, NOT a task-oriented, mechanistic strategy.

🍴 Nutrition Tip

Feeding a cognitively impaired older adult:

- Establish a pleasant dining environment.
- Approach the client in a gentle, nonthreatening manner.
- Introduce the older adult to his or her dining companions.
- Use a large cloth napkin rather than a bib.
- Present one course of the meal at a time with the appropriate eating utensil.
- Guide the older adult to feed him- or herself, offering assistance as required.
- Avoid the use of negative labels like "uncooperative"; rather, try to understand the meaning behind the client's behavior.

Data from Kayser-Jones, J., & Schell, E. (1997). The mealtime experience of a cognitively impaired elder: Ineffective and effective strategies. *Journal of Gerontological Nursing*, 23(7), 33–39.

5. For the client with Parkinson's disease, massage the facial and neck muscles before meals to reduce rigidity and enhance chewing and swallowing abilities.
6. Maintain accurate intake and output (I&O) records for the client with an acute neurologic disorder. Document and report immediately any unexpected mismatch in the I&O. For example, clients with acute neurologic disorders may develop a serious neurologic condition called diabetes insipidus, whereby large volumes of dilute urine are produced. This situation requires immediate medical treatment.

🍴 Nutrition Tip

Feeding a client with dysphagia:

- Stay with the client.
- Maintain the bed in high Fowler's position, making certain the client has not slipped down in bed.
- Offer semisolid foods, and avoid thin liquids.
- Encourage the client to tip chin *down* (flex the neck) to encourage food to enter the esophagus.
- Allow adequate time for feeding—DO NOT RUSH!

7. Because the older adult with a neurologic deficit is often dependent on those at home for meal selection and assistance, review the Food Guide Pyramid (Chapter 6) with the client and caregivers.
8. Implement nursing interventions aimed at reducing the risk of constipation related to weakened abdominal muscles and adverse effects of medications. Commonly employed interventions include encouraging fluid intake, increasing fiber consumption, enhancing mobility, and judiciously using stool softeners or laxatives.

Interventions to Promote Rest and Sleep

1. Provide a quiet environment to promote uninterrupted sleep.
2. Assist the client with acute CVA to find a comfortable position for sleep. Position the client on the unaffected side. Carefully use pillows and trochanter rolls to support any paralyzed extremity. Position any paralyzed extremity very carefully, as it may have abnormal sensations.
3. Provide passive range-of-motion exercises to alleviate muscle rigidity that may interfere with restful sleep.
4. Offer pain management interventions to the client with CVA or Parkinson's disease. Range of motion, careful positioning, or the use of heat may help. If these interventions are ineffective, consult with the physician or advanced practice nurse about the possibility of administering pain medications.
5. Encourage the client with Parkinson's disease who has difficulty sleeping at night to discuss medication therapy with his or her physician. For some individuals, an extended-release form of medication may improve nighttime sleep by decreasing skeletal muscle activity at night.
6. Employ nursing interventions designed to decrease agitation in the client with Alzheimer's disease to promote rest. Interventions that reduce physical expressions of agitation include massage, foot acupressure, and music therapy. If the client is on the medication donepezil (Aricept), administering it at bedtime can promote sleep.

GATHERING DATA FOR EVALUATION

Your role in helping to evaluate and modify the care plan for the older adult with an acute or chronic neurologic disorder is crucial. Your observations and data gathering regarding the older adult's neurologic status will provide crucial information in charting the course for successful nursing interventions.

As always, evaluate the care plan using the client outcomes as your guide. Outcomes that are very objective will make evaluation of progress easier. For example, one outcome identified for the nursing diagnosis, Risk for Injury, reads, "Client will experience no injury." This outcome can be easily evaluated at the bedside through your assessment and observations. In the evaluation column, you can write, "8/27: No injury noted," followed by your initials.

Evaluation of outcomes may also require you to be knowledgeable about the client's baseline. For example, one outcome written for the nursing diagnosis, Constipation, states, "Client will maintain regular bowel evacuation." Although a bowel evacuation every 3 days is certainly regular, it may be insufficient for an individual who is accustomed to a "once-a-day" pattern.

In addition, your evaluation should take into consideration individual interventions employed. Consider the nursing diagnosis, Anxiety. It would be helpful to document on the care plan which nursing interventions were most helpful in reducing the client's anxiety.

Summary

- The brain and spinal cord undergo neuron loss with age; the brain decreases in size and weight, and neurotransmitter production is reduced.
- Older adults demonstrate slower movements, delayed response time, slower reflexes, difficulty with fine movement, and perhaps senile tremor. Long-term memory tends to be better preserved than short-term memory.
- Learning complex information may take more time for the older adult. Life-long patterns of intelligence and personality remain stable.

- Functioning of the ANS is less efficient with age; thus, maintenance of homeostasis is more difficult.
- Dementia is never considered normal aging of the brain.
- The first step in assessment of the mental acuity of an older adult is to create a comfortable environment to encourage the best possible performance.
- Document the client's LOC, level of orientation, and mental status. The MMSE may be used. Assess and document pupillary response.
- Check for movement and strength in all extremities; note tremulousness at rest, gait, balance, coordination, and sensory/perceptual functioning.
- CVA is the third leading cause of death among Americans. Older adults are at increased risk for stroke, especially men. Rehabilitation can be painful, lengthy, and frustrating. Other risk factors include hypertension, cardiovascular disease, atherosclerosis, obesity, stress, smoking, high blood cholesterol, clotting disorders, and diabetes mellitus.
- CVA develops from interruption of blood flow to the brain. Ischemia and necrosis of brain tissue occur. Signs and symptoms can range from headache and blurred vision to coma and death, and depend on whether the right or left brain hemisphere is affected. Thrombolytic therapy has been shown to be effective for clients experiencing CVA from thrombosis or embolism. When thrombolytic therapy is administered within 3 hours of the onset of symptoms, brain tissue can be saved.
- Assist the emergency team with stabilizing the client who experiences a CVA. Attend first to the ABC's of emergency care. Other treatments include close monitoring and frequent measurement of vital signs.
- Parkinson's disease is a disorder of the central nervous system that affects one's ability to move about normally. Signs and symptoms of the disease usually appear between the ages of 50 and 70. The cause of Parkinson's disease is unclear and there is no known cure.
- The part of the brain affected by Parkinson's disease is the substantia nigra, which is responsible for the production of dopamine.

The four classic signs are tremor, rigidity, bradykinesia, and postural instability.

- Drug therapy for Parkinson's disease is aimed at controlling the symptoms. Levodopa/carbidopa (Sinemet) is often the first drug to be employed. Tolcapone (Tasmar) is a newer drug that enhances the effectiveness of Sinemet. New surgical procedures may help.

- Dementia refers to loss of short-term and long-term memory, as well as other cognitive deficits that occur gradually and worsen over time. The older adult may lose the abilities to perform self-care activities, to recognize familiar surroundings, and to recognize familiar faces. The most common form of dementia is Alzheimer's disease.

- It is important to differentiate delirium from dementia. Delirium is temporary disorientation, is usually treatable, and can be the short-term result of a number of factors.

- The major risk factor for Alzheimer's disease is aging. The exact cause is unknown. Primary abnormalities include the proliferation of tangles and plaques, and neuron loss. Initially, signs are subtle; later, more severe deficits become apparent, and in the final stage, the client is dependent on others for care.

- No known treatment will prevent or cure Alzheimer's disease, although certain medications, known as cholinesterase inhibitors, may slow the progression of symptoms. The two newest drugs used are donepezil (Aricept) and rivastigmine (Exelon).

- Nursing diagnoses are unique to the individual client. Once the nursing diagnosis is established, outcomes must be set. It is important that they be realistic, measurable, and individualized.

- Interventions to promote safety include the following: closely monitor LOC and vital signs of the client with an acute neurologic disorder; never offer oral food or fluids until swallowing has been tested; turn the bedridden client every 2 hours; and teach the client techniques for safe ambulation.

- Interventions to promote health education include the following: help identify individuals at risk for CVA; educate the public about the need for emergency medical attention if signs and symptoms of CVA occur; offer support; assist in the development of a teaching plan; and educate caregivers about ways to facilitate communication with the Alzheimer's disease client.

- Interventions to promote lifestyle modification include the following: encourage clients at risk for CVA to modify risk factors; assist the post-CVA client in identifying home areas that require modification; identify ways to arrange the environment to facilitate self-care; encourage self-care within the client's ability, to promote independence; and assist the older adult with memory impairment in developing strategies to help compensate.

- Interventions to promote mobility include the following: begin rehabilitation techniques; perform range-of-motion exercises; and elevate the arm of the client who has experienced a CVA. Consider the possibility of pain in a cognitively impaired older adult.

- Interventions to promote nutrition include the following: assist the client in maintaining good nutrition; weigh the client weekly; monitor the older adult at mealtime and provide assistance, as needed; use an individualized approach; massage the facial/neck muscles of the Parkinson's disease client before meals; maintain I&O records; review the Food Guide Pyramid with the client; and implement interventions to reduce the risk of constipation.

- Interventions to promote rest and sleep include the following: provide a quiet environment; assist the client with acute CVA to sleep on the unaffected side; provide passive range of motion; offer pain management interventions; encourage the client to discuss medications with the physician; and attempt to decrease agitation in the client with Alzheimer's disease.

- Evaluation should be aimed directly at the outcomes, and should take into consideration the effectiveness of individual interventions.

STUDY QUESTIONS

Multiple-Choice Review

1. Which of the following accurately describes normal changes of aging in the central nervous system?
   1. Neurons are lost in the brain but not the spinal cord.

2. Neurotransmitter production increases.
3. Fine motor movement becomes more difficult.
4. Long-term memory is not as sharp as short-term memory.

2. To obtain the best possible result from your neurologic assessment of the older adult, you should:
   1. Keep the pace relatively fast, to keep his or her attention.
   2. Perform the assessment in a room with fluorescent lighting.
   3. Perform the entire assessment in one sitting.
   4. Make certain the older adult is comfortable and well rested.

3. According to experts, the number one modifiable risk factor for CVA is:
   1. Smoking.
   2. Hypertension.
   3. Male sex.
   4. Diabetes.

4. The four classic signs of Parkinson's disease are:
   1. Tremor, rigidity, bradykinesia, and postural instability.
   2. Tremor, rigidity, bradykinesia, and forgetfulness.
   3. Numbness in fingertips, rigidity, bradykinesia, and postural instability.
   4. Tremor, rigidity, bradycardia, and postural instability.

5. Mr. Tagg is a 70-year-old gentleman who was recently diagnosed with Alzheimer's disease. He pays his bills on time and lives independently. He experiences mild forgetfulness; however, it has not compromised his safety. He has lost interest in attending family functions. What stage of the disorder is Mr. Tagg probably in?
   1. Stage 1
   2. Stage 2
   3. Stage 3
   4. Stage 4

Critical Thinking

1. The wife of your client recently diagnosed with Alzheimer's disease says to you, "Why should we try those new drugs? They will only slow down this terrible disease and put us through more torture!" How should you respond to this question?

2. Claire was diagnosed 3 years ago with Alzheimer's disease. She formerly was a nurse, but quit working after she had trouble remembering how to perform medication calculations. She still lives alone, but was unable to find her way home yesterday. She had quite a scare last week, as she forgot to turn her stove off after preparing lunch. Identify priority nursing diagnoses for Claire.

3. Mrs. Nguyen is an older adult with dementia who resides in the long-term care facility where you work. At mealtime, she usually makes a mess, spilling large quantities of food on herself and her surroundings. She tries to use various inappropriate items to feed herself, such as her knife or the menu card. Recently, she has started mixing all food items together into an unpleasant-looking mess. Describe some possible causes of the problem and nursing interventions you could employ.

4. Your older adult client who was recently diagnosed with Parkinson's disease informs you that he is considering taking up cigarette smoking because he read that "it could help." How would you respond to his statement?

Resources

Internet Resources

Alzheimer's Association
www.alz.org
Alzheimer's Disease Education and Referral Center
National Institute of Aging:
www.alzheimers.org
National Institute on Neurological Disorders
www.etb.ninds.nih.gov
Stroke Risk Screening Tool
www.destroke.org (click on "prevention")

Organizations

Alzheimer's Association
919 North Michigan Avenue, Suite 1000
Chicago, IL 60657-1676
(800) 272-3900

American Parkinson's Disease Association
60 Bay Street, Suite 401
Staten Island, NY 10301
(800) 223-2372

National Stroke Association
8480 East Orchard Road, Suite 1000
Englewood, CO 80111-5015

Selected References

Barker, E. (1999). Brain attack! A call to action. *RN, 62*(5), 54–57.

Brockington, C. D., & Lyden, P. D. (1999). Criteria for selection of older patients for thrombolytic therapy. *Clinics in Geriatric Medicine, 15*(4), 721–739.

Clifford, T. J., Warsi, M. J., Burnett, C. A., & Lamey, P. J. (1998). Burning mouth in Parkinson's disease sufferers. *Gerodontology, 15*(2), 73–78.

Dellasega, C. (1998). Assessment of cognition in the elderly: pieces of a complex puzzle. *Nursing Clinics of North America, 33*(3), 395–405.

Doraiswamy, P. M. (2000). Update on pharmacotherapy for Alzheimer's disease. American Association for Geriatric Psychiatry 13th Annual Meeting. Available at http://www/medscape.com/medscape/CNO/2000/AAGP/AAGP-06.html Accessed 11/26/00.

Ebersole, P., & Hess, P. (1998). *Toward healthy aging.* St. Louis: Mosby-Year Book.

Epstein, D. K., & Connor, J. R. (1999). Dementia in the elderly: An overview. *Generations, 23*(3), 9–16.

Farlow, M. R. (1999). Therapeutic advances for Alzheimer's disease and other dementias. *Medscape Neurology Treatment Updates.* Available at http://www.medscape.com/Medscape/Neurology/TreatmentUpdate/1999/tu03/pnt-tu03.html Accessed 12/4/99.

Favre, J., Burchiel, K. J., & Hammerstad, J. (2000). Outcome of unilateral and bilateral pallidotomy for Parkinson's disease: Patient assessment. *Neurosurgery, 46*(2), 344–355.

Follett, K. A. (2000). The surgical treatment of Parkinson's disease. *Annual Review of Medicine, 51*, 135–147.

Folstein, M. F., Folstein, S. E., & McHugh, P. R. (1975). "Mini Mental State": A practical method for grading the cognitive state of patients for the clinician. *Journal of Psychiatric Research, 12*, 189–198.

Ford, B. (1998). Pain in Parkinson's disease. *Clinical Neuroscience, 5*(2), 63–72.

Fratiglioni, L., & Wang, H. X. (2000). Smoking and Parkinson's and Alzheimer's disease: Review of the epidemiologic studies. *Behavioral Brain Research, 113*(2), 117–120.

Galloway, S., & Turner, L. (1999). Pain assessment in older adults who are cognitively impaired. *Journal of Gerontological Nursing, 25*(7), 34–39.

Gerdner, L. A. (1999). Individualized music intervention protocol. *Journal of Gerontological Nursing, 25*(10), 10–16.

Hendryx-Bedalov, P. M. (2000). Alzheimer's dementia: Coping with communication decline. *Journal of Gerontological Nursing, 26*(8), 20–24.

Hodgson, B. B., & Kizior, R. J. (1999). *Saunders nursing drug handbook.* Philadelphia: W. B. Saunders.

Honey, C. R., Stoessl, A. J., Tsui, J. K., Schulzer, M., & Calne, D. B. (1999). Unilateral pallidotomy for reduction of parkinsonian pain. *Journal of Neurosurgery, 91*(2), 198–201.

Jacobson, D. (2000). Unmasking Alzheimer's. *UCSF Magazine, 20*(1), 17–23.

Jann, M. W. (2000). Rivastigmine, a new-generation cholinesterase inhibitor for the treatment of Alzheimer's disease. *Pharmacotherapy, 20*(1), 1–12.

Kayser-Jones, J., & Schell, E. (1997). The mealtime experience of a cognitively impaired elder: Ineffective and effective strategies. *Journal of Gerontological Nursing, 23*(7), 33–39.

Kelly-Hayes, M., & Phipps, M. A. (1999). Preventive approach to poststroke rehabilitation in older people. *Clinics in Geriatric Medicine, 15*(4), 801–817.

Kurlowicz, L., & Wallace, M. (1999). The mini-mental state examination (MMSE). *Journal of Gerontological Nursing, 25*(5), 8–9.

Leira, E. C., & Adams, H. P. (1999). Management of acute ischemic stroke. *Clinics in Geriatric Medicine, 15*(4), 701–720.

Lewis, S. M., Heitkemper, M. M., & Dirksen, S. R. (2000). *Medical-surgical nursing: Assessment and management of clinical problems.* St. Louis: Mosby.

Matteson, M. A., McConnell, E. S., & Linton, A. D. (1998). *Gerontological nursing: Concepts and practice.* Philadelphia: W. B. Saunders.

Mazzoni, P. (2000). Movement disorders: New and clarified options for treatment. Proceedings from the 52nd Annual Meeting of the American Academy of Neurology. Available at http://www.medscape.com/medscape/cno/2000/AAN/Story.cfm?stort_id=1213 Accessed 8/17/00.

Milisen, K., Foreman, M. D., Godderis, J., Abraham, I. L., & Broos, P. L. O. (1998). Delirium in the hospitalized elderly: Nursing assessment and management. *Nursing Clinics of North America, 33*(3), 417–436.

Monahan, F. D., & Neighbors, M. (1998). *Medical-surgical nursing: Foundations for clinical practice.* Philadelphia: W. B. Saunders.

Rowe, M., & Alfred, D. (1999). The effectiveness of slow-stroke massage in diffusing agitated behavior in individuals with Alzheimer's disease. *Journal of Gerontological Nursing, 25*(6), 22–34.

Schweiger, J. L., & Huey, R. A. (1999). Alzheimer's disease: Your role in the caregiving equation. *Nursing99, 29*(6), 34–41.

Stocchi, F., Barbato, L., Nordera, G., Berardelli, A., & Ruggieri, S. (1998). Sleep disorders in Parkinson's disease. *Journal of Neurology, 245*(Supplement 1), 5–8.

Sutherland, J. A., Reakes, J., & Bridges, C. (1999). Foot acupressure and massage for patients with Alzheimer's disease and related dementias. *Image: Journal of Nursing Scholarship, 31*(4), 347–348.

Tandberg, E., Larsen, J. P., & Karlsen, K. (1998). A community-based study of sleep disorders in patients with Parkinson's disease. *Movement Disorders, 13*(6), 895–899.

III

Promotion of Psychosocial Health for the Older Adult

Promoting Psychosocial Health and Wellness

SIGNE S. HILL and HELEN STEPHENS HOWLETT

OBJECTIVES

After completing this chapter, you will be able to:

- Define emotional well-being as it applies to the older adult.
- Discuss the psychosocial characteristics of centenarians.
- Identify the importance of family as related to role change and loss.
- Describe how powerlessness, alcohol abuse, and depression are threats to psychosocial wellness in the older adult.
- Examine the nursing role in promoting psychosocial wellness in the areas of sexuality, pet therapy, music therapy, volunteer programs, senior centers, and humor and spirituality.

CHAPTER OUTLINE

KEY TERMS

Activity theory
Alcohol-dependent
Alcoholic
Anxiety

Busyness
Centenarians
Continuing stressors
Continuity theory

Denial	Oldest old
Disengagement theory	Projection
Displacement	Regression
Dysthymic	Role reversal
Emotionally	Selective memory
Exploiting age or illness	Selective sensory intake
Gerotranscendence	Socially
Idealization	Somatization
Illusion	Spirituality
Integrity vs. despair	Subintentional suicide
Intellectually	Young old
Multitasking	Zoonotic

CASE STUDY

Mattie was 59 years old when her husband died a painful death. She was glad when he died. During his final hours of life, she related incident after incident of how he had hurt her feelings. She had kept these feelings in during their 30+ years of marriage. Her anger intensified through the years, as she waited for a time she could tell him, without fear of retaliation.

After the death of her husband, Mattie felt energized and almost happy. She purchased a home in the country, applied for a job in a nearby mental health facility for clients with chronic mental illness, took training to become a nurse's aide, and made client care the center of her life. She also enrolled for driving instruction, purchased a car, and for the first time in her life felt totally in charge of her life. Sometimes she would travel to neighboring towns for a day trip or invite a friend or two to join her for a longer adventure. Family and friends were amazed at how well she coped with her husband's death. For the most part, Mattie experienced a sense of emotional well-being. Had the aggressive verbal attack on her husband at the time of his death dealt with the underlying problems? Was the one-way communication enough to resolve the core issues? Was her sense of relief temporary or permanent? Would the feelings intensify again and show up at a future time? Throughout this chapter, we will examine different aspects of Mattie's story to illustrate psychosocial concepts of aging.

PSYCHOSOCIAL HEALTH

Mattie met basic criteria for psychosocial health. She was in touch with reality and able to cope with activities of daily living, and she functioned within the rules of society. **Emotionally,** Mattie had dealt with the loss of her husband through a direct angry outburst. **Intellectually,** she had made a life-changing decision to begin a new career. **Socially,** she changed her environment by purchasing her own home and enhanced her independence by learning to drive and owning her own car. Mattie reestablished contact with former friends to create an active social life. **Spiritually,** her life was on hold because she questioned whether God would allow so many bad things to happen to her.

Mattie was soon to be influenced by psychosocial changes shared by other older adults.

Everything went reasonably well until age 65, when she faced retirement. Although older adults usually fare well with retirement, Mattie's retirement was mandatory. When her employer told her that he would be calling her back to work part-time, she assumed this would be without pay. No way was anybody going to take advantage of her when she had always put so much into her work. When the calls came, she abruptly turned each opportunity down. Only much later did she learn from a former employee that she would have been paid for her work. By that time, Mattie's personal habits had begun to deteriorate. The daily walk to and from work had kept her muscles flexible, to say nothing about the stretching involved in client care. The facility had made food available to employees for a modest price. She had eaten with fellow employees of her choice, so the eating time not only provided nourishment but was a social occasion as well. Once she was on her own, cooking for one person held minimal interest. Mattie literally retreated to her rocking chair next to her heating stove. Her main companions were the coffee pot on the stove, radio talk shows, and assorted television programs, including soap operas and game shows. Mattie's sleep patterns changed, and she slept for short periods around the clock. At no point did she feel rested. She began to turn down opportunities to socialize with friends and family members who had been a part of her life. How did Mattie's psychosocial changes relate to those faced by other older adults?

Personality traits became even more ingrained, resulting in less flexibility in problem solving and behavior. Older adults become more of whatever they were before. Mattie verbally made it clear that if she could not do what she wanted to do, which was work for pay with clients she loved, she would do nothing. "No one can make me do anything," she said. This statement turned out to mean more than anyone, including her family members, could have realized.

The use of defense mechanisms can help an older adult adjust to changes of aging, but they can also interfere with this adjustment. Negative use of defense mechanisms made Mattie's life increasingly difficult. Mattie developed a variety of illnesses during the next years of her life. Common defense mechanisms are defined in Table 12–1. As you read the information in this table, see if you can identify which defense mechanisms Mattie used and how she used them.

Table 12–1	
COMMONLY USED DEFENSE MECHANISMS	
Defense Mechanisms	**Definition**
Denial	Unpleasant realities are denied and kept out of conscious awareness
Projection	Attributing one's own feelings, actions, and behaviors to others
Regression	Behaving in a helpless or childlike manner
Somatization	Complaining of physical symptoms to gain attention
Displacement	Taking out feelings on someone less threatening (e.g., a grandchild)
Idealization	Overestimating an admired aspect or attribute of another
Selective memory	Recalling only positive or negative aspects of a situation
Exploiting age or illness	Gaining advantage, attention, or favors based on age or illness
Busyness	Keeping stressful feelings and thoughts temporarily in check
Selective sensory intake	Responding only to what you can deal with

WELLNESS

The wellness-illness continuum is a popular way to think about mental illness and mental wellness. The continuum, an imaginary line with mental health on one end and mental illness on the other end, changes for individuals on a daily basis according to what is going on in life. The ideal is to be past the center point and as close as possible to mental wellness (health) on any given day. Think about the course of Mattie's life. Where on the illness-wellness continuum do you see her at the time you were first introduced to her and at this time?

According to Erik Erikson's theory of personality development, the stage or task of the older adult is **integrity vs. despair**. The age involved is usually from 65 years to death. Integrity means that the person has developed a sense of self and an understanding of his or her personal motivation. Older adults accept the human life cycle and are able to look back with satisfaction on their own achievements. They are able to accept assistance if needed and they adjust, or substitute, when losses occur. They have developed a wisdom that permits them to accept both past failures and future limitations. They are also able to help the younger generation to view life realistically and to finally accept death with dignity. The significant person during this stage of development *is* the older adult. Despair means that the older adult is dissatisfied with the way in which he or she has lived life, is disgusted with the series of missed opportunities, and sees him- or herself as a failure. Ultimately, an older adult in this state faces death with fear. An actual dread of death, once identified, may be a sign of depression.

A newer theory of personality development differs from Erikson's theory in that the person is not looking back. Lars Tornstam's theory of **gerotranscendence** shows that life crisis accelerates the process of personality development. The changes cannot be explained away as symptoms of illness or depression or as the result of psychiatric medications. People with a high degree of gerotranscendence have the following characteristics: a higher degree of self-controlled social activity, a higher degree of life satisfaction, and greater satisfaction with social activities. They are also less dependent on social activities for their well-being and have more active and complex coping patterns (Tornstam, 1999-2000).

Psychosocial theories of aging, which were briefly discussed in Chapter 1, have been used to explain how the older adult responds or should respond to the psychological challenges of aging. The **disengagement theory** indicates that the older adult and society mutually disengage (pull away) from each other. The **activity theory** supports the continuation of activities and hobbies, as well as substitution when necessary, in order to sustain interest in, and quality of, life. The **continuity theory** suggests that older persons become even more predictable based on their previous patterns of involvement in life. Another possibility that has been discussed in the news media is that perhaps pessimists live longer because they never expect things to go right and are always on the alert for another loss. Mattie certainly fit into this last category. She also fit into the disengagement theory, especially when viewed as selective disengagement. Could it be that one theory does not fit all older persons and that there is more to be learned?

PSYCHOSOCIAL CHARACTERISTICS OF CENTENARIANS

The **young old** are older adults up to age 75 years. The **oldest old** are persons age 75 years and older. The age 75 years plus is the most rapidly growing age group in our population, and this trend is expected to continue. **Centenarians,** who are the oldest old adults, are 100 years of age and older. Interest in the study of centenarians has been generated by the recent increase in their number. A major study conducted by the University of Georgia investigated 11 areas: basic personal information; family longevity; social and environmental support; personality, stress and coping; life satisfaction and morale; physical health; mental health; nutrition and dietary patterns; intelligence and cognition; reminiscence; and religiosity (Poon et al., 1992). The most important characteristics of centenarians included optimism, engagement, hope, and the ability to cope with loss. According to records, the oldest living person is at least 121 years old.

Centenarians have escaped the usual causes of earlier deaths, notably those related to the cardiovascular system and cancer. However, with aging, the incidence of chronic disease including dementia (see Chapter 11) increases. The ongoing myth is that all centenarians are robust, that is, they experience good mental and physical health. This is usually not true. Approximately one third of centenarians fit this category. The other two thirds are described as "housebound" or "bedfast" (Smith, 1997).

Mattie did not permit herself to be happy or pleased for any length of time. She often said, "when something good happens, you can be sure that something bad will happen soon." Mattie involved herself in selective engagement; for example, she did not turn down a game of cribbage or a chance to try out a new restaurant. Even after she had agreed to participate in an activity or to visit someone, she would often cancel at the point of getting ready to leave. She was never hopeful that things were going to turn out or that she would be able to enjoy herself. The one hope that Mattie had was a secret that was revealed only when her death became imminent: "I wanted to live until I was 85, so that I would be older than Mandy when she died at 84 and one half"!

THE IMPORTANCE OF FAMILY

There is a myth that older adults in our society are abandoned by their families and spend their remaining years alone in nursing homes. According to the 1990 census: of older men, 75% live with their spouses, 18% live alone or with nonrelatives, and 7% live with other relatives; of older women, 39% live with spouses (women live longer than men), 43% live alone or with nonrelatives, and 18% live with other relatives. Furthermore, today, more families than ever before are involved in the care of older family members. Approximately two million women who have children and work outside the home also care for older adult family members.

Mattie's family was no exception to the trend. Although her family lived a good distance from her, they visited frequently and assisted with chores, repairs, and appointments, and did whatever Mattie requested of them. There were times that they wished she had been one of those persons who had a pleasant personality all of her life and became even more pleasant with age. Mattie

had always harbored underlying disagreeable feelings and, as she aged, she was less able to hide them. She had never been a warm person and made it clear which family members she favored. The female grandchildren and great-grandchildren experienced most of her wrath (displacement). When confronted, she would accuse them of lying (projection). Mattie especially favored a particular grandson, and he could do no wrong in her eyes (idealization). All memories of him were held in great favor with enhancements to make the memories even more positive (selective memory). Adult family members found ways to deal with her negative responses, knowing that these changes were related to her sense of despair about her childhood and her adult life. The younger members tried hard to please and accepted the explanation that Mattie's behavior was not about them.

Role Change

When psychosocial and physical changes take place slowly, it is easier for the older adult to adapt to these changes. In the intellectual realm, decreased verbal ability and changes in pitch, loudness, and voice tone may be so subtle that they go unnoticed. A compound set of verbal or written instructions may have to be repeated or broken down into steps. There may be a slower response in following verbal directions and/or in comprehending the scope of the immediate situation. As one ages, risk taking is less common and the person feels more vulnerable. Anxiety-provoking situations are more likely to affect memory and the ability to learn. Long-term memory is the least affected in the older adult. The person can usually remember details about grade school but is unable to recall what he or she had for breakfast. Many older persons compensate for unreliable short-term memory by preparing to-do lists so that they do not forget the important tasks for each day. Mastering new skills may take more time as one ages. Daily chores and ordinary intellectual tasks such as paying bills are not hampered by normal age-related changes. There is a relationship between retaining intellectual skills, level of education attained, and continued stimulation. Mattie's choice of watching daily game shows enabled her to participate in the show actively. She would try to come up with the correct answer before the contestant could answer the question. Mattie deliberately made this choice, knowing that her social isolation could take a toll on her intellectual ability.

Because so much value is placed on independence in our culture, it is difficult to age gracefully and accept help when it is needed. There may be a **role reversal** between spouses related to mental or physical illness. When Mattie's husband became seriously ill, he was angry with her for assuming responsibility for the finances. He had always made all of the financial decisions with the exception of the money that she earned. Her husband paid all the bills, but would not give her any spending money except for groceries. Getting an outside job was her major strike for independence. Mattie would save her earnings until she had enough money to get what she really wanted. For example, she had bought an electric stove to replace the old gas stove that came with the apartment, and she had a long fur coat made for herself. Mattie liked the sense of power that came with managing the finances, and she discovered that she had a way with numbers. She even began to invest the money, and the savings gradually increased. There was no way that she was going to share that power again with anyone until the very end.

Even with her success in managing money, other past decisions affected her ability to trust those around her. Major vision changes made her suspect that things were being removed from her home without her permission. This increased her determination that no one in the family would tell her what to do in regard to living arrangements and personal care issues. She carefully checked her house and garage after someone had visited to see if something was missing. Mattie occasionally forgot that she had given an item as a gift and would accuse the person of stealing.

Loss

For many older adults, most **continuing stressors** relate to losses. Mattie lost the job that had given new meaning to her life. In the process, she lost her reason for exercise, good food, and casual companionship. She also lost the opportunity to learn through doing her work and attending required in-service programs. *Become a nonperson*

The next major loss in her life was the death of her dog, Rufus. "He never judged me and I could always tell my troubles to him. He never told me what I should do, and it was okay with him if I made mistakes. Rufus would just snuggle up and love me anyway." Because of deep issues of lacking trust in herself, she did not feel this same level of comfort with most family members.

When Mattie's eyesight began to fail, she compensated for her concern about safety by driving to the railroad yard parking area and taking a bus into town to do her errands. This method worked for her for a couple of years. When the surgeries on her eyes were unsuccessful, she had to begin to rely on family members to take her to buy groceries and do errands. This did not go over well with her. Her family wanted her to surrender her driver's license because she would periodically sneak to the grocery store by herself. Her vision at this stage was dim, at best. She confided that the best time to drive was in the morning because a film settled over her eyes in the afternoon.

The losses related to neurosensory changes create anxiety in older adults. Changes in vision combined with perceptual changes make it difficult for the older person to quickly identify the names on street signs, whether the person is driving or acting as the navigator for a spouse or friend. Looking to one side and then the other to locate a sign or place can cause the car to go in the opposite direction (change in proprioception). The person is thus more vulnerable to accidents. Changes in sight hinder one's ability to locate items at different levels in the grocery store. The person often ends up with something that is in a similar package but is not the correct item. In the hospital or other facility, older adults may have difficulty finding their rooms or the bathroom. Reading the newspaper, a favorite magazine, or instructions for taking a medication becomes a chore. Most print whether on a menu or in a favorite book is not meant for challenged eyes. It becomes difficult to dial phone numbers, and no one may think of getting a telephone with extra large numbers. Mattie was fortunate that a grandson knew these were available and purchased such a telephone for her. He also bought her a digital clock with very large numbers that she could even see in the night. He recognized that there were times that she would not be sure what time of the day it was when she awakened. He found her a watch with large numbers that was useful both at home and when going out.

Fortunately, Mattie's hearing remained keen. Loss of hearing can result in an **illusion** (misinterpretation) of sounds, especially in the night. The person begins to worry that someone is trying to break in when no one is there. It becomes difficult to take part in a meaningful conversation. Others may think that the errors are funny, and the person may withdraw from further attempts because of humiliation. Doctors' appointment times and dates may not be heard properly, resulting in missed opportunities for diagnosis and treatment. Assessment questions may be misunderstood. Older adults with hearing difficulties may find that people do not speak directly to them but instead ask a relative or staff member who is near them how they are doing. The onset of nonperson status is a grim reality for some older adults. Mattie made sure that her presence was known. She would tell the doctor or nurse, "Ask me; I know the most about me."

When Mattie began to show symptoms of serious illness, she either refused to go to the doctor or, when appointments were scheduled, would change her mind. Because she was 5 feet 6 inches tall and 240 pounds, no one was going to pick her up and take her in. A sitdown strike had begun. Mattie used denial as a major defense mechanism during this period of time. "I don't have anything wrong with me. Seeing the doctor is a waste of time and money." To her way of thinking, if you didn't admit to something (or could avoid diagnosis), then it didn't exist. The loss of physical strength and stamina and the increased bouts of diarrhea and constipation made her even more irritable toward those around her.

Mattie's friends seemed to be taking turns dying. She cared for one long-time friend in her home for a time and saw her through her death. Mattie tried to attend the funerals of the "good friends" and stayed away from the funerals of "not so good" friends. "It doesn't help much," she said. "Preachers talk too long about nothing and leave important stuff out about the person." She would sometimes comment that there was hardly anybody left that she knew.

THREATS TO PSYCHOSOCIAL WELLNESS IN THE OLDER ADULT

What constitutes a threat to psychosocial wellness for the older adult is largely dependent upon how they have responded to their own stages of growth and development, beginning with infancy. " . . . Mastery of developmental tasks through adolescence plays a key developmental role in determining how resourceful healthy elders are in their daily activities" (Zausznieski & Martin, 1999). You may know an older adult who views mental and physical changes with a sense of curiosity, for example, "I noticed during the past couple of days that I can't just whip out of bed anymore. It makes me dizzy. Guess my body is telling me to take my time." Alternatively, older adults may notice that they cannot always trust their own memory: "I write everything on my calendar and look at it first thing every morning. I missed some meetings before I began using a calendar." Problem-solving skills continue to be important, as is the desire to learn about age-related changes and to make the necessary adjustments.

Powerlessness

There is plenty of evidence that, with aging, the older adult faces increased **anxiety** (sense of impending doom). As his or her world narrows owing to age-related changes and losses, everyday issues take on a significance that they did not hold previously. Mattie experienced numerous events that increased her sense of powerlessness. She had initially redeemed a sense of power by taking on a job that she loved and did well. Both the clients and the head nurse praised her for her conscientious work. She achieved status by improving the care of the clients for whom she was responsible. The clients had fewer acute psychotic episodes than had been recorded for several years. Losing the job was an automatic loss of status for Mattie. She also experienced loss of identity.

Loss of her job also put Mattie on a fixed income. She began to limit payments and purchases to only what was needed, knowing that there would be no extra money coming in. This probably played a role in limiting her outings with friends, thereby limiting her social life even more severely. There was no hope that this would ever be different.

Mattie's sense of powerlessness increased as her physical strength decreased. She had always taken pride in how she dressed and how she looked. This became increasingly difficult for her to do. It no longer was an easy fix to put rollers in her hair and comb it out just so. She finally got a wig to wear when going out. Her make-up became limited to powder and lipstick. Finally, even that took too much effort. When people dropped in unexpectedly, she was sure they were thinking, "Poor Mattie—she doesn't have it any more," and that made her unhappy. Ultimately, she simply wore a housedress around the clock, changing it only as necessary. Her many lovely nightgowns stayed clean and folded in the drawer.

Mattie had always been fussy about her personal cleanliness, a personality trait that had developed because being clean was not a part of her childhood. She had suffered from being teased in grade school because of body odor. As soon as she was old enough to take care of herself, she vowed nothing like this would ever happen again.

It was difficult for Mattie to ask for help when getting into and out of her tub. It was even more difficult to not meet the standards she had set for herself. After being unable to get out of the tub one day, she let the water out, reached for towels to cover her, and went to sleep. When Mattie awakened, she refilled the tub, recalling that her granddaughter when first learning to swim had demonstrated how water made the body more buoyant. A reminder from a child had saved the day! When her family arrived to take her out to dinner, she was dressed and ready. Later that evening, she told the story and said she guessed she did need "a bit of help."

Multitasking had been a way of life for Mattie for as long as she could remember. This characteristic, which is common for most women, enabled Mattie to have several projects going on at the same time (multitasking), and to get them done as planned. She knew that her arthritis was slowing her down, but what she did not count on was her short-term memory playing tricks on her. Mattie would plan to do something, and

along the way she would do other tasks that needed to be done. When she arrived in the room she was heading for, she could not remember why she was there. Mattie would backtrack to where she started from and repeat the task out loud so that she would not forget again. Playing this game with herself worked for a while. She would determine in advance which jobs she wanted to do, count the number of tasks, and keep the number in mind as she went along. Finally, it was safer to just focus on a single task at a time. This latter development occurred just after the time she put her frying pan on the heat of the stove and heard the mailman. She got engrossed in going through the mail, and the pan overheated. Mattie was grateful that she had not put the oil in the pan. That could have caused a fire.

Mattie was also proud of her home in the pines and the yard she had pampered. Many of the additional trees were ones that she had dug up from the woods and replanted. She had faithfully watered them to get them to grow. Mattie had cleared away underbrush and other vegetation. She put up birdhouses and bird feeders. An occasional bear would come and feast on the oatmeal that she cooked for him. As time went on, Mattie could no longer rake and mow her lawn. Although others would do it, she made it clear that they did not do it quite right. At least by assertion, she was trying to maintain some sense of power.

Although Mattie had been admitted to the hospital several times in her life, her experience during diagnostic testing for what was to be her final surgery was trying. Hospital sheets gave her a rash, and even after a change to Ivory-washed linens, this took a while to clear up. Her son brought in her down quilt and pillow, so she could sleep.

Mattie was physically uncomfortable and emotionally stressed in the hospital. Everything felt like it was no longer under her control. Pain was not being controlled to her satisfaction. When she rang for a nurse, she had to wait before getting to the bathroom. For years, her bladder had kept her going frequently around the clock. Urinating into a bedpan was no small chore, and trying to place it just right did not work.

The morning after her admission to the hospital, a family member walked in to find two nurses giving her a bed bath. One was on each side of the bed. Mattie's covers were pulled to the end of the bed and there wasn't a bath blanket in sight. Even the privacy curtain had not been drawn! Was Mattie in control? Did she have any power? Not likely. The family member interceded quickly, but the damage had already been done. It was at that point that her son decided someone would be with Mattie 24 hours a day.

Mostly, she feared that she had inoperable cancer and would die as her husband and many friends had done, with severe pain. It turned out that she was correct. When the doctor explained the results of the tests, Mattie's defense mechanism of selective sensory intake kicked in. This helped to stabilize her during both surgery and the recovery period. Mattie felt so much better after her palliative surgery that she was able to maintain the defense mechanism until her condition began to deteriorate. This gave her a way to regain some power until she absolutely had to deal with reality. This began a more peaceful time during which she visited places with meaning, requested help in doing some long-term planning, and began to accept help from her family. Many other changes continued to instill a sense of powerlessness. Mattie expressed this feeling as irritation. For example, it was difficult for her to get into and out of a car. She made sure that she wore something slippery to facilitate rotating out of the seat. In some ways, her limited eyesight made what she could not accomplish less annoying. She could chide a family member who was cleaning that it really did not need to be done. It was an interesting time during which she was losing power and trying to find ways to regain it.

Alcohol Abuse

Another important threat to psychosocial wellness for the older adult is alcohol abuse. In *Healthy People 2010*, the Surgeon General has addressed alcohol and substance abuse issues as target areas for improvement. Selected objectives related to alcohol abuse can be found in Box 12–1.

Dulling chronic pain is often a reason for getting involved in drinking alcohol. Mattie had osteoarthritis that caused pain with any kind of movement. She had the perfect set-up for alcohol abuse. An interest of Mattie's that she continued

---

> **Box 12–1 *Healthy People 2010* Objectives Related to Alcohol Abuse**
>
> - Reduce deaths and injuries caused by alcohol- and drug-related motor vehicle crashes.
> - Reduce the number of cirrhosis deaths.
> - Reduce alcohol-related hospital emergency department visits.
> - Reduce intentional injuries resulting from alcohol- and illicit drug–related violence.
> - Reduce the proportion of persons engaging in binge drinking of alcoholic beverages.
> - Reduce average annual alcohol consumption.
> - Reduce the proportion of adults who exceed guidelines for low-risk drinking.
> - Reduce the treatment gap for alcohol problems.
> - Increase the proportion of persons who are referred for follow-up care for alcohol problems, drug problems, or suicide attempts after diagnosis or treatment for one of these conditions in a hospital emergency department.
>
> Data from U.S. Department of Health and Human Services, *Healthy People 2010* website http://www.health.gov/healthypeople. Washington, DC: U.S. DHHS, 2000.

---

to pursue after retirement was making wine. She had a large chokecherry tree in her yard and learned to make sweet wine from the berries. Mattie used the bottles of wine for gifts, but there was also a time she thought the wine might ease her joint pain. Mattie could do her drinking privately and in secret, as older women tend to do. She liked the taste of her wine but discovered quickly that the wine aggravated her joints even more. Mattie described it by saying, "it goes right to my knees." A brief trial of this form of self-medication was enough. However, Mattie's reliance on Vicodin and aspirin is another story.

The estimate of older adults involved in heavy drinking (12 to 21 drinks per week) is about 3% to 9% (Older Adults and Mental Health, 2001). Approximately four times more men than women are involved in heavy drinking. The number for both men and women is expected to increase as Baby Boomers age. Older adults do not fit the usual description of alcohol abusers because the standard description is based on young men. Older adults usually are no longer in the work force and are not operating vehicles on a regular schedule. Their responsibilities have changed, and there may be no "boss" to evaluate reliability. Drinking activity is often more solitary and hidden, especially for the women involved. Alcohol abuse can mimic chronic disorders, or the older adult may have a chronic disease unrelated to alcohol.

> ## ⚠ Signs and Symptoms Tip
>
> Signs and symptoms of alcohol abuse in older adults:
>
> - Falls or small accidents
> - Injuries
> - Self-neglect
> - Confusion
> - Abdominal complaints
> - Uncontrolled hypertension
> - Ecchymosis
> - Insomnia
> - Weight loss
> - Vague physical complaints
> - Chronic depression
> - Tension headaches
> - Memory loss
> - Fatigue

Nurses sometimes forget to ask about alcohol use. Some nurses assume that their older clients do not drink. A home health practical nurse told a story of how she was alerted to drinking problems in the housing complex for older adults. She had been making regular visits there for a long time and never suspected a problem. The nurse was having a drink one evening with her friend who was a garbage hauler. He always had some stories to tell, but on this particular evening, he made a comment about the large number of beer, wine, and booze bottles deposited in the senior housing trash each week. The nurse was definitely interested and discussed this information at the next staff meeting.

The home health nursing staff decided to add questions about alcohol use to their assessment of all older adults, including those who lived in their own homes. They specifically asked, "Do you drink alcohol"? If this question was answered affirmatively, they asked about the type of alcohol, when it was consumed, and how much and how often each day. Every vague answer was followed by a request for specific information. This was a small, close-knit community in which people knew a lot about each other. The nurses were not prepared for what they learned. The number of older adults abusing alcohol was large, and the attitude regarding intervention was, "Leave me alone. I have worked hard all of my life, and what I do with the rest of my time is my own business." Up to this time, no one had aggressively sought information about drinking patterns and intervention. This was about to change.

Shared information revealed that a common area of concern for older clients was medication. Needs ranged from discussing medications with their physicians to understanding directions about their use; drug interactions such as additive effects when certain medications are combined with alcohol and other adverse effects were other areas of interest. A workshop on medication for older adults was planned. Information about combining medications and alcohol was included. Presenters would also include information on age-related changes in the liver that made it less efficient in detoxifying alcohol and other drugs. This seemed to be a perfect way to reach many older adults. The trick would be to get them there. Patterns of attendance at other meetings had proved that food and transportation were the enticements. Workshop invitations encouraged older adults to bring their spouses or family members who helped them with their doctors' appointments and medications. The turnout was better than anticipated. Getting direct advice on what to do was an important aspect of the workshop, which was followed by smaller-group community meetings to provide information on available services, costs of services, and which were covered by health care policies. Attendees learned how to access services such as Alcoholics Anonymous and psychotherapy. The tone of the presenters was empathetic and never judgmental.

Older adults who are involved in alcohol abuse fit into one of two major categories. They either started abusing alcohol many years ago, or they just started drinking within the past few years. The older adult may be alcohol-dependent, or may be an alcoholic. The individual who is addicted (alcoholic) will experience physical withdrawal symptoms when alcohol consumption is stopped. The alcohol-dependent older adult will not have such a physical withdrawal effect.

Reasons vary as to why older adults use alcohol (*The Brown University GeroPsych Report*, 1998). A common reason is related to attempts to self-medicate. Anxiety related to losses is a reality, plus there is the realization that the loss is often permanent. Drinking initially decreases anxiety. Alcohol also sedates the person who is having trouble getting to sleep. However, alcohol prevents the person from going through the needed sleep cycles in order to wake up rested. Alcohol is also used to blur the feelings associated with depression. It reduces inhibition and, for a while, makes things funnier, brighter, and more loving. For the shy person, socialization becomes easier. In a social setting, alcohol breaks down barriers of race, culture, social class, and religion. An older adult who was asked why he spent so much of his time at the club drinking said, "Where else can I find so much laughter and companionship? The judge, a councilman, the top surgeon, a construction worker, a truck driver, and I are all at the same table laughing and having a good time. No one cares about anybody's race, religion, finances, or ethnic background." It works for a while, until the effect of alcohol begins to take a toll.

Older adults who are isolated and lonely are also candidates for alcohol abuse. Their spouse or partner may have died. Family members may live far away. Driving or other means of transportation may no longer be readily available. Reading and other hobbies may not hold interest, or the older adult may be limited by mobility and eyesight. Sexual problems may exist. Some have retired directly to their easy chairs and television. Others have arrived there because of the limitations imposed by a chronic disorder. For some, a few drinks can make a mediocre television program look pretty good. Furthermore, time seems to pass more easily with no need for the older person to think about it.

Conflicting information in the media provides a reason for some older adults to start drinking. Although media messages suggest "if you do not drink, don't start," a far more forceful message is about the possibility that one drink a day is good for the heart. If there is heart disease in the family, the older adult may interpret this as being worth a try. Perhaps the individual does stay with the one drink a day, perhaps not.

Women seem to be more susceptible to the effects of alcohol. There is speculation that this is related to a decrease in alcohol dehydrogenase, which breaks down alcohol in the body. The higher body fat–to–body water ratio in women is thought to result in a higher blood alcohol level after a smaller amount of alcohol. Women begin drinking hard liquor sooner than do men, who often begin by drinking beer. Older women are also more likely to develop serious illness such as liver disease sooner (Ludwick et al., 2000).

For both men and women, it is thought that alcohol is an underlying cause of many physical and psychosocial disorders. It is associated with an increased risk of oral, pharyngeal, and esophageal cancers. Other important conditions related to alcohol intake include liver disorders; hypertension, stroke, and heart failure; brain shrinkage of the prefrontal and frontal lobes (especially in men who experience chronic alcoholism); alcohol personality disorder; depression; anxiety disorders; sexual disorders; and cognitive disorders. Calcium metabolism is impaired, thereby increasing the risk of osteoporosis. The immune system is depressed, making the older adult susceptible to infections such as pneumonia, flu, and tuberculosis. Thermoregulation, which is already compromised in the older adult, is further affected by alcohol. The older adult becomes even more susceptible to hypothermia. Consider the possible consequences of this for the older adult who has turned down the thermostat to reduce heating costs.

Physical and psychosocial disorders related to drinking alcohol affect the client's state of psychosocial health and wellness. Emotional changes can range from mellowness to rages. Paranoid responses are common. Intellectually, the person exhibits a decreased ability to process information. Confusion is common, as are forgetfulness and poor judgment. Socially, the person may withdraw and may be unable to continue meaningful relationships. Family problems increase. Poor balance and gait can lead to falls and other injuries. Drinking often replaces meals, leading to malnutrition and related physical and psychological problems. Spiritually, the older adult may feel out of touch and may dis-continue previous spiritual practices that brought comfort.

Depression Not normal ī aging

Depression in the older adult is often dismissed as aging, senility, or a dementia. Depression often remains undiagnosed, even though assessment tools like the Geriatric Depression Scale are available. For example, the older adult with mild to moderate symptoms of Alzheimer's disease may deny both cognitive and depressive symp-toms (Shau-Haim et al., 1997). Frequently, the presenting complaint relates to a physical illness or to chronic pain. Depression does not look the same in the older adult as it does in the younger person.

> ### ⚠ Signs and Symptoms Tip
>
> Signs and symptoms of depression in older adults:
>
> - Pseudodementia
> - Chronic pain
> - Anxiety disorder
> - Alcohol and/or other substance abuse
> - Somatization

There is actually far more information avail-able about identifying and treating depression in children and younger adults. Many older adults prefer to seek medical help from their primary physician, and make frequent visits for physical complaints when they are depressed. Assessing activities of daily living (ADLs), mood, feelings, or behavioral changes may not be part of the protocol. It is common practice to limit client office visit time. Referral to specialists may not be as readily available because of cost-cutting practices in a specific clinic or by an insurance company. Some policies still disconnect the mind from the rest of the body as far as avail-ability of psychiatric services is concerned. In-formation about available services may actually be suppressed. For example, a health educator for a county health department received a por-tion of her salary from the local medical clinic.

Part of her responsibility to the clinic was to write a weekly column in the local newspaper on health and illness issues and how to access ser-vices. She would always submit her article to the clinic director for review. When she decided to do a series on mental illness that encouraged clients to discuss such problems as depression with their doctor, she was told to drop the idea. However, the health educator felt that the infor-mation was important because of the number of older adults in the community, and she wrote the article anyway. Information on signs, symp-toms, and possible treatment was included. The newspaper published the first article and then mysteriously did not have available space until she began writing about physical illness again. The newspaper editor would offer no additional information. Finally, a person on the clinic board explained that psychiatric care is not cov-ered by the major health maintenance organiza-tion (HMO) in the area.

Clients may also be intimidated by fear of stigma related to psychiatric diagnosis and treat-ment. Stigma is still a reality as far as mental illness is concerned (Bauer & Hill, 2000). One at-titude that remains is that depression is brought on by the person, and it can be remedied by "pulling yourself up by the bootstraps." It is still regarded by some as a weakness of character, rather than an illness. Depression is increasingly referred to as a physical illness regardless of its cause. This makes treatment more acceptable to some older adults; also, the physical emphasis is true for certain depressions.

In a nursing home setting, basic care is often provided by a nursing assistant who is not trained to identify symptoms of depression. The licensed practical nurse/licensed vocational nurse (LPN/LVN) charge nurse may have been educated in a program with no mental (psychiatric) nursing theory and clinical experience. The registered nurse (RN) supervisor is often too busy to do a comprehensive psychosocial assessment of all clients. The ideal of having a geropsychiatric nurse on staff is possible for a limited number of agencies. Physician consultations are often dependent on information provided by the charge nurse, and the focus remains on physical com-plaints. One psychiatrist who consulted at a nursing home complained that his biggest prob-lem was related to the fact that nurses did not understand how psychotherapeutic drugs worked. When adverse effects began to develop (and they do appear earlier than the therapeutic effects of the drug), the charge nurse would call the primary physician who would usually discontinue the drug without consulting the psychiatrist. No wonder your instructors quiz you about the effects and adverse effects of each medication you give. Your responsibility to keep your knowledge current does not end at graduation.

Looking back, Mattie probably had a **dysthymic** (less severe, more chronic, low-grade) depression much of her life. She had a depressed mood most of the day for more days than not. She was able to function and hold responsible jobs throughout her life, but never felt real joy or satisfaction in regard to herself and her life. Mattie may have experienced major depression at different periods of her life, then returned to the dysthymic state upon recovery. Symptoms such as deepening mood, loss of interest and pleasure in activities, insomnia, weight gain, slowing of activity, fatigue, a sense of worthlessness and guilt, and indecisiveness about obtaining medical care certainly signal a major depression. Did anyone pick up on Mattie's depression? Not really. Her rare visits to her doctor or surgeon were related to serious physical ailments, and were often followed by surgery. Her family provided the follow-up care and had mostly adjusted to her moods. They saw this behavior as her personality. Mattie saw it as her life.

Mattie was not alone in experiencing depression. An estimate of older adults with mild depression who live in the community is about 8% to 20%. The rate increases to over 30% for those who live in nursing homes and similar facilities. Associated risk factors include previous depressive episodes, family history of depression, previous suicide attempt, female gender, heavy use of alcohol, illness, and certain medications. Other triggers for depression include losses (previously discussed), such as death of a loved one (including a pet), financial worries, and certain illnesses (Box 12–2). Depression often increases the severity of other illnesses, or makes the older adult more vulnerable to illness. The older adult with depression might fail to fill a prescription or to take the required medication. Both self-neglect and the effect of depression on body systems weaken the natural defense mechanisms.

> ### Medication Safety Tip
>
> Drugs that may cause depression:
>
> - Antihypertensive agents (e.g., propranolol)
> - Systemic corticosteroids (e.g., prednisone)
> - Antiparkinsonian medications (e.g., levodopa)
> - Narcotic analgesics (e.g., fentanyl)
> - Sedative hypnotics (e.g., zolpidem)

The risk of suicide is approximately six times greater for the white man over 80 years old than for any other age group (Older Adults and Mental Health, 2001). Many of these suicides are directly related to depression. The lethality of the method chosen indicates that the person intended to commit suicide. When assessing for depression, it is important to ask if the person has considered suicide and, if so, to determine their method and plan. The method and plan alert you to the seriousness.

Long-standing self-destructive behavior is sometimes referred to as **subintentional suicide** and is not counted as a part of suicide statistics. Mattie's behavior was long-standing self-destructive behavior. Mattie also had periods in her life when she may have considered active suicide. She also had the means. Mattie had purchased a small handgun to protect herself from intruders. She slept with the handgun by her side each night. What may have kept Mattie from going through with a plan was the self-challenge to live longer than Mandy.

> ### Box 12–2 Illness That Can Cause Depression in Older Adults
>
> Hypothyroidism
> Diabetis mellitus
> Stroke (especially left hemisphere)
> Parkinson's disease
> Alzheimer's disease
> Myocardial infarction
> Head injury
> Central nervous system tumors
> Infections (especially viral)
> Cancer
> Multiple sclerosis

The irony of undiagnosed depression of older adults is that it is a treatable disorder. If the depression is medication-related, discontinuing or changing the medication will solve the problem. If it is illness-related, as with hypothyroidism, treating the disorder usually relieves the depressive symptoms. For other types of depression, antidepressants and electroconvulsive therapy (ECT) are the most common therapies. Because of age-related physical changes, older adults are initially treated with a small dose of medication that is titrated carefully until the therapeutic dose is achieved. The nurse must know about and be alert for the adverse effects associated with a specific medication. The older adult is far more sensitive to the untoward effects of antidepressant medications than is the younger patient, and some antidepressants must be used with great caution. ECT does not cause the adverse effects associated with medication. If it has been successful during previous depressive episodes and the older adult does not have a physical disorder that will be adversely affected by the treatment, ECT may be a treatment choice. It is considered the fastest-acting, most efficient therapy available without the adverse effects of medication. Temporary memory loss is the most consistent adverse effect. If the older adult has not had a previous depressive episode, medication is often prescribed first.

Psychotherapy is highly recommended to accompany the medical treatment, which relieves symptoms of depression. The medical treatment alone does not resolve the underlying issues that helped to create the depression. Group psychotherapy involving other older adults is preferred. Older adults find out that they are not the only ones with morbid (dark) thoughts and feelings. Most important is that they problem-solve together and assist each other with possible solutions to the underlying problems.

Clients who are not able to participate in group therapy sessions have been shown to respond favorably to the efforts of empathic staff members. The effect of the caregiver's touch cannot be overemphasized. How a person is touched either validates or invalidates the client as a human being. Using gentle touch when providing routine care, doing range-of-motion exercises, and giving a soothing backrub or footrub is much more than a mechanical function. Clients often report that the final footrub in the evening soothes them into peaceful sleep. Music chosen according to the client's personal taste adds to the therapeutic effect. Aromatherapy with essential oils, such as lavender, is gaining greater acceptance for its calming effect in many facilities for older adults.

PROMOTION OF PSYCHOSOCIAL WELLNESS IN THE OLDER ADULT

Psychosocial wellness is a reality for the majority of older adults. Lifestyle choices are used to modify the potential risks associated with aging. There is a common thread in the characteristics that these older adults seem to share. First, their life has not been without personal crisis, but they have had the ability to face and solve the problems encountered. They have built up a supportive network of people who are really there for them (Figure 12–1). They are careful to stay away from destructive people and situations, especially when recovering from a crisis. They are able to get past their feeling of being a victim and take charge of what happens to them. Overall ability to solve novel problems (sometimes called *fluid IQ*) may decrease with age. This tendency can be countered through training in problem solving and the development of cognitive skills strategies. Ongoing training of older adults involves contact with members of their support system as they discover ways to help each other and to deal with whatever they are facing, along with more formal learning provided through workshops.

These individuals are also considered tough in the sense that they look at incidents in their life as challenges to be met and to overcome. Although they tend to remain healthier by refusing to adapt to a victim mode, this does not mean that they are free from chronic disorders. One difference is that they do not see themselves as their disease; for example, they would not say, "I'm diabetic." When pressed, they are more likely to say, "I *have* diabetes." Older adults with this characteristic have solid commitments to certain areas of their lives. These might include family, personal wellness, special organizations, church, volunteer programs, enrichment classes, music, theater, travel, and so forth.

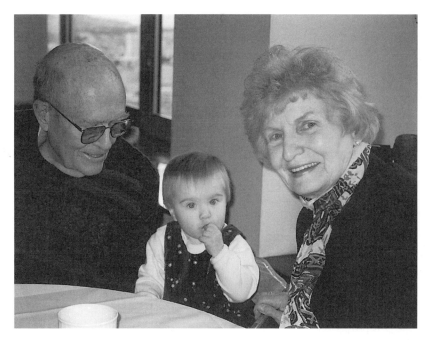

Figure 12–1. The rewards of grandparenting in one's later years.

Older adults who are psychosocially well also recover from, or adjust reasonably well to, crisis and change in their life. A history of being flexible in life serves them well as challenges continue to emerge. When old ways of dealing with issues fail, they look for alternative, novel ways of overcoming and dealing with new challenges. They continue to regard life as holding purpose and meaning. They live their lives with as much meaning as possible each day, rather than constantly focusing on what the future will hold.

Sexuality

Humans are sexual beings from birth to death. Infants discover early the pleasure of touching their genitals. As older adults are dying, touching their genital area is a natural self-comforting reaction. Because of all the myths, taboos, and rules that are culturally driven, many older adults who are dying are prevented from soothing themselves in this manner. Some care facilities have been known to tie the wrists of the older adult to the bedrail to prevent them from touching their genitals as they are dying. Most health care facilities today have rules regarding the use of restraints.

However, a policy alone without staff understanding of growth and development is insufficient to cause meaningful change.

Sex refers to the physical, erotic, and genital relationship. Sexuality is everything else—thoughts, feelings, experiences, emotions, values, and fantasies as they relate to being male or female. It is further personalized by how we communicate the way we feel about ourselves through words, posture, clothing, actions, and attitude. Sexuality includes how we relate to members of the opposite or same sex, and how we respond to the messages they send. Sexuality is a part of our lives from birth to death.

Many of you will work in facilities that provide care for older adults. Now is the time to examine your feelings, attitudes, and values about sex. Once this is clear in your mind, consider sex and the older adult. Older adults continue to be interested in and to enjoy sex. For some, sex may not occur as often or with youthful intensity, but it continues to be a source of satisfaction and promotes a sense of psychosocial well-being. With aging, sexuality continues to be a part of the human reality. Older adults, regardless of sexual orientation, continue to hug, hold hands, kiss, touch, flirt, and dress to attract as ways of expressing sexuality.

Mattie shared a gentle intimate relationship for a time. Sam's wife of many years had died and he missed her deeply. Mattie and Sam had known each other for as long as they could remember. They were neighbors out in the country and began to get together to share a meal or to go on a day trip. The time together translated into laughs about old times, and gradually they grew closer. Although both had grown children, none of the children attempted to interfere with the relationship. Their relationship continued until he became ill and died. Unlike the death of her husband, Mattie responded to this loss with sadness.

Sexuality is expressed in many ways. An older adult in his 70s proudly showed his most recent snapshots. The first picture was of his lovely wife who had died several years ago. The others were photographs of beautiful women that he had taken during a recent trip to Brazil. He explained that he always appreciated looking at beautiful women. Since his wife died, he had traveled throughout the world as a way to fill his loneliness. Whenever he saw a really beautiful woman, he would ask to take her picture; that was all. As he left the train, he was seen giving an appreciative look to a beautiful woman. The gentleman he shared the pictures with (an older adult) gave him a thumb's up.

What will be your response when you walk into a room or dayroom and see that a client is masturbating? What if a client reaches to touch your breasts or your genitals? How about the client who insists on patting your buttocks? How will you respond to the client who asks you to stimulate him/her during a shower, tub bath, or bed bath? What are you going to do when you are doing a room check and find two clients engaged in intercourse? How will you react when you find your client reading sexually explicit magazines or watching an erotic video? And how will you respond to the client who tells you that you are really "hot" and that he/she is ready for the date you've been hinting about? At this point, go back to the beginning of the paragraph. Imagine the same scenes, but with someone in your own age group. Is there a change in your internal reaction and self-talk?

Granted, much of this behavior is based on the life-long need for closeness—to be touched, held, and valued. One client said it quite well: "It's like my skin gets so hungry and no one wants to touch old people." Sometimes caregivers have set the stage for the client's behavior. Think about a time when you may have heard someone kidding a client about going on a date. The banter may come off as lighthearted and funny. However, if the client is experiencing cognitive impairment, they may be taking the conversation seriously. Finding out that he/she is mistaken is both embarrassing and a rejection. The client may begin to avoid staff. How staff members dress has an impact as well. A professional look is hard to mistake and gives the client a sense of safety. Suggestive clothes give a different message, a mixed message, whether the staff member is male or female.

Think and talk about how you will deal with the older adult when similar situations occur. Which behaviors are best ignored? When will you suggest a more private area for the client to continue what he/she was doing? *When is the behavior an attack that must be stopped immediately so that no harm occurs?* When does a situation enhance the client's well-being? When does the client need to be reported? When would a community meeting with staff and clients be appropriate? When do you simply leave the client alone to complete whatever is going on? Which behaviors will cause you to say "No, you may not do that (or will not do that)"? Will what you hear and see be passed on as institutional gossip? When must something be passed on to the charge nurse?

Tunstull and Henry (1996) did something unique because of their concern that the sexuality of their nursing home residents was at times a problem for the staff. They developed a seven-session support group called the Intimacy Group. The group involved both staff and residents and focused on intimacy and friendship as well as sexuality. A group dinner involving staff and residents supported the theme of intimacy and friendship. Staff interventions included role modeling and education. Resident interventions included personal counseling sessions, provision of privacy, help with grooming, medical evaluation, and interdisciplinary care planning. These clinicians concluded that much of what they did could work elsewhere, with modifications appropriate to meet each facility's needs.

Loss of libido and impotence (now called erectile dysfunction, or ED) are often brushed off as, "What do you expect? You're up there in years."

This loss can create problems in intimate relationships and, in some cases, accusations of unfaithfulness. Remember to check out adverse effects of the medications you give to your clients. The physician may be able to substitute a medication without disrupting the therapeutic effect. Sometimes a physician will specifically order a medication that is effective therapeutically and also decreases libido, in order to decrease inappropriate sexual acting out.

Viagra (sildenafil citrate) reversed impotence in about 50% to 80% of the men in a study undertaken by the manufacturer and the FDA. The men in the study had either illness-related impotence or impotence due to psychological causes. The most common adverse effects were headache, facial flushing, and indigestion. Some men had blurry vision or saw everything tinged blue.

The manufacturer warns against taking Viagra in conjunction with nitroglycerin or other nitrate medications that are used to relax blood vessels and lower the blood pressure of men with angina and other circulatory problems. The combination can lower blood pressure drastically and could be fatal. Viagra is also discouraged for clients who have had a heart attack, stroke, or serious arrhythmia within the past 6 months, who have significantly low blood pressure or blood pressure higher than 170/110, who have a history of heart failure or coronary heart disease causing unstable angina, or who have retinitis pigmentosa. Sometimes, a man may experience a prolonged, painful erection, which requires medical attention. Viagra has also emerged as a street drug.

Medication Safety Tip

A life-threatening abuse of Viagra combined with "poppers" (amyl nitrate) is being used to enhance sexual performance. The severe decrease in blood pressure can be fatal. The addition of amphetamine provides a triple threat. The combination of amyl nitrate, which lowers blood pressure, and amphetamine, which increases blood pressure and respiration, can lead to cardiac arrest.

Source: *Psychopharmacology Update*, October 1998, 9(10), 2–3.

Pet Therapy

Mattie would have told you that it is often easier to talk to an animal than to a human. A pet provides unquestioning emotional support. Hospitals and long-term care units that have not incorporated pet therapy as part of treatment are surprised to learn that pet therapy has a long history. The York Retreat, started in the late 1700s for the mentally ill, had small animals like chickens and rabbits that the clients helped care for. As a result, harsh treatments of the day and control methods such as restraints were used with less frequency. Florence Nightingale, as early as 1860, was said to have advocated a small pet as a companion for someone ill, especially if it was a long-term illness.

Observational evidence shows that clients respond physically in positive ways to the presence of pets. The greatest response is to personal pets, whether in critical care units or in a nursing home setting. However, there is also a positive response to carefully chosen pets that are part of an animal therapy program established for a facility. A protocol is established and followed, and clients are the beneficiaries of the program. There has been no increase in **zoonotic** (animal-borne) illness with the introduction of carefully screened pets. When blood pressure has been monitored as a measure of effectiveness, both the systolic and diastolic rates have shown a decrease, as have respirations. Withdrawn clients often respond to a dog or cat, and the animal becomes the catalyst for therapy. Dogs and cats are also used to encourage range of motion and strengthening of muscles. This is done through play with the animal. An animal therapist who regularly takes one or more of her well-trained dogs into the rehabilitation unit tells the story of a man who was refusing to cooperate with the therapists. She walked in with her Russian wolfhound and asked if he would like to pet him. He gave a curt response, "Get out of here"! She agreed, but gave the dog a hand signal to stay. The pet therapist explained that the dog was refusing to go, but she would be back for him shortly. By the time she got back to the client's room, he was petting the dog and laughing. It was the breakthrough the staff needed.

Pet therapy also decreases tension, induces relaxation, and stimulates interest in surroundings.

Clients with pets seem to recover more quickly and are thought to live longer. Owners who are able to have their pets with them when they are dying look peaceful. This may be related to having their dog or cat next to them and being comforted by touch. This was true for Mattie who had been given an older dog about a year before she died. Having the dog gave her responsibility. He also provided incentive for movement during feeding, going outdoors, and brushing. Duke was always close to her, and she naturally reached out to pet him. If she didn't, Duke would manage to find her hand. He was a source of laughter for Mattie and never far away. As Duke gave to her, she also gave to him.

The Eden Alternative, developed by Dr. William Thomas and others in 1991, is a way to change nursing homes into habitats for human beings. While serving as medical director for a nursing home, Dr. Thomas realized that quickly visiting clients and ordering medication did not effectively relieve the symptoms of illness. The three major issues of helplessness, loneliness, and boredom were identified as a common denominator of traditional nursing homes. The core concept for the Eden Alternative is that long-term care facilities for the elderly should be seen as habitats for human beings, rather than institutions for the frail and elderly. The introduction of children, animals, birds, and plants in a natural setting stimulates interest and provides an opportunity for clients to participate in their care. In this setting, clients give as well as receive care. The Eden Alternative is considered a process, not a program. It requires the participation of all staff members and clients to help it grow and evolve (Thomas, 1996).

Music Therapy

Everyone has some connection to music. It seems to reach clients when other methods fail. It is a mistake to assume that the same kind of music relaxes everyone. Music that relaxes one client may be stressful to another client. Remember too that, like your own taste in music, what the client wants to hear may vary according to the time of day and what is happening.

Some clients may not be able to tell you verbally what music they want to hear and will signal you nonverbally with their behavior. Music is used successfully to calm and reduce agitation in clients who have Alzheimer's disease. Music also helps the client sleep by increasing the secretion of melatonin, which is secreted mostly at night and provides sleeping and healing effects.

Sing-along has become increasingly popular in nursing homes. When the songs are familiar, they bring joy, increase sociability, foster contact with reality, enhance cognitive skills, develop listening skills, and promote attention span and expression of feelings. Music is used as a motivator for exercise, coordination, and strength. The beat becomes the focus for whatever is being done. Self-pity and physical complaints are known to decrease when the music is based on the client's wishes. For Mattie, religious music was a way to get in touch with her spirituality.

Volunteer Programs

Volunteerism is a way to stay engaged in life and maintain higher cognitive and physical functioning. Major motivators are an enhanced sense of purpose; giving back to society; the desire for personal growth; following through on an interest; continuing productivity; and the need for structure in daily life (Bradley, 1999–2000). For the long-term volunteer, there is also a relationship to improved physical health. Persons most likely to be involved in volunteerism are younger older adults who are well educated and better off financially. Some older adults see volunteerism as a life-long commitment. One older adult, Pat, said, "When I was growing up, my brothers and I were already expected to volunteer. Our father would periodically remind us that we had a responsibility to give back to our community. You work hard, you receive, and you also give back." She is quick to point out to committee members not doing their share of the work that volunteer commitment is no different than a commitment to work for pay.

Because of the costs, many health and social programs for older adults would not be possible without volunteers. The most common roles assumed by volunteers (more women than men) are those of ongoing support provider and lay educator or facilitator. Examples of programs in which older adults can volunteer include hospice; grief counseling; home safety checks; feeding, reading to, and rocking preemies; teaching memory skills and other older adult health-related classes; senior food programs; meal delivery; tutoring students; and much more. Volunteering helps one to maintain a sense of self-worth by continuing to do work that enhances the lives of others. Those who volunteer experience a sense of belonging and community. The physical activity enhances muscle strength and mobility, thus decreasing the likelihood of illnesses related to sedentary lifestyle. As people live even longer, most older old adults still prefer to live outside of institutions. Examples of volunteer specialty programs available to support living at home include The Faith in Action and The Senior Companion Program. The Faith in Action uses church volunteers and, through the generosity of start-up funds from the Robert Wood Foundation, involves nearly 450 churches, synagogues, and social service agencies. Depending on the geographic area, volunteers perform services such as delivering medications and groceries to isolated older adults. The Senior Companion Program, started in 1974 and managed by the Federal Corporation for National Service, is one of the oldest volunteer programs. The original idea—to help the poor by hiring them for a small stipend to do chores for home-bound older adults—has continued to expand. The cost to the taxpayers is a fraction of what it costs to provide nursing home care for older adults (Rowe, 1997).

Senior Centers

Title 111 of the Older Americans Act of 1975 directed the development of comprehensive and coordinated services to serve the needs of older adults. A 1997 amendment identified senior centers as service delivery focal points. The plan was to deliver services to *all* adults, including those at risk. In reality, the services provided vary according to center budgets, competency of staff members, location of the center, and whether there is transportation available. The activities, trips, recreational programs, and services have added enrichment to the lives of older adults who are capable of going to the center. Some centers have added teleconferencing programs for home-bound older adults, Internet through Senior Net, and interactive television programs.

While Mattie was still working, she visited the senior center closest to her. There was no bus pick-up service as an option for those located outside the city limits. Mattie did not say why she decided to stop going after just two visits. She hinted that she did not fit in, and that was the end of it for her.

Humor

Humor is a powerful communication tool, whether it is used to lighten up a serious situation or as a way to express hostility. The latter is the most difficult to counter because the individual responds with, "I was just kidding," or, "Can't you take a joke?" The recipient of the joke or slight is further humiliated or angered when trying to explain how the message came across to him or her—a no-win situation.

The timing of humor, its appropriateness, and the person involved are important aspects of humor. Older adults have a genuine ability to laugh at themselves and are the first to share jokes about aging. More and more, long-term care facilities are including humor classes for their clients. Class often starts with clients sharing a favorite joke or a recent cartoon. Humor relieves stress and is connected physically to a client's state of wellness. Laughter releases endorphins, a natural analgesic. It also increases adrenaline in the brain and enhances memory and learning. Clients have gone so far as to surround themselves with humor (funny movies, videos) as a way to help them heal. Humor is also a way of gaining perspective about a situation that feels overwhelming. Sometimes, exaggerating a situation completely out of proportion while imagining outlandish endings results in laughter. This is what worked with Mattie.

As Mattie's health continued to decline, she began to talk about how the doctor lied to her when he said she would be all right. Her daughter had accompanied her to doctor visits before and after the surgery. She gently corrected Mattie. In time, Mattie was able to acknowledge what she had really heard. As visits continued, it was time to introduce the topic of Mattie's wishes for her funeral. This is where good humor came into play and saw her through until she died. Mattie responded by saying she didn't care "I'll be dead anyway and won't know." When the response was, "Of course you will, Mother. Your spirit will be hovering over the coffin with finger pointed, saying 'I don't like the coffin, I don't like the flowers, I don't like the clothes I'm wearing, I never wore my hair like that, I always hated those songs, and what on earth is the preacher talking about? And furthermore, who ever thought of feeding this stuff to people after the funeral?'" Mattie began to laugh for the first time in months: "You're right. That sounded just like me. Okay, I'll think about this." Over a period of weeks, Mattie planned every step, with the exception of what she was going to wear from her waist down. The laugh line up to 2 days before her death was, "I still haven't decided, but no one will know that I'm buck-naked from the waist down!" This humorous approach may not work with someone else as it did with Mattie. You must know the older adult well before attempting to use it.

Spirituality

Spirituality is unique to each older adult. It includes a personal belief of how the person came into being, what sparked the breath of life into their physical being, the meaning of life, how to live life, and the meaning of death. Belief is influenced by culture, life experiences, and other personal factors. All people are considered to be spiritual whether or not they have a religious affiliation. Religion is the attempt to give structure to spirituality—to provide specific rules, rituals, and guidelines for living.

Older adults, especially women, are considered to be highly spiritual and religious. Some studies have shown a connection between spiritual well-being and a sense of purpose in life, positive self-worth, and physical and emotional health. Observations suggest that older adults recover more rapidly from a physical or emotional crisis when they feel connected to a higher power. They also face death as a continuing part of the life cycle.

Even though spiritual assessment is part of the nursing process, spiritual intervention continues to be neglected by nurses. More and more, nursing textbooks are addressing spiritual need as a part of holistic care. Putting theory into action remains difficult for some nurses. Part of this is related to the fear of imposing personal beliefs. A larger issue is lack of knowledge about the beliefs, practices, and rituals of religions other than

their own. Take time to learn about the practices of all the religions represented in the area in which you live and work. Remember to examine your personal belief system. When you understand, value, and respect your spirituality, differences are no longer threatening.

Nurses are busy with all that they must accomplish in the course of a day. Sometimes, it seems that there is no time for spiritual assessment and intervention. Think about what you talk about to your client during the time you are giving care. Any client contact provides time to use the nursing process. Spiritual assessment involves open-ended questions about strength, hope, and the meaning of life. General questions to include in a spiritual assessment by the nurse can be found in Box 12–3.

Your job is not to take over for the client and become his or her spiritual leader. Neither is it your job to make clients dependent on you as their source of spiritual inspiration. Part of your responsibility may be to contact the client's spiritual leader with his or her permission. Some realistic interventions are provided in Box 12–4 for your consideration and further development.

Mattie, as you recall, had put her spiritual beliefs on hold. As it turned out, the time that she spent sitting alone looking out at her beautiful yard with birds and other wildlife provided opportunity for introspection. Remember too that she listened to the radio at night and watched television during the day. She gradually began to check out early-morning religious programs on both radio and television. Mattie would mention that she liked so-and-so, but not someone else,

---

Box 12-3 | Questions to Ask in a Spiritual Assessment

- What is your source of strength when you face a serious illness (or loss)?
- What gives you a sense of hope in dealing with challenging situations?
- Who is your source of inspiration?
- Are there any spiritual or religious practices that you have not been able to continue since your illness?
- How can we assist in meeting your spiritual needs?

Box 12–4 Spiritual Care Interventions

- Ask open-ended questions.
- Actively listen to the client. Sit beside the client.
- Be aware of nonverbal messages from the client.
- Experience the feelings of the client but avoid adopting those feelings for yourself (empathy).
- Expect to learn from clients.
- Stay with the client after the person has received an unfavorable diagnosis.
- When appropriate, offer to pray with clients.
- After assessing the situation and when appropriate, offer to read scripture or other special reading to clients.
- Assist the client to participate in religious rituals.
- Protect the client's religious articles.

Data from Hill S. S., & Howlett H. S. (2001). *Success in practical vocational nursing from student to leader.* Philadelphia: W. B. Saunders.

and "Oh yes, the music." Programs became important enough for her to turn on even when family was visiting. Her spiritual life had been given a second chance.

Interesting changes began to emerge slowly. Even though Mattie's physical illness continued to become more serious, she began to recover emotionally. It was as though she was learning that just because she had pain, she did not have to contribute to her own pain. Mattie began to find ways to give back to life in subtle ways. She expanded the kinds of programs she listened to, and began to share new information that she thought would be helpful to the one with whom she was conversing. Mattie began to develop an appreciation for how much life had taught her, and how much new knowledge she was continuing to gain.

There was a sense of urgency when she would say, "I know so much and I have so little time to teach it to others." Mattie was gifted with her hands. She had, for example, made lifelike wood fiber flowers for weddings and for homes. When Mattie went on her sitdown strike, the materials just sat there for years. One weekend when a granddaughter arrived for a visit, she was surprised to find the boxes of materials on a card table. "I know you asked me a long time ago to teach you how to make flowers. If you're still interested, we can do it." Mattie had begun to shift her focus to the needs of family and those dearest to her. A serene kind of happiness began to follow.

When Mattie began to take a second look at her spirituality, she also set the stage for accepting help more graciously. Her son brought a hot meal to her every night. It was a social occasion when they ate together. Her appetite had dwindled, so there was enough left each time for lunch the next day. Finally, she asked if she could come and live with him, and she did so for the last 2 weeks of her life. During that time, she continued to plan her funeral, and chose the verses to be read and songs to be sung. The verses and songs were the ones that had given her comfort: "I always liked . . . ." Mattie also took it upon herself to call her two granddaughters to ask if they would sing these songs at her funeral. Not only did she acknowledge the beauty of their voices but was able to let them know that she loved them. During each of the conversations, Mattie began to cry for the first time in years. She confided that the tears were for herself and the people she was leaving.

Mattie made clear what had annoyed her at other funerals and asked that these pet peeves be avoided. Also, in case you think Mattie had mellowed beyond recognition, not so. The day before she died, Mattie said with an unusual amount of strength in her voice, "I can't wait to see Joe (her husband). I've got a few more things to say to him!"

Her physician made a home visit when additional symptoms emerged. This time, she listened carefully and asked about her prognosis. Based on the prognosis, Mattie chose not to have further treatment. Mattie also asked for medication that would relieve her pain. This she received, as prescribed, around the clock. Mattie died where she wanted to, in her son's home, under his watchful eye. She died peacefully one morning just as the sun was rising. Mattie was 85 years old.

Summary

- Psychosocial health relates to the emotional, intellectual, social, and spiritual characteristics of an older adult.

- They are in touch with reality, able to cope with activities of daily living and to function within the rules of the society in which they live.
- Psychosocial health does not mean the absence of physical illness.
- Location on the wellness-illness continuum varies according to how the individual copes with daily challenges.
- Many theories attempt to explain what normal aging is. No one theory fits perfectly.

- The most important characteristics of centenarians include optimism, engagement, hope, and the ability to cope with loss. They consider themselves healthy and practice moderation in eating and drinking. A majority see themselves as being religious and tolerant of the views of others, and they practice forgiveness of themselves and others.
- The myth persists that older adults are abandoned by their families and live their remaining years in nursing homes.

  - Of older men, 75% live with spouses, 18% live alone or with nonrelatives, and 7% live with other relatives. Similarly, of older women, 39% live with spouses, 43% live alone or with nonrelatives, and 18% live with other relatives. More families than ever are involved in the care of older adults.
  - Giving up long-time personal roles is difficult.
  - Continuing stress for an older adult is related to loss.

- A threat to psychosocial wellness is largely dependent on one's response to all other stages of growth and development.

  - Powerlessness is related to the loss of anything that provided support to personal identity, status, financial security, social contacts and independence, and so forth.
  - Alcohol is used to dull chronic pain, to self-medicate, or to cope with isolation and loneliness. More men drink heavily than do women, but women are more susceptible to the physical effects of alcohol.
  - Depression unrecognized and untreated is related to increased physical illness and suicide. The rate of suicide is approximately

six times greater for white men over 80 than for any other age group.

- Nurses can play a significant role in promoting psychosocial wellness of the older adult.

  - Nursing skill is based on knowledge of self, scientific knowledge of age-related changes, and appreciation of the older adult as a work in progress.
  - Sex and sexuality continue as a vital part of life for older adults. Staff needs to be respectful of age-appropriate behavior and to set limits on inappropriate or harmful behavior.
  - Pet therapy is widely used because of its healing effect both physically and mentally.
  - Music therapy, when based on need and individual taste, is a way of touching the very core of an older adult. Music calms and reduces agitation in the client with Alzheimer's disease. It is also a catalyst for activity, socialization, increased cognition, and uplifted spirit.
  - Volunteer activities provide a way for older adults to stay engaged in life, and make it possible for senior programs and activities to continue when that would otherwise not be possible because of cost.
  - Senior centers focus on senior services but best serve those who are able to come to the centers. Some centers have staff and finances that permit them to assist frail, home-bound adults.
  - Humor is a powerful communication tool. Different types of humor are appropriate to different situations. Laughter increases endorphins and adrenaline.
  - Many older adults consider themselves highly spiritual and religious. There is a connection between spiritual well-being and a sense of purpose in life.

STUDY QUESTIONS
Multiple-Choice Review

1. Which of the following defines emotional well-being as it applies to the older adult?
   1. Serene and easy to manage with age
   2. Well off financially because of investments

3. Able to adapt to age-related changes
4. Remains fiercely independent

2. According to the Georgia Centenarian Study, which characteristics accurately reflect centenarians?
    1. Free of illness, robust, hardy
    2. Optimistic, hopeful, engaged
    3. Mental health, family support, hope
    4. Family longevity, intelligence, good morals

3. What is the role of families in the continuing care of older adults?
    1. Oldest child primary caregiver
    2. Visit parents in nursing homes
    3. Limited to occasional visits
    4. More involved than ever

4. How does depression become a threat to psychosocial wellness for the older adult?
    1. Underlying cause of illness and suicide
    2. Difficulty pulling themselves "up by bootstraps"
    3. Depression in older adults is chronic in nature
    4. Lack of compliance results in hospitalization

5. Why is the nursing role significant in promoting psychosocial wellness in the older adult?
    1. Nursing process can uncover many problems that the nurse can respond to.
    2. Nurses are taught to do all forms of therapy in the absence of specialists.
    3. Nurses are taught to respond to their feelings in making client care decisions.
    4. Nurses can choose to use their own value system in issues of spirituality and sex.

Critical Thinking

1. While on a holiday to visit relatives in Europe, you are taken aside by an older cousin who begins to berate the "tragic care of the older adults in your country." Using the skills and concepts learned in nursing, explain how you would deal with this situation.

2. Upon graduation, you have acquired a job as the office nurse for a gerontologist. The physician has informed you that you will accompany her on daily rounds. She expects you to be alert to atypical signs and symptoms in the older adults that you visit. What is your response to the physician? What will you be looking for? Which of the skills that you have acquired while in school will be the most valuable?

3. Two nurses' aides and an LPN are giggling about something in the hallway. As you get closer, they include you in their joke. It turns out that Mrs. French found her way to the second floor and into her husband's bed. One of the night staff found them performing oral sex. The staff member scolded Mrs. French and escorted her back to her room. Mrs. French was angry, especially because "we weren't through." What is your part of this conversation? What are some steps that you would take, based on what you have learned about the sex and sexuality of older adults?

4. Shortly after you graduate, you move to a more remote area of the country. You expect to find backward conditions in the small nursing home, the only immediate place of employment. Although staff is not especially welcoming of you, the clients have a lot of freedom and seem happy. People wander in and out, and bring family pets. There are resident birds, a cat and a dog, and lots of plants throughout the home. Music is playing much of the time. Children of different ages are involved in assorted projects with the clients. You are worried about sanitation, but no one seems to be picking up anything significant from people or pets. Why do you think that staff does not accept you? What ideas do you have for dealing with your own discomfort? What do you bring to contribute to the care of the clients?

Resources

Internet Resources

Alcoholics Anonymous
www.alcoholics-anonymous.org
www.alcoholics-anonymous.org/ectroff.html (main offices by state)

National Institute of Mental Health
www.nimh.gov/home.htm

National Clearinghouse for Alcohol and Drug Information
www.health.org

Organizations

Alliance for Psychosocial Nursing
6900 Grove Road
Thorofare, NJ 08094
(856) 848-1000

American Psychiatric Nurses Association
Colonial Place Three
2107 Wilson Blvd, Suite 300-A
Arlington, VA 22201
(703) 243-2443

Selected References

Bauer, B. B., & Hill, S. S. (2000). Older adults and mental health. In *Mental Health Nursing, An Introductory Text.* Philadelphia: W. B. Saunders.

Bauer, M. (1999). Their only privacy is between their sheets: *Journal of Gerontological Nursing, 25*(8), 37–42.

Benefits of animal-assisted therapy are widespread. (1998). *AACN News, 15*(9), 6.

Bradley, D. B. (Winter 1999–2000). A reason to rise each morning: The meaning of volunteering in the lives of older people. *The Gerontologist, xxiii*(4), 45–50.

Browning, M. A. (1995). Depression, suicide, and bereavement. In M.O. Hogstel (Ed.), *Geropsychiatric Nursing* (2nd ed, pp. 117–170). St. Louis: Mosby.

Carlsen, M. B. (Winter 1999–2000). The sustaining power of meaning. *The Gerontologist, xxiii*(4), 10–14.

Carson, V. B. (2000). Unique attributes of successful travelers: personal strengths. In *Mental health nursing: The nurse-patient journey* (2nd ed, pp 187–199). Philadelphia: W. B. Saunders.

Chlan, L. (1999). Music therapy in critical care: Indications and guidelines for intervention. *Critical Care Nurse, 19*(3), 35–41.

Cobb, M., & Robshaw, V. (Eds.). (1998). *The spiritual challenge of health care.* Philadelphia: Churchill-Livingstone.

Davis, C., Leveille, S., Favaro, S., & LoGerfo, M. (1998). Benefits to volunteers in a community-based health promotion and chronic illness self-management program for the elderly. *Journal of Gerontological Nursing, 24*(10), 16–23.

Ebersole, P., & Hess, P. (1998). *Aging today: Toward healthy aging* (5th ed.). St. Louis: Mosby.

Ebersole, P., & Hess, P. (1998). *Intimacy, sexuality, and aging: Toward healthy aging* (5th ed.). St. Louis: Mosby.

Editorial (1997). Spirituality and aging. *Journal of Gerontological Nursing, 23*(7), 7–8.

Eliason, M. J. (1998). Identification of alcohol-related problems in older women. *Journal of Gerontological Nursing, 24*(10), 8–14.

Gibson, M. C., Bol N., Woodbury M. G., et al. (1999). Comparison of caregivers', residents', and community-dwelling spouses' opinions about expressing sexuality in an institutional setting. *Journal of Gerontological Nursing,* 25 (4): 30–39.

Giuliano, K. K. (1999). Implementation of a pet visitation program in critical care. *Critical Care Nurse, 19*(3), 43–50.

Healthy People 2010 objectives related to substance abuse. Available at http://www.health.gov/healthypeople/Document/tableofcontents.htm Accessed 1/24/01.

Hill, S. S., & Howlett, H. S. (2001). Spiritual caring, spiritual needs, and religious differences. In *Success in practical/vocational nursing from student to leader.* Philadelphia: W. B. Saunders, pp. 152–167.

Hogstel, M. O., & Weeks, S. M. (2000). Mental health. In A. G. Lueckenotte (Ed.), *Gerontologic Nursing* (pp. 256–280). St. Louis: Mosby.

Holtz, C. S. (1999). Acknowledging the whole person: Culture, ethnicity, and religion. In S. R. Tyson (Ed.), *Gerontological nursing care* (pp. 89–110). Philadelphia: W. B. Saunders.

Isaia, D., Parker, V., & Murrow, E. (1999). Spiritual well-being among older adults. *Journal of Gerontological Nursing, 25*(8), 15–21.

Johnson, B. K. (1996). Older adults and sexuality: A multidimensional perspective. *Journal of Gerontological Nursing, 22*(2), 6–15.

Johnson, C. L. (1994). Introduction: Social and cultural diversity of the oldest-old. *International Journal of Aging and Human Development, 38*(1), 1–12.

Jorgenson, J. (1997). Therapeutic use of companion animals in health care. *Image: Journal of Nursing Scholarship, 29*(3), 249–254.

Kavanaugh, K. M. (Winter 1996–1997). The importance of spirituality. *Perspectives, 24*(2), 29–35.

Kurlowicz, L. (1999). The geriatric depression scale (GDS). *Journal of Gerontological Nursing, 25*(7), 8–9.

Lau, M. (2000). Sound health. *Nurseweek, 13*(8), 27.

Ludwick, R. E., Sedlack, C. A., Doheny, M. O., & Martsolf, D. S. (2000). Alcohol use in elderly women. *Healthy People 2000, 26*(2), 44–49.

McCurren, C., Dowe, D., Rattle, D., & Looney, S. (1999). Depression among nursing home elders: Testing an intervention strategy. *Applied Nursing Research, 12*(4), 185–195.

Miller, C. A. (2000). Update on drugs for emotional pain in elders. *Geriatric Nursing, 21*(3), 164–165.

Murray, C. K. (1995). Addressing your patient's spiritual needs. *AJN, 95*(11), 160–161.

Nurse care by phone improves outcomes for depressed patients. *Archives of Family Medicine/MedscapeWire,* August 18, 2000. Available at http://nurses.medscape.com/MedscapeWire/2000/0800/medwire.0818.Nurse,html Accessed 1/23/01.

Older Adults and Mental Health. Mental health: A report of the surgeon general. Available at http://www.surgeongeneral.gov/library/mentalhealth/chapter5/sec1.html#topper; http://www.surgeongeneral.gov/library/mentalhealth/chapter5/sec2.html#topper; http://www.surgeongeneral.gov/library/mentalhealth/chapter5/sec5.html#topper; http://www.surgeongeneral.gov/library/mentalhealth/chapter5/sec6.html#topper; http://www.surgeongeneral.gov/library/mentalhealth/chapter5/sec7.html#topper. Accessed 1/23/01.

O'Neil, D. P., & Kenny, E. K. (Third Quarter, 1998). Spirituality and chronic illness. *Journal of Nursing Scholarship, 30*(3), 275–280.

Poon, L. W., Clayton, G. M., Martin, P., et al. (1992). The Georgia Centenarian Study. *International Journal of Aging and Human Development, 34*(1), 1–17.

Pressley, L. (May 1999). Your best friend may be making you better! *Today's Health,* pp. 4–6.

Prouix, D. (1998). Animal-assisted therapy. *Critical Care Nurse, 18*(2), 80–84.

Rowe, J. (1997). Some other ways volunteers assist "aging in place." *U.S. News & World Report,* December 30, 1996/January 5, 1997.

Ryden M. B., Pearson, V., Kaas, M. J., et al. (1999). Nursing interventions for depression in newly admitted nursing home residents. *Journal of Gerontological Nursing, 25*(3), 20–29.

Shua-Haim, J. R., Sabo, M. R., Comsti, E., & Gross, J. S. (1997). Depression in the elderly: Hospital medicine. Available at http://www.medscape.com/quadrant/HospitalMedicine/1997/v33.n07/hm3307.03.shua/hm3307.03.shua.html

Smith, D. W. E. (1997). Centenarians: Human longevity outliers. *The Gerontologist, 37*(2), 200–207.

Straus, C. (1999). How much is too much? An alcohol Q&A. *Today's Health*, May 1999.

Summary statement of the American College of Cardiology and the American Heart Association on the use of sildenafil (Viagra™) in patients at clinical risk from cardiovascular effect. *Medscape Wire*, August 10, 1998. Available at http://www.medscape.com/MedscapeWire/1998/08.98/news.0810.summary.html Accessed 1/23/01.

The Brown University GeroPsych Report. (1998). *2*(10),1–8.

Thomas, W. H. (1996). *Life worth living* (p. 66). Acton, MA: VanderWyk & Burnham.

Tolley, M. (1997). Power to the patient. *Journal of Gerontological Nursing, 23*(10), 7–12.

Tornstam, L. (Winter 1999–2000). Transcendence in later life. *Generations, xxiii*(4), 10–14.

Tunstull, P., & Henry, M. E. (June 1996). Approaches to resident sexuality. *Journal of Gerontologcal Nursing, 22*(6), 37–42.

Utiger, R. D. (1998). A pill for impotence. *New England Journal of Medicine, 338*(20), 1458–1459.

Viagra™ combined with nitrates may be lethal: *Medscape Wire*, August 10, 1998. Available at http://www.medscape.com/MedscapeWire/1998/08.98/news.0810.viagra.html Accessed 1/23/01.

Viagra and poppers: A "dynamite combination." (October 1998). *Psychopharmacology Update, 9*(10), 2–3.

Whall, A. L. (1999). Missed depression in elderly individuals. *Journal of Gerontological Nursing, 25*(6), 44–46.

Wright, K. B. (1998). Professional, ethical, and legal implications for spiritual care in nursing. *Image: Journal of Nursing Scholarship, 30*(1), 81–83.

Zauszniewski, J. A. (1997). Teaching resourcefulness skills to older adults. *Journal of Gerontological Nursing, 23*(2), 14–20.

Zauszniewski, J. A., & Martin, M. H. (1999). Developmental task achievement and learned resourcefulness in healthy adults. *Archives of Psychiatric Nursing, xiii*(1), 41–47.

IV

Special Challenges in Care of the Older Adult

Protecting the Vulnerable Older Adult

MARY ANN MATTESON

OBJECTIVES

After completing this chapter, you will be able to:

- State the ethical principles related to care and protection of the vulnerable older adult.
- Trace the events leading up to the development of guidelines for restraint reduction.
- Identify the types of restraints used in the care of vulnerable older adults.
- Discuss the hazards of restraining vulnerable older adults.
- Examine alternatives to restraint use in older adults.
- Identify the types of abuse in older adults.
- Discuss assessment and interventions for abuse and its prevention in older adults.

CHAPTER OUTLINE

KEY TERMS

Abuse
Autonomy
Beneficence
Chemical restraint
Confidentiality

Duty
Ethical dilemma
Fidelity
Justice
Loyalty

Neglect

Nonmaleficence

Physical restraint

Primary prevention

Secondary prevention

Values

Veracity

CASE STUDY

Mrs. Jones is an 87-year-old woman admitted to a nursing home for rehabilitation after hospitalization for a hip fracture. Before fracturing her hip, she had been living alone in a small apartment. She had long suffered from diabetes, hypertension, and poor eyesight. Her daughter, who was Mrs. Jones's primary caregiver, had pleaded with her to move to an assisted living center, but Mrs. Jones was determined to live on her own. Mrs. Jones had fallen many times in her home, but this was the first time she had had a serious injury. When she was in the hospital, she had many episodes of acute confusion and agitation; on several occasions, wrist and chest restraints were placed on her to keep her from getting out of bed. In the nursing home, Mrs. Jones had continued episodes of confusion and agitation, and she spoke endlessly about going home.

Mrs. Jones's son and daughter had sharp disagreements about how much input Mrs. Jones should have in decision making regarding her care, particularly in relation to risk-benefit issues such as living at home, the use of restraints and/or feeding tubes, and pain and comfort measures. Her son wanted her to return home, but her daughter wanted her to go to an assisted living facility. The daughter had been primarily responsible for Mrs. Jones's care because she lived nearby, whereas the son lived some distance away. The daughter was also concerned about safety issues such as falls, as well as proper nutrition and pain medication.

This situation, like many similar situations, presents many issues and problems that are challenging to patients, family members, and caregivers. How much decision making should be left to the patient, who may be chronically ill and not well oriented? When should a family member step in, and which family member has the authority to make decisions? How do you as a nurse participate in decision making as an advocate for the older patient? Issues facing nurses in resolving ethical problems include control, legal issues, failure, coercion, obligation, advocacy, respect, and cost (Beckel, 1996).

ETHICAL PRINCIPLES

Ethical principles are the basis for decision making and for protecting vulnerable older adults. As an advocate for older clients, you need to be aware of the process of ethical decision making.

Values form the basis of ethical principles in nursing care, which in turn form the laws governing nursing practice. Specific values and their related ethical principles include freedom (**autonomy**) doing good (**beneficence**), doing no harm (**nonmaleficence**), fairness (**justice**), and being true (**fidelity**).

Autonomy. Freedom, power, and choice are words frequently used in relation to the ethical principle of autonomy. Laws that uphold the principle of autonomy are made to enforce and protect the individual's power to decide and to do what is wanted. However, laws also place limits on an individual's power to act, restricting the actions of clients, as well as families and caregivers. For example, freedom to decide among older adults is related to their general condition, whereas a nurse's freedom to provide certain types of care of patients is limited by law.

Beneficence. In Latin, *bene* means "good," and *ficence* means "to do or make." Thus, the value underlying the ethical principle of beneficence is doing good or caring for the client. Nurses are legally mandated to do good, and this value above all others characterizes nursing. Most caring promotes life, either extending or improving the quality of life. The dilemma arises when it is unclear whether care is actually doing good or no harm. In these cases, the benefit (beneficence) is weighed against risk of harm (nonmaleficence).

Nonmaleficence. In Latin, nonmaleficence is made up of three words: *non* meaning "not," *mal* meaning "bad," and *ficence* meaning to "do or make." The **duty** to do no harm is mandated of all people, not just health care professionals. It is the basis of all criminal law. However, nurses are held to a higher standard when providing care because not only must you do no harm, but you also must meet a standard of care (do good) required by licensure law.

Justice. The ethical principle of justice requires treating people fairly under the law, which means applying the same process to everyone, without bias. It does not mean giving all people the same things; it does mean treating all the same. Justice can refer to treating individuals fairly (individual autonomy) or doing good for the group (social justice). Conflict may arise in ethical decision making between those who believe in individual autonomy and those who believe in social justice.

Fidelity. Fidelity, or being true, incorporates keeping promises (**loyalty**), keeping secrets (**confidentiality**), and telling truth (**veracity**). In the nurse-client relationship, you are required to be true to your older clients. To be true means being faithful, telling the truth, and maintaining confidentiality. In addition, fidelity is reflected in the Code of Ethics of the American Nurses Association. The code mandates nurses to protect the public from misinformation and misrepresentation and to maintain the integrity of nursing (Hall, 1996).

Mrs. Jones's situation presented **ethical dilemmas** that involve many of the values just described. How much autonomy and freedom to choose care should Mrs. Jones possess? Who should be responsible for making decisions? Beneficence versus nonmaleficence (or doing good versus doing no harm, or the balance of risk versus benefit) in health care decision making is another major ethical dilemma. How safe would Mrs. Jones be if she were living alone? To what extent does the use of restraints and medication benefit or harm her? These are not easy questions to answer, and often the family members turn to the nurse for clarification and support.

RESTRAINT USE

A major ethical dilemma occurs when there is a question of whether to restrain or not to restrain a vulnerable older adult. Older patients are more likely to be restrained than younger patients, probably because of their greater likelihood of confusion and falling. The most common reasons given for using protective restraints with older clients in hospitals or nursing homes are protection of the client, equipment, or others from harm; prevention of falls from bed or chair; and prevention of wandering (Table 13–1). The most common precipitating events for the use of restraints involve patient attempts to get out of bed or resistance to treatment while confused or disoriented. Categories of restrained residents and the associated problems and difficulties are: (1) ambulation (falling, balance problems); (2) behavioral (agitation, combativeness, restlessness); (3) positioning (in chair, wheelchair, or bed); (4) wandering (outside the building, into other residents' rooms); (5) jeopardizing life support (catheters, feeding tubes, intravenous lines); and (6) new admissions (behavioral problems, wandering)

Table 13–1	
CATEGORIES OF RESTRAINED RESIDENTS	
Category	**Difficulties/Problems**
Ambulation	Falling, balance problems
Behavioral	Agitation, combativeness, restlessness
Positioning	In chair, wheelchair, or bed
Wandering	Outside the building, into others' rooms
Jeopardizing life support	Catheters, feeding tubes, intravenous lines
New admissions	Behavioral problems, wandering

From Cohen, C., et al. (1996). Old problem, different approach: Alternatives to physical restraints. *Journal of Gerontological Nursing, 22*(2), 23–29.

(Cohen, Neufeld, Dunbar, Pflug, & Breuer, 1996). Restraints restrict an individual's movement and are classified as either physical or chemical.

Types of Restraints

Physical Restraint. **Physical restraints** consist of vest, waist, wrist, or ankle ties. Wrist and ankle restraints may be made of soft material or leather. Anything that restricts movement, such as geriatric chairs, siderails, or even an overbed table, can be considered a physical restraint. If a client is able to apply or release a safety device by himself or herself, then it is not considered a restraint.

Chemical Restraint. **Chemical restraints** are primarily psychotropic medications that are given to subdue agitated or confused clients. Psychoactive drugs should never be used for purposes of discipline or convenience; rather, they should be used only if there exists a great risk of self-injury or injury to others. In the past, the most commonly prescribed psychoactive medications were haloperidol (Haldol), thioridazine (Mellaril), and lorazepam (Ativan). Newer neuroleptic drugs such as risperidone (Risperdal) and olanzapine (Zyprexa), which have fewer adverse effects, are now being used.

> ### Medication Safety Tip
>
> *Any* psychoactive drug has the potential for producing adverse effects and untoward reactions.

Hazards of Restraining Older Adults

Restraints seldom eliminate the risk for injury and may actually cause or worsen problems. Clients are often able to untie physical restraints and wriggle out of them, resulting in falls from wheelchairs and beds. In addition, accidental strangulation can occur when some forms of physical restraint, particularly a vest restraint, are used. Physical restraints also may cause damaging psychological adverse effects in older clients, such as feelings of anger, discomfort, resistance, and fear. Behaviors noted include loss of self-image,

growing dependency, increased confusion and disorientation, regressive behavior, and withdrawal. Chemical restraints have the potential for causing adverse effects and even untoward reactions, such as greater confusion, agitation, and an increased number of falls.

In Chapter 1, we discussed the Omnibus Reconciliation Act (OBRA) or Nursing Home Reform Act of 1987. One reason this law was enacted was to protect older adults residing in nursing homes from unnecessary restraint. OBRA specifies that nursing home residents have the right to be free from any physical or chemical restraints for the purposes of discipline or convenience. In addition, **a physician's order is required for restraint use, and the order must specify the duration and the circumstances under which the restraints may be used.**

According to OBRA regulations, the only people who should be restrained are those who:

- Have a history of severe falls or an extremely high risk of taking a fall that is life-threatening.
- Are neurologically, orthopedically, or muscularly impaired and need postural support for safety or comfort, or both.
- Experience any of a number of mental dysfunctions that may cause patients to be a serious hazard to themselves, objects, or others.
- Have life-threatening medical symptoms; a restraint is used temporarily to provide necessary treatment.

The problem of restraint use in acute care settings is now being addressed. In 1996, the Joint Commission on Accreditation of Healthcare Organizations (JCAHO) issued guidelines for clients in accredited institutions, including hospitals. These compel organizations to limit restraint use to appropriate or justified situations. The guidelines are similar to the OBRA guidelines for nursing homes; however, reasons for restraint use and possible alternatives in acute care settings may be different from those in nursing homes. More attention needs to be directed toward finding alternatives to the use of restraint in acute care hospitals; nurse researchers are investigating situations and solutions related to restraint use (Cruz, Abdul-Hamid, & Heater, 1997; Kanski, Janelli, Jones, & Kennedy, 1996; Ludwick & O'Toole, 1996; Matthiesen, Lamb, McCann, Hollinger-Smith, & Walton, 1996).

If physical restraint is used, the least restrictive device is best. For example, a mitt is preferable to a wrist restraint that limits movement. The restrained client should be checked frequently, at least every 15 to 30 minutes. A client who is agitated or combative must be monitored continuously. You should make sure that the client's condition is good and that the restraint is used properly, providing adequate protection and comfort. Physical restraints must be removed **every two hours** for 10 minutes to provide for range of motion, toileting, nourishment, and restorative activities such as physical therapy, ambulation, and cognitive activities. After being apprised of the risks and benefits, the older adult and/or family, not the nurse, should decide whether or not physical restraint should be used.

Benefits of Restraint Reduction

The reasons for restraint use are largely based on myths and misconceptions about their benefits. Nurses' concerns for safety and control of behavior form a foundation of belief for restraint use that stands in contrast to the efficacy and ethical arguments against use. For example, it has been commonly believed that restraints protect clients, prevent falls and injuries, decrease staff needs and costs, and prevent lawsuits. However, just the opposite is true. Restraints can be dangerous, costly, and require more care, whereas restraint reduction may provide greater safety and enhance cost-effective care. Table 13–2 provides a few examples of the refuted restraint misconceptions. A risk-free alternative to restraints probably does not exist; however, restraints are not risk free either. Thus we must weigh the risks versus benefits of restraint reduction (Mayhew, Christy, Berkebile, Miller, & Farrish, 1999).

Alternatives to Restraint

It is important for you, the licensed practical nurse/licensed vocational nurse (LPN/LVN), to identify older clients at risk for restraint. Close observation of the older adult can decrease or eliminate the need to use physical restraint. Several alternatives to restraint include physical therapy, sitting and talking to clients for short periods, and asking staff to be responsible for wanderers in small blocks of time. Specific suggestions for alternatives to restraints include the following:

- Provide general comfort measures, including proper positioning, therapeutic touch, massage, or acupressure when appropriate.
- Provide companionship and supervision by involving staff, family, friends, or volunteers, especially at night.
- Distract the client's attention with television, radio, tape player, or other activities.
- Place objects in the environment so that they are easily accessible and safe, e.g., call bell within reach, adequate lighting, bedrails down, mattress on the floor, and so forth.
- Arrange the room and bed so that the client is within sight of the nursing staff.

Careful nursing care, administrative support, an interdisciplinary approach, education of staff and families, and organizational promotion of dignity and quality of life are measures that can effectively reduce the use of restraints.

ABUSE OF OLDER ADULTS

Abuse of older adults is an important social problem, causing unnecessary pain and suffering for many. It consists of destructive behavior directed toward an older adult, occurring within the context of a trusting relationship, that is of sufficient intensity and/or frequency to produce unnecessary suffering, injury, pain, loss, and/or violation of human rights, as well as poorer quality of life (Fulmer & Paveza, 1998).

Types of Abuse

Abuse is defined as the willful infliction of physical pain, injury, or debilitating mental anguish; unreasonable confinement; or the willful deprivation of services necessary for the maintenance of physical or mental health. Abuse of older adults encompasses physical, psychological, financial, and social abuse or violation of an individual's rights. *Physical abuse* usually includes beatings, withholding of personal or medical care, or failure to supervise an impaired person adequately to prevent injury. *Psychological* or *emotional abuse* involves instilling fear through verbal assaults or demands to perform demeaning tasks, making threats, or isolating an older adult. *Financial abuse* includes theft or mismanagement of money or personal belongings. *Social abuse* or *violation of rights* involves being forced out of one's home, or

Table 13–2
EXAMPLES OF LITERATURE REFUTING RESTRAINT MISCONCEPTIONS

Misconception	Literature
Restraints protect patients and are for their own good.	One-hundred-twenty-two restraint-related deaths have been reported.[1] Longer than 4 days of physical restraint is the strongest predictor of nosocomial infection and pressure sores.[2]
Restraints prevent falls and injuries.	Studies report that 13% to 47% of patients who fall are restrained.[3] Seventeen percent of serious fall-related injuries occurred in restrained patients, versus 5% in unrestrained patients.[4] England, known to use fewer restraints, has a fall/fracture rate of 0.7% to 1.7% compared with the United States' rate of 1.8% to 3.8%.[5]
Reducing restraint use increases staff needs and costs.	More than half of nursing homes surveyed reported no additional expense with restraint reduction.[6] Residents who were physically restrained required more care.[7]
Restraints prevent lawsuits and malpractice claims.	Lack of restraints was a factor in only a few court cases; false imprisonment and assault charges pose a greater risk.[8] Lawsuits for serious physical injury caused by misapplication of restraints are more common.[9]

1. Miles, S. H., Irvine, P. (1992). Deaths caused by physical restraints. *The Gerontologist, 32,* 762–766.

2. Lofgren, R. P., MacPherson, D. S., Granieri, R., Myllenbeck, S., Spralka, M. (1989). Mechanical restraints on medical wards: are protective devices safe? *American Journal of Public Health, 79,* 735–738.

3. Mion, L. C., Strumpf, N., NICHE Faculty. Use of physical restraints in the hospital setting: implications for the nurse. *Geriatric Nursing, 15,* 127–132.

4. Tinetti, M. E., Liu, W. L., Ginter, S. F. Mechanical restraint use and fall-related injuries among residents of skilled nursing facilities. *Annals of Internal Medicine, 116,* 369–374.

5. Rubenstein, H. S., Miller, F. H., Postal, S., Evans, H. B. Standards of medical care based on consensus rather than evidence: the case of routine bedrail use for the elderly. *Law and Medical Health Care, 11,* 271–276.

6. Mahoney, D. F. Analysis of restraint-free nursing homes. *Image, 27,* 155–160.

7. Phillips, C. D., Hawes, C., Fries, B. E. Reducing the use of physical restraints in nursing homes: will it increase costs? *American Journal of Public Health, 83,* 342–348.

8. Blakeslee, J. A., Goldman, B. D., Papougenis, D., Torell, C. A. Making the transition to restraint-free care. *Journal of Gerontological Nursing, 17*(2), 4–8.

9. Johnson, S. H. The fear of liability and the use of restraints in nursing homes. *Law and Medical Health Care, 18,* 263–273.

From Mayhew, P. A., Christy, K., Berkebile, I., Miller, C., & Farrish, A. (1999). Restraint reduction: research utilization and a case study with cognitive impairment. Geriatric *Nursing, 20*(6):305–308.

being denied the opportunity to exercise rights as an adult.

Neglect

Neglect refers to a lack of the services necessary to maintain the physical and mental health of older adults who live alone or who are unable to provide self care. Neglect may be committed by oneself or another. *Passive neglect* describes the legitimate inability of the caregiver to perform caregiving activities, such as bathing, dressing, or changing an incontinent older adult. *Active neglect* implies that a caregiver is intentionally withholding food or services to harm an older adult. *Self-neglect,* in which an older adult refuses medical care, services, or money, presents another form of neglect that is fraught with ethical problems. Older adults, unlike children, can choose their own lifestyle, and the right to self-determination is given up only when they are legally declared incapable or incompetent.

Legal Requirements for Reporting Abuse

Abuse of older adults has gone largely unreported in the past. Now that all 50 states have passed mandatory reporting laws and have instituted adult protective service (APS) programs, abuse of older adults has been increasingly recognized as a social problem. State APS statutes provide APS agencies with the authority to investigate cases of mistreatment; in some states, they fund services to alleviate the abusive or neglectful situation. Mandatory reporting laws require the disclosure of suspected mistreatment of older adults despite the adult victims' wishes. In addition, APS agencies must investigate reported mistreatment cases by interviewing victims and others who may be knowledgeable about the case. Unfortunately, both professionals and the public continue to underreport cases of abuse. Reasons cited include denial, reluctance to report abuse, and lack of awareness of abuse laws (Capezuti, Brush, & Lawson, 1997).

Nursing Assessment and Intervention for Abuse and Neglect

Abuse and neglect can be difficult to determine because older adults who are abused or neglected may demonstrate signs and symptoms similar to the signs and symptoms of many common medical conditions. Nevertheless, when working with older adults, whether in the hospital, nursing home, clinic, or home setting, nurses should be alert for signs and symptoms of abuse or neglect. Common indicators of abuse and neglect of the older adult include injuries, untreated medical problems, poor hygiene, and malnutrition (Table 13–3).

Assessment and treatment of abuse and neglect consist of five components: identification, access and assessment, intervention, follow-up, and prevention.

In *identification*, nurses must be aware of potential abuse and always observe for it in the older adult who cannot care for himself or herself. Older adults who are the most likely victims of abuse and neglect are socially isolated women who retain some independence and on whom the abuser is dependent financially. Other risk factors for elder abuse are advanced age, a history of significant conflict between a parent and child, alcohol abuse in either the caregiver or the older adult, and a history of abuse. Older adults who are most at risk for neglect are those with dependency needs related to confusion, immobility, and personal hygiene. In addition, individuals with disorders associated with multiple disabilities, both physical and emotional, such as Parkinson's disease, Alzheimer's disease, and stroke, are thought to be at high risk.

Access to the older adult must be obtained before *assessment* can take place. Access may be particularly difficult if an older adult is living independently at home because adults who are considered competent have the right to make their own personal care decisions. Once access is obtained, assessment should focus on the following questions:

1. Is the older adult in immediate danger of bodily harm?
2. Is the older adult competent to make decisions regarding his or her own care?
3. What is the degree and significance of the older adult's functional impairments.
4. What specific services might help to meet the client's unmet needs?
5. Who in the family is involved in the abuse or neglect, and to what extent?
6. Are the patient and family willing to accept intervention?

Intervention is based on the findings of the assessment. The major goals of intervention are protection of the older adult and prevention of further episodes of abuse or neglect. The intervention process should be based on ethical decision making, particularly in regard to risk-benefit. For example, when decisions such as remaining in the home are considered, the risk of staying in the current situation should be weighed against the benefits of alternative situations. Depending on the situation, suggested interventions may provide support services (home health aide, homemaker/chore services,

Table 13–3
HIGH-RISK SIGNS AND SYMPTOMS OF ELDER MISTREATMENT

Abuse	Unexplained bruises
	Repeated falls
	Laboratory values inconsistent with history
	Fractures or bruises in various stages of healing
	Any report by a patient of being physically abused should be followed up immediately.
Neglect	Listlessness
	Poor hygiene
	Evidence of malnutrition
	Inappropriate dress
	Pressure ulcers or urine burns
	Reports of being left in an unsafe situation
	Reports of an inability to get needed medications
Exploration	Unexplained loss of social security or pension checks
	Any evidence that material goods are being taken in exchange for care
	Any evidence that elder's personal belongings (e.g., house, jewelry, car) are being taken over without consent or approval of elder
Abandonment	Evidence that someone has "dropped off" elder at the emergency room or the family unit with no intention of coming back for him or her
Other High-Risk Situations	Drug or alcohol addiction in the family
	Isolation of the elder
	History of untreated psychiatric problems
	Evidence of unusual family stress
	Excessive dependence of elder on caretaker

From Stone, J. T., Wyman, J. F., & Salisbury, S. A. (1999). *Clinical Gerontological Nursing* (2nd ed.). Philadelphia: W. B. Saunders, p. 670.

transportation, medical/nursing care, counseling, respite care) to the family to minimize the opportunity for abuse, or may explore alternative living arrangements (other family, foster care, congregate living, nursing home). In addition, intervention, such as counseling or job training, may be directed at the abuser.

Careful *follow-up* is indicated in all situations of neglect or abuse of the older adult, even if interventions are accepted, because the risk for further abuse remains.

Prevention efforts are most effective when they are implemented earlier rather than later. Early efforts (**primary prevention**), designed to foster well-being, include interrupting the cycle of family violence, promoting effective family communication, increasing family understanding of the aging process, and maximizing nonfamily natural helping networks for dependent older adults. Later efforts (**secondary prevention**), directed toward early detection and treatment, include identifying older adults at risk for self-neglect or abuse, identifying families at risk for abuse and neglect, monitoring high-risk situations, counseling, and recommending substance abuse programs. When abuse and neglect have been chronic and ongoing, efforts are aimed at reducing morbidity (*tertiary prevention*) through the use of adult protective service programs (e.g., placement, guardianship) and family counseling, and by maximizing support from sources other than the primary caregiver (Hogstel & Curry, 1999). Further examples of primary, secondary, and tertiary prevention can be found in Table 13–4. In summary, it is better to prevent abuse and neglect of the older adult than to treat it (Matteson, McConnell, & Linton, 1997).

CASE STUDY

Mrs. Johnson is a 79-year-old woman who lives with her 81-year-old husband in a small, older home. They have lived in their home for 40 years. They have several children and grandchildren who try to help them out as best they can, but they all live far away. Both are in failing health, and Mr. Johnson is disabled and in a wheelchair as a result of a previous stroke. Mrs. Johnson makes a good effort but has difficulty taking care of him because of her failing eyesight and restricted movement from arthritis. They have few resources to keep them living independently, but they refuse any outside help. Their living conditions are unsafe and unsanitary.

Table 13–4

IDEAS FOR REDUCTION OF ELDER ABUSE AND NEGLECT

A classic prevention model, in which three levels of preventive efforts are defined, is a framework that suggests different strategies for reducing the prevalence of elder abuse. Each level of prevention is described, followed by a list of ideas for reduction of elder neglect and abuse at each level.

Primary Prevention

Efforts designed to foster well-being, such as the introduction of healthful lifestyle teaching in elementary school to promote activity and better nutrition.

Primary Prevention and Elder Abuse

1. Projects to interrupt cycles of family violence
2. Projects that increase family communication effectiveness
3. Projects that increase family understanding of the aging process
4. Projects that maximize nonfamily natural helping networks for dependent elders
5. Gray Panther, American Association of Retired Persons, National Council on the Aging efforts to enhance the image/status of the elderly

Secondary Prevention

Efforts directed toward early detection and treatment of disease before adverse effects have been felt. An example is hypertension and diabetes screening.

Secondary Prevention and Elder Abuse

1. Identifying elderly at risk for self-neglect or abuse
2. Identifying families at risk for elder abuse or neglect
3. Identifying communities at risk for elder abuse or neglect (migrant communities; communities that are over- or underpopulated with old people; certain ethnic groups, e.g., WASP women or blacks; mentally retarded elders; bag ladies; SRO occupants; nursing home chains with ageist corporate philosophies)
4. Monitoring of high-risk situations—advocacy groups, ombudsman programs
5. Counseling or therapy for those showing signs of neglect or abuse
6. Substance abuse programs

Tertiary Prevention

Efforts aimed at reducing morbidity from existing disorders, such as rehabilitation after cerebrovascular accidents or myocardial infarction.

Tertiary Prevention and Elder Abuse

1. Adult protective services programs—placement, guardianship
2. Family counseling
3. Maximizing support from sources other than the primary caregiver

From Matteson, M. A., McConnell, E. S., & Linton, A. D. (1997). *Gerontological Nursing* (2nd ed.). Philadelphia: W. B. Saunders, p. 632.

Mr. and Mrs. Johnson's situation could be called an example of self-neglect. They have difficulty accepting the fact that they are no longer able to care for themselves. They refuse to leave their home or accept outside services. This case presents the ethical dilemma of autonomy versus beneficence. Mr. and Mrs. Johnson are both cognitively oriented and mentally alert and have the right to choose their own living situation and to refuse care. However, how do we weigh their freedom to choose against the obligation to do good for them? To what degree is this a case of self-neglect, and when do we step in and report this case to adult protective services? There is no easy answer to this question, and we must look at our own values, as well as the values of older clients and their families, to make a just decision.

Summary

- The care and protection of vulnerable older adults challenge nurses to examine their own values and ethics.
- Ethical principles are based on values and include autonomy, beneficence, nonmaleficence, justice, and fidelity.
- The use of restraints presents an ethical challenge for caregivers; patients and families must be apprised of the risks and benefits of restraint use in order to be involved in decision making about their use.
- Abuse of older adults includes physical, psychological or emotional, financial, and social abuse.
- Neglect may be self-neglect or neglect by families or caregivers.
- Nurses must examine their own values, as well as the values of older clients, their families, and society, when participating in ethical decision making.

STUDY QUESTIONS

Multiple-Choice Review

1. Beneficence is an ethical principle that means
   1. Doing no harm.
   2. Doing good.
   3. Treating people fairly.
   4. Maintaining confidentiality.

2. Older people are frequently restrained because they
   1. Say nasty things to caregivers.
   2. Tend to be cranky.
   3. Are likely to be confused.
   4. Are sexually uninhibited.

3. One alternative for restraint use is
   1. Placing objects out of reach of the older patient.
   2. Providing companionship.
   3. Keeping the room quiet by turning off the TV or radio.
   4. Restricting food and fluids.

4. An indication that an older person is at risk for abuse is
   1. Alcohol abuse.
   2. Living with the family.
   3. Financial dependence on a son or daughter.
   4. Dynamic personality.

5. The first action that should be taken when a vulnerable adult is at risk for abuse and neglect is
   1. Identification.
   2. Access.
   3. Assessment.
   4. Intervention.
   Follow up
   Prevention

Critical Thinking

1. What are the main ethical principles involved in the care of vulnerable older adults?
2. For what reasons are older adults restrained?
3. What are the hazards of restraint use?
4. What alternatives may be used for restraint use?
5. How do you identify older adults who are at risk for abuse and neglect?
6. What actions should be taken when vulnerable adults are at risk for abuse and neglect?

Resources

Internet Resources

Children of Aging Parents
www.careguide.net/careguide.cgi/caps/capshome.html

Family Caregiver Alliance
www.caregiver.org

National Center on Elder Abuse
www.elderabusecenter.org

Association for Protection of the Elderly
www.apeape.org

Organizations

Center for Devices and Radiological Health
5600 Fishers Lane (HFZ-250)
Rockville, MD 20857

The Food and Drug Administration
Consumer Information
Telephone Number: (301) 443-3170
Toll Free Telephone Number: 1 (800) 283-7332

Selected References

Beckel, J. (1996). Resolving ethical dilemmas in long-term care. *Journal of Gerontological Nursing, 22*(1), 20–26.

Capezuti, E., Brush, B. L., & Lawson, W. T. (1997). Reporting elder mistreatment. *Journal of Gerontological Nursing, 23*(7), 24–32.

Cohen, C., Neufeld, R., Dunbar, J., Pflug, L., & Breuer, B. (1996). Old problem, different approach: alternatives to physical restraints. *Journal of Gerontological Nursing, 22*(2), 23–29.

Cruz, V., Abdul-Hamid, M., & Heater, B. (1997). Research-based practice: reducing restraints in an acute care setting—Phase 1. *Journal of Gerontological Nursing, 23*(2), 31–40.

Department of Health and Human Services. (1991). *Potential hazards with protective restraint devices.* Rockville, MD: Food and Drug Administration, pp. 3–4.

Fulmer, T., & Paveza, G. (1998). Neglect in the elderly patient. *Nursing Clinics of North America, 33*(3), 457–466.

Generations. (Fall 1998). Ethics and aging: Bringing the issues home. *Journal of the American Society on Aging, 22*(3).

Generations. (Summer 2000). Abuse and neglect of older people. *Journal of the American Society on Aging, 24*(11).

Hall, J. K. (1996). *Nursing ethics and the law.* Philadelphia: W. B. Saunders.

Health Care Financing Administration. (1994). *Surveyor guidebook on dementia: Evaluating compliance with regulatory requirements.* Department of Health and Human Services, Washington, DC.

Hogstel, M. O., & Curry, L. C. (1999). Elder abuse revisited. *Journal of Gerontological Nursing, 25*(7), 10–18.

Kanski, G., Janelli, L., Jones, H., & Kennedy, M. (1996). Family reactions to restraints in an acute care setting. *Journal of Gerontological Nursing, 22*(6), 17–22.

Ludwick, R., & O'Toole, A. W. (1996). The confused patient: Nurses' knowledge and interventions. *Journal of Gerontological Nursing, 22*(1), 44–49.

Mayhew, P. A., Christy, K., Berkebile, J., Miller, C., & Farrish, A. (1999). Restraint reduction: research utilization and a case study with cognitive impairment. *Geriatric Nursing, 20*(6):305–308.

Matteson, M. A., McConnell, E. S., & Linton, A. D. (1997). *Gerontological nursing: Concepts and practice.* Philadelphia: W. B. Saunders.

Matthiesen, V., Lamb, K. V., McCann, J., Hollinger-Smith, L., & Walton, J. C. (1996). Hospital nurses' views about physical restraint use with older patients. *Journal of Gerontological Nursing, 22*(6), 8–16.

Middleton, H., Keene, R. G., Johnson, C., Elkins, A. D., & Lee, A. E. (1999). Physical and pharmacologic restraints in long-term care facilities. *Journal of Gerontological Nursing, 25*(7), 26–33.

Tatara, T. (1995). *An analysis of state laws addressing elder abuse, neglect, and exploitation.* Washington, DC: National Center on Elder Abuse.

End-of-Life Care

MARY ANN MATTESON

OBJECTIVES

After completing this chapter, you will be able to:

- State the meaning of quality of life and well-being.
- Discuss pain and symptom management at the end of life.
- Identify issues related to end-of-life decision making.
- List three types of advance directives.
- Describe the principles of palliative care and hospice.
- Examine the process of dying.
- Discuss the impact of dying on the client and family.

CHAPTER OUTLINE

KEY TERMS

Advance directives

Do not resuscitate

Durable power of attorney

Hospice

Living wills

Medical directives

Palliative care

Quality of life

Well-being

TECHNOLOGICAL ADVANCES: CAN WE LIVE FOREVER?

Most people who are young and in good health would like to live forever. Even many older adults who are frail, dependent, and suffering want to prolong their lives. Fear of death, the pain of leaving loved ones, and the unknown all contribute to the desire for preservation of life at any cost. Technological advances in health care have developed at a fast pace because of clients' and loved ones' fight against death.

But, **quality of life** can diminish when we do everything possible to sustain life at any cost. This issue becomes extremely important in the care of older adults, that is, people who have lived long lives and can anticipate few years ahead of them. Thus, when caring for people at the end of life, we must consider both their quality of life and **well-being,** particularly in relation to their own desires and wishes.

QUALITY OF LIFE

Quality of life is related to the concept of well-being. Well-being is defined as the state of being healthy, happy, and prosperous; it is made up of physical, psychological, social, and spiritual dimensions. Physical well-being is achieved primarily through symptom and pain management. Psychological and social well-being involve peace of mind and relationships with family and friends. Spiritual well-being is the sum of physical, psychological, and social well-being. It is the affirmation of life in a relationship between God, or some higher power, self, community, and environment that nurtures and celebrates wholeness. *The goal of nursing care at the end of life is to preserve quality of life and well-being to ease the transition into death.*

NURSING INTERVENTIONS TO IMPROVE QUALITY OF LIFE

Pain and symptom management are integral for maintaining quality of life at the end of life. If pain and symptoms of illness are not under control, a person cannot achieve well-being. Pain may be acute or chronic; other symptoms of illness may include dyspnea, fatigue, and nausea. Pain and symptoms each have physiologic,

sensory, and affective components that are unpleasant, subjective experiences and may not be related to the underlying illness. Your role as a licensed practical nurse/licensed vocational nurse (LPN/LVN) is extremely important, as good nursing care can help alleviate pain and other symptoms, while promoting well-being and quality of life.

Nursing home residents frequently do not receive the pain and symptom relief necessary to maintain their comfort and well-being. Researchers have found that more than one quarter of residents with cancer pain—especially blacks and the oldest old—are not given any pain medication. Older adults are particularly vulnerable to inadequate treatment of pain for many reasons. Their experience of the pain may be altered owing to age-related changes. The nursing staff may have misconceptions that older adults have a high pain tolerance, that pain may be a part of normal aging, or that older adults cannot tolerate opioids. In addition, pain often goes unrecorded in nursing homes, partly because of the staff's inability to assess pain in residents unable to speak, and because of residents' reluctance to complain of it. Pain is now considered a fifth vital sign. It is important to remember that pain is a subjective experience and is not necessarily related to the severity and type of disease or condition. Caregivers should assume that residents are in pain and should include pain and comfort measures as part of the routine care of all nursing home residents.

As is true for pain, the severity of other symptoms, such as dyspnea, nausea, and fatigue, that are common in terminal illness cannot always be predicted from objective assessment. To effectively manage symptom discomfort, it is important that the following factors be assessed:

- Character of the discomfort
- Location
- Onset
- Severity
- Duration
- Aggravating factors
- Alleviating factors
- Impact on daily living, including relationships with others and ability to sleep, eat, work, and exercise.

Interventions for pain and symptom management may include:

- Medications—narcotics (if monitored carefully), anti-inflammatories
- Exercise—active and passive range of motion; breathing exercises
- Physical modalities—applications of heat and cold, massage, positioning

- Environmental manipulations—room arrangements, room temperature, types of bed covers
- Cognitive strategies—relaxation, distraction, guided imagery

RESPECTING AN OLDER ADULT'S RIGHT TO CHOOSE

CASE STUDY

Mr. Smith suffered a right brain stroke and had been living in a nursing home for 5 years. He had left-sided paresis and was legally blind; he was incontinent of bowel and bladder and unable to swallow, so he had a gastric tube for feeding and a catheter for urination. His hearing and mental abilities were intact. Mr. Smith's skin became very jaundiced one day, about the same time he pulled out his gastric tube, thinking that it was the nurses' call bell. There was discussion among the family members about whether to intervene because his quality of life seemed very poor. He was virtually bedridden. He could not read his favorite books and magazines, see his favorite television shows, or snack on his favorite foods, which had given him so much pleasure. Who would want to live like that? Mr. Smith's wife finally asked the physician to discuss options for care with Mr. Smith, particularly in regard to reinserting the feeding tube and pursuing diagnostic interventions for the jaundice. The physician agreed, although he was uncomfortable with these issues knowing that Mr. Smith didn't realize that end-of-life choices were the subject of the discussion. After the physician left, Mrs. Smith asked him what he wanted to do. Mr. Smith asked his wife what were the consequences of not putting the tube back, and she told him that he would die. Mr. Smith vehemently said, "Put the tube back in!"

Older adults are frequently unable or unwilling to initiate discussions regarding end-of-life decisions, and health care providers and family members often are reluctant to discuss these issues. In addition, studies have found that nurses, physicians, and family members frequently are unable to predict what an older person would choose, as in Mr. Smith's case. Older people who are competent to make decisions should be able to accept or decline potentially beneficial medical care during the days, months, and sometimes years prior to death.

Upholding the end-of-life choices of competent older adults is difficult; however, respecting the desires of those who are no longer able to state their wishes is even more difficult. In 1991, the Omnibus Reconciliation Act (also known as the Patient Self-Determination Act; see Chapter 1) became effective. This act is designed to allow clients to guide their medical treatment should they become incapacitated. It requires that all institutions that participate in Medicare reimbursement provide written information to clients concerning their rights to accept or refuse treatment, including information about the right to make advance directives. Institutions must determine if a client has an advance directive and document this in the patient's record (Perrin, 1997).

ADVANCE DIRECTIVES

Advance directives are designed to: (1) protect the moral and legal rights of the client to self-determination, (2) diminish uncertainty about what a client would want done, and (3) reduce conflict among decision makers (Pellegrino, 1992). The two most common types of advance directives are instructional directives, such as living wills, and proxy designations, such as the durable power of attorney. Every state has legislation detailing the types of advance directives permitted in that state, as well as statutes that designate relatives as proxy decision makers when no advance directive exists. It is important to be familiar with the type of advance directives used in your state.

Living Wills

Living wills are documents in which clients express their health care wishes should they become terminally ill and lose the ability to make decisions (McKee, 1999). Appendix B provides an example of a living will in Florida. As with most living wills, the wording is relatively general with no specific definitions provided for "life-prolonging procedures" or "the performance of any medical procedure deemed necessary to provide me with comfort and care and to alleviate pain." Because these statements are open to interpretation, the document has presented many problems, particularly in determining which specific care measures should be provided. Most people are fairly clear about whether or not they want cardiopulmonary resuscitation (CPR), but other measures that may or may not provide comfort such as artificial respiration, certain types of medications like antibiotics, and supplemental nutrition and hydration need to be clarified.

Medical Directives

Medical directives were developed in the 1980s as an attempt to overcome the problems associated with the living will. They provide specific directions regarding various health care measures that people would desire, such as CPR, mechanical ventilation, food or nutrition, and antibiotics, in such circumstances as irreversible coma or brain damage with or without a terminal illness. Copies of the most recently updated medical directives are available from Emanual and Emanual, Massachusetts General Hospital (see resources for address). The majority of older adults are able to differentiate their preferences in the various scenarios given. Disadvantages of using a medical directive are that the actual situation may differ from that presented in the directive and not all patients want directives followed strictly. In addition, new therapeutic options may not be considered in the directive, as well as the fact that the

interests of a patient may change over time or in a given situation.

Durable Power of Attorney

Many older adults would rather choose a family member as proxy to make health care decisions than make them themselves. The **durable power of attorney** for health care allows the individual to designate a person to make decisions under specific circumstances such as incompetence, incapacity, or terminal illness (Appendix B). It is important that a person's wishes be communicated to the proxy before the need arises so that the relative can make the right decisions. In many cases, however, a relative must obtain durable power of attorney after the older adult becomes incapacitated. This presents a complicated situation for family members who may have differing ideas about the care that should be provided.

Do Not Resuscitate (DNR) Orders

DNR orders refer to CPR. CPR is much less likely to succeed in very old or very sick clients than in witnessed arrests where a cardiac arrest is observed, sudden death in young people, and drowning. However, almost all hospitals and nursing homes in the United States have policies requiring that CPR be done on all clients who die—for any reason, of any age, with any condition. Unless there are specific orders written to the contrary, CPR is automatic.

"Do not resuscitate" does not mean "do not care" or "do not treat." People may receive other types of treatment and palliative care, even when a DNR order exists. Clients with a DNR order deserve your best nursing care. In addition, a living will does not justify an automatic DNR. A DNR should be written when either the client refuses CPR or the physician assesses that CPR would be futile, but the decision must involve the client and/or the family.

PALLIATIVE CARE AND HOSPICE

Palliative care and **hospice** are terms that are often used interchangeably to describe a philosophy or system of care that facilitates quality of life and death with dignity in people who are terminally ill. Hospice care is designed to provide comfort and support to clients and their families when a life-limiting illness no longer responds to cure-oriented treatments. Support services are provided by a multidisciplinary team of health care providers who have expertise in pain control, symptom management, and comfort measures, as well as in the ability to meet the psychological, social, and spiritual needs of clients and their families.

Generally, people with terminal cancer and a prognosis of 6 months or less are referred to hospice care; however, hospice services are not limited to those with end-stage cancer. Many hospices offer palliative care to people with diagnoses such as cardiac, pulmonary, or liver disease; AIDS; or dementia that are life-limiting but without a specified prognosis (Kazanowski, 1997).

Hospice is not a place. Eighty percent of hospice care is provided in the home and in nursing homes. Inpatient units are sometimes available to assist with caregiving. For example, a terminally ill client may wish to be admitted to an inpatient hospice unit on a short-term basis for pain control measures, or to give his or her family respite. In addition, trained volunteers are an integral part of hospice service. Volunteers provide more than 5 million hours of care and service in the United States annually.

Hospice care neither prolongs life nor hastens death. It deals with the emotional, social, and spiritual impact of the disease on the client and the client's family and friends. Clients and families who choose hospice are at the core of the hospice team and are at the center of all decision making. Hospice follows the philosophy that when family members experience the dying process in a caring environment, it helps counteract the fear of their own mortality and the mortality of their loved one. Hospice offers a variety of bereavement and counseling services to families before and after a client's death.

DEATH AND DYING

Each encounter with death is a signal of our own mortality. Although death is a natural part of life and is expected with aging, the actual dying process can be very difficult for caregivers. We must be sensitive to the needs of the dying and their family members, as well as our own attitudes surrounding death.

Some common signs and symptoms of impending death are:

- noisy and moist breathing
- urinary incontinence, or urinary retention
- pain
- restlessness and agitation
- dyspnea
- nausea and vomiting
- sweating (diaphoresis)
- jerking, twitching, and plucking
- confusion

In the last 48 hours, clients usually lack appetite and thirst, taking in small amounts of liquids and foods. They often complain of dry mouth, which is unrelated to thirst. When clients stop taking foods and fluids, consideration should be given to discontinuing artificial hydration. This is especially true if pneumonia is present (occurring in 90% of patients under hospice care) because hydration can increase the presence of respiratory secretions and can prolong the dying process. Pain medication should be given until the end. Both bladder and bowel continence may be lost, and clients previously able to walk can no longer get out of bed. Clients with previous vigorous cough begin to have diminished cough and increased adventitious breath sounds ("rattles"). They may drift into and out of consciousness. After hunger and thirst have faded, speech may be lost, followed by sight. Hearing is the last sense to leave the client.

Many dying clients experience pre-death visions, which may occur in both oriented and disoriented clients. Pre-death visions are almost always about people and usually include dead relatives, guardians/angels, or babies. The visions may be pleasant for clients but can be upsetting for families. Treatment, like neuroleptics such as Haldol, should not be prescribed. Confusion and agitation may also occur prior to death. If the confusion and agitation appear to be disturbing to the client, family members may become upset. Sedation may be given; however, clearing both the confusion and the agitation is difficult.

As the client's needs change during the last 48 hours, so do the needs of the family. As death nears, the family increasingly assumes the role of "client." As the reality of impending death becomes clear, fears of dying and death may become overwhelming. Family members may experience guilt or doubt over medical decisions to treat or not to treat. Many family members feel an intense need to "do something." However, as they see the dying person move beyond everyday concerns, caregivers may come to realize that they no longer know what the dying person's needs are.

During the last 48 hours of life, family members must establish a new relationship with the dying loved one. Redefining the relationship is part of the grief process. Family members may no longer be able to establish a verbal link with confused or unresponsive clients, and verbal communication becomes "one-way." It is important to encourage this communication, and to continue to explain all aspects of the nursing care you are providing to the client, because hearing is the last sense to go. Following the death, most people continue this one-way communication without the presence of a physical body.

You can bring comfort to family members by discussing with them the kind of care that will be given, including maintaining a pain-free state, offering frequent mouth and skin care, providing privacy, and offering support—both spiritual and professional. Helping family members to be involved in providing appropriate care and comfort measures such as mouth swabbing, hand holding, and gentle talking to the dying can both aid the dying person and provide an opportunity for the family to enter into behavior that can be comforting. These actions facilitate the grieving process.

When the actual death occurs, it is a time to be a silent witness while quietly providing support. Some family members may become anxious and flustered and want to begin funeral arrangements immediately. Sometimes it is a good idea to suggest that they take a few minutes to sit quietly and catch their breath because there will be plenty of time to make the arrangements. But it is of utmost importance that you be sensitive to the family's psychological needs and religious and cultural traditions surrounding death.

Summary

- Nurses are in a unique position to provide care and support to older adults and their families at the end of life.
- Older adults should have the right to choose how they will be treated when terminally ill;

nurses should be advocates for clients and their families in helping them to carry out their wishes.
- Advance directives, including living wills, medical directives, and durable power of attorney, provide options for making one's wishes known.
- Palliative care and hospice promote comfort and dignity for the dying and provide support for grieving family members.
- Above all, nurses should respect the needs and cultural traditions of older adults and their families during the dying process.

STUDY QUESTIONS

Multiple-Choice Review

1. A goal of end-of-life nursing care is to
   1. Preserve quality of life and well-being.
   2. Prolong life at any cost.
   3. Keep family members away from the dying patient.
   4. Avoid dealing with religious aspects of dying.

2. When caring for an older person in pain, it is important to remember that
   1. Old people do not experience pain.
   2. Pain is not always directly related to the disease process.
   3. Pain should be objectively measured only by the nurse.
   4. Older people are frequently overtreated for pain.

3. Decisions about end-of-life care for an older adult who is alert
   1. Should be made by a family member.
   2. Should be made by older clients themselves.
   3. Should be made by the physician.
   4. Should be made by the guardian.

4. Hospice care is
   1. Provided only for cancer clients.
   2. A place where people go for treatment.
   3. A way to end life quickly.
   4. An approach to care that involves the emotional and spiritual aspects of dying.

5. During the last 48 hours of the process of dying,
   1. Clients should be given IV fluids if they stop taking fluids orally.
   2. Pain medication should be withdrawn.

3. Clients should be given a neuroleptic agent such as Haldol (haloperidol) for visual hallucinations.

4. Family members must establish a new relationship with the dying person.

Critical Thinking

1. You are caring for an older adult who is in the process of dying. A registered nurse (RN) who has floated to your unit is reluctant to administer the IV medication for pain because it is a narcotic, and expresses fears that the client will become addicted. How should you respond to the RN?

2. Describe what the hospital of 2050 might look like. Describe hospice care in 2050.

3. What is meant by the phrase, "pain is the fifth vital sign"?

4. What is the difference between a Living Will and a Durable Power of Attorney for Health Care?

Resources

Internet Resources

National Hospice Association
www.nho.org
www.noh.org/database.htm (hospice locations)
Hospice Association of America
www.nahc.org/HHA/home.html
The Hemlock Society
www.hemlock.org
Choices in Dying
www.choices.org

Organizations

Hospice Foundation of America
2001 S St. N.W., Suite 300
Washington, DC 20009
1-800-854-5312

AARP
601 E Street N.W.
Washington, DC 20049
1-800-424-3410
AARP Webplace

Choice in Dying
200 Varick Street
New York, NY 10014
1-212-366-5540

Emanual, L. L., & Emanual, E. J.
The Medical Directive
General Internal Medicine Unit
Massachusetts General Hospital
32 Fruit Street
Boston, MA 02114

Selected References

Hall, J. K. (1996). *Nursing: Ethics and law.* Philadelphia: W. B. Saunders.

Kazanowski, M. (1997). A commitment to palliative care. *Journal of Gerontological Nursing, 23*(3), 36–42.

McKee, R. J. (1999). Clarifying advance directives. *Nursing 99, May,* 52–53.

Morse, J. M. (2000). On comfort and comforting. *American Journal of Nursing, 100*(9), 34–38.

Pellegrino, E. D. (1992). Ethics. *Journal of the American Medical Association, 268*(3), 354–355.

Perrin, K. O. (1997). Giving voice to the wishes of elders for end of life care. *Journal of Gerontological Nursing, 23*(3), 18–27.

The SUPPORT Principal Investigators. (1995). A controlled trial to improve care for seriously ill hospitalized patients. *JAMA, 274,* 1591–1598.

V

Management Skills in Care of the Older Adult

Leadership Role of the LPN/LVN

HELEN STEPHENS HOWLETT and SIGNE S. HILL

OBJECTIVES

After completing this chapter, you will be able to:

- Explain the LPN/LVN expanded role.
- Using your state's nurse practice act, identify the conditions under which you may assume a charge nurse position in extended care.
- Describe similarities and differences of leadership and management.
- Compare and contrast characteristics of leaders and followers.
- Recognize three styles of leadership: autocratic, democratic, and laissez-faire.
- Discuss examples of situational leadership.
- Explain the LPN/LVN charge nurse's role in assignment and delegation.
- List ten suggestions for legally defensible documentation.
- Identify examples of verbal and nonverbal assertive communication.
- Use the nursing process to manage conflicts.

CHAPTER OUTLINE

KEY TERMS

Aggressive communication

Assertive communication

Assigning

Autocratic

Collaborate

Compromise

Delegating

Democratic

Expanded role of the LPN/LVN

Formal authority

Informal authority

Laissez-faire

Leadership

Leadership style

Lose-win

Management

Objective entry

Passive communication

Situational leadership

Win-lose

Win-win

CASE STUDY

Some of the nursing assistants from East and West wings of Sunnyside extended-care unit were on their morning coffee break. There was quite a bit of conversation going on as the aides discussed Matt Moatevatore, the new LVN charge nurse for East and West wings on the day shift.

"He sure is different from Theresa Tanque," sighed a nursing assistant from East wing. "Do you remember how each day with Theresa as charge nurse seemed like a day in basic training? She just barked and ordered us what to do. If things were not done her way and in her time frame, she would sarcastically let us know and humiliate us. She never gave us credit for anything. We never could make suggestions about what we thought would improve how we cared for clients."

A nursing assistant from West wing offered a different point of view: "At least Theresa was better in code situations than Jan Gelifisch, the charge nurse who replaced her. We do not have a lot of codes around here, but when we do, it is helpful to have someone give orders and tell you what to do the way Theresa did. Jan ran codes as if we were having a staff meeting and she was afraid to offer any input for fear she would be stepping on our toes."

The West wing nursing assistant continued, "This new charge nurse, Matt, is a pleasure to work with. He is concerned about getting the work done, but he is also respectful and does not talk down to you. He even asked me for suggestions as to how to improve Mr. Crist's bathing routine!" The East wing nursing assistant was quick to add, "and when we had that crisis on east wing on Wednesday, he gave brisk orders and the situation was taken care of quickly. When it was over, he actually gathered us together and asked for suggestions for improvement if the situation should ever arise again! And he thanked us for acting quickly. It is about time we had a charge nurse who treats us like the team members we want to be."

The purpose of this chapter is to help you understand the differences among the three charge nurses discussed here. It provides the opportunity for you to think about your development into the type of leader, in any nursing setting, who will receive positive feedback from team members, such as Matt received in the previous case study.

UTILIZATION OF THE LPN/LVN IN EXTENDED CARE

Although LPN/LVNs could be hired to provide direct client care in extended care, these nurses are frequently utilized as charge nurses in this setting. After a summer on long-term care, an RN from Pennsylvania stated "the units of this home were run mostly by LPNs" (Fauber, 1999).

A job analysis of newly licensed LPN/LVN practice is conducted every 3 years by the National Council of State Boards of Nursing (NCSBN). The latest Job Analysis was conducted in 2000. A majority of study participants reported working in long-term care facilities. Forty-one percent (41%) of study participants indicated that they had administrative responsibilities. Sixty-three percent (63%) of this group stated administrative responsibilities were their primary position. Administrative responsibilities included titles of Unit Manager, Team Leader, Charge Nurse, and Coordinator (National Council 2001). In the 2000 study, LPNs/LVNs with administrative responsibilities represent an eleven percent (11%) increase since the 1997 Job Analysis. The long-term care/extended care unit continues to be a growing site of employment for LPNs/LVNs. The complete 2000 Job Analysis may be obtained from the National Council.

The Expanded Role of the LPN/LVN

The charge nurse position in extended care is an example of the **expanded role of the LPN/LVN**. In their expanded role, LPN/LVN charge nurses supervise, direct, and guide the care given by nursing assistants on assigned units and wings. The current Nurse Practice Act of your state's Board of Nursing provides legal definitions of the exact role and boundaries of the charge nurse position and how best to function in this expanded role, including educational requirements for this position according to site of employment.

Value of the Extended-Care Clinical Rotation

You will encounter the older adult frequently throughout the student PN/VN experience. You will work with older adults as clients on the medical-surgical floor or in the extended-care unit, in the community, and in outpatient centers and mental health facilities, and as family members in pediatrics or maternity departments. Your clinical experience at the extended-care facility will focus on learning about the care of the older adult who is completing rehabilitation and who has chronic health problems. In addition to learning about the older adult client at this site, you will be able to observe LPN/LVNs functioning in their expanded role as charge nurses. The topics of leadership and management for the LPN/LVN in this chapter are discussed in the context of the LPN/LVN in the extended-care facility who is functioning in the expanded role of charge nurse.

Expanded Role as LPN/LVN Charge Nurse

Some Nurse Practice Acts stipulate that an LPN/LVN should accept the charge nurse position only if prepared to competently perform the assignment based on education, training, and experience beyond the basic practical/vocational nursing curriculum. Learning the leadership and management skills for the charge nurse role requires much more than taking one course or reading one chapter. Such activities will not turn you into a leader and manager.

Becoming a leader and manager requires the ongoing development of skills that grow over time and with experience. This chapter provides basic information about the role of the LPN/LVN in leading and managing. (A more detailed "how to" approach can be found in Hill and Howlett, 2001.) As a student PN/VN, you can most effectively acquire leadership and management abilities by developing strong nursing skills, time management strategies, stress management techniques, assertive behaviors, and solid communication skills. Also, enhanced self-assessment skills and the ability to accept constructive evaluative comments will benefit you in future nursing positions, including that of LPN/LVN charge nurse.

LEADERSHIP/MANAGEMENT ROLE OF THE LPN/LVN IN THE LONG-TERM CARE FACILITY

Leadership

Leadership is achieved when the supervising LPN/LVN charge nurse influences nursing assistants in such a way that clients receiving nursing care reach their desired outcomes. The focus of leadership is on persuading or influencing others. Human relationship skills, which are the primary tools of an effective leader, include communication, assertiveness, conflict resolution, stress reduction, and the ability to treat team members with sensitivity and respect. Good human relationship skills help the LPN/LVN to interact in a positive, effective manner with team members, clients, and families.

Nobody is born a leader. Leadership comprises skills that can be enhanced through experience. Some of you started to develop leadership skills before you entered the LPN/LVN program. All of you have been given the opportunity to acquire leadership skills from the day the nursing program began.

Not all nurses who have studied leadership are effective leaders. On the other hand, some nurses who have never taken a formal leadership course are excellent leaders. In fact, some of the great leaders, such as Napoleon and Julius Caesar, have become famous because of their ability to lead, but they never had formal learning in the subject. The authority that leaders possess is not attained simply because they accept a particular position or job title; rather, it is achieved when the leader earns the respect of those around him. For this reason, it is called **informal authority**.

All LPN/LVNs need to develop leadership skills. Some LPN/LVNs will use these skills in direct client care, and others will apply them in management positions. Box 15–1 includes examples of leadership behaviors that enhance the effectiveness of the LPN/LVN who is involved in direct client care or is in a management position. However, to be an effective leader in a charge nurse position, an LPN/LVN also must acquire strong management skills.

Management

Management for the LPN/LVN charge nurse involves directing the nursing assistants under his or her supervision to achieve specific client outcomes by providing safe, timely, and cost-effective nursing care. Such management includes control of resources, including equipment, supplies, time, and ancillary services. Tools of the effective LPN/LVN nurse manager include time

Box 15–1 Leadership Behaviors of the LPN/LVN Involved in Direct Client Care or Management

- Acknowledges a team member's extra effort
- Displays enthusiasm for suggestions to improve client care
- Displays self-confidence
- Displays sensitivity to feelings of team members
- Maintains a professional image
- Manages personal stress
- Mentors team members new to practical/vocational nursing
- Motivates nursing assistants to provide safe nursing care for clients
- Participates in team efforts
- Prevents/stops the spread of rumors
- Problem-solves about obstacles to smooth unit functioning
- Provides constructive evaluation directly to team members
- Provides positive feedback to team members for a job well done
- Role-models wellness

management, strong basic nursing skills, and the ability to organize. The most important resource of the LPN/LVN charge nurse is *people*. A successful manager also possesses the excellent human relationship skills of a leader. Whether working at the bedside, in a clinic setting, within the community, or as a charge nurse with groups of patients and nursing assistants in extended care, LPN/LVNs need to effectively manage resources.

Although the authority of a leader that is bestowed by followers can be informal, the LPN/LVN charge nurse in an extended-care setting works most effectively by conveying the **formal authority** that is accepted to be part of the job.

When the LPN/LVN demonstrates capability as a manager, efficiency of nursing assistants in an extended-care setting is enhanced. But the LPN/LVN who has strong leadership skills, especially human relationship skills, gets the job done in the most efficient *and* effective manner, and everyone involved can enjoy the experience that much more. Team members experience a sense of pride and accomplishment as client outcomes are met.

Box 15–2 Management Behaviors of the LPN/LVN Charge Nurse

- Assigns clients according to team members' strengths and needs for challenge
- Collaborates with team members
- Communicates expectations clearly for team members
- Controls stress level in clinical area
- Delegates duties within legal parameters
- Exhibits strong clinical skills while assisting team members
- Interprets facility and unit policies to team members
- Manages clinical time effectively
- Manages personal anger
- Offers team members constructive evaluation
- Reduces conflicts effectively

Box 15–2 presents examples of management behaviors exhibited by an effective LPN/LVN in the charge nurse position. By comparing Boxes 15–1 and 15–2, you can see how the concepts of leadership and management overlap.

Characteristics of Leaders

The quality of leadership provided by an LPN/LVN cannot be predicted from a cluster of personal traits alone. One positive characteristic of LPN/LVN charge nurses is their ability to persuade the nursing assistants under their supervision to provide the nursing care that will help clients to reach established outcomes. When a nurse leads, then someone has to follow. Leaders know they are leading when clients are meeting established outcomes and team members find the work environment satisfying. Do not ask yourself how you rate as a leader; instead, ask your followers to rate you. As you read the characteristics of effective LPN/LVN charge nurses listed in Box 15–3, focus on those traits that would also characterize a good follower. Keep in mind that you, as LPN/LVN charge nurse, are also a follower when you take direction from your supervisor, who is most probably a registered nurse.

Leadership Styles

Leadership style refers to the manner in which LPN/LVN charge nurses relate to nursing

assistants under their supervision in order to influence them to work toward meeting client outcomes. The focus of leadership is to establish a work environment that will encourage the team to be productive and to meet client outcomes. Leadership style comprises two important concepts: *task* and *relationship*. Task refers to the work that needs to be done on a particular shift. Outcomes and tasks are specified on individual client care plans. Relationship refers to the human relationship skills discussed earlier in this chapter. Human relationship skills involve treating others as you would like to be treated. There is a link between the leadership style of a supervising LPN/LVN charge nurse and the level of job satisfaction of nursing assistants.

Specific leadership styles can be classified as autocratic, democratic, and laissez-faire. As you read about the three styles of leadership in the following paragraphs, it may be helpful for you to review the discussion of the LPN/LVN charge nurses presented in the Case Study at the beginning of this chapter.

Autocratic Style of Leadership

The primary focus of the **autocratic** style of leadership is concern for the task, not for the manager's relationship with the staff. This leadership style focuses on achieving results. Employees' needs are not a priority. When the aggressive, autocratic style is used, the LPN/LVN charge nurse

Box 15–3 Characteristics of an Effective LPN/LVN Charge Nurse

Acts as a mentor	Impartial
Assertive	Investigative
Caring	Knowledgeable
Coaching	Organized
Collaborative	Perceptive
Communicative	Problem-solving
Courageous	Respectful
Creative	Self-directed
Curious	Skilled
Empathic	Thinks critically
Enthusiastic	Trustworthy
Flexible	

decides what needs to be done and how it is to be done. This LPN/LVN charge nurse supervises nursing assistants by giving orders. Input is not sought from the team. The autocratic style is efficient, and work gets done quickly. Examples of situations in which the autocratic style of leadership is successful include codes, crisis situations, and emergencies. A consistent autocratic approach in all situations can breed hostility among nursing assistants toward the charge nurse. Theresa Tanque's aggressive approach (discussed in the Case Study) earned neither the approval nor the respect of nursing assistants.

Laissez-Faire Style of Leadership

The **laissez-faire** style of leadership is the opposite extreme of the autocratic style. The primary focus of this passive leadership style is the relationship of the LPN/LVN charge nurse and team members. The motto is, "No conflict, peace at any price." When the laissez-faire style is used, nursing assistants are free to function with little input from the charge nurse. Because of the permissiveness of this charge nurse and the lack of communication of expectations, the shift may take its own direction, and there is no concern about whether client outcomes will be reached. The ideal situation for an effective laissez-faire method of leadership occurs when a team is composed entirely of members who have consistently demonstrated an excellent knowledge base, strong self-direction, and good problem-solving skills. However, if all team members do not have these skills, the laissez-faire style of leadership could create an unsafe environment for the client, wherein team members struggle awkwardly without direction and client outcomes continue to go unmet. Jan Gelifisch's passive, laid-back attitude might be enjoyed at first, but eventually it would wear thin with nursing assistants under her supervision.

Sometimes when an LPN/LVN charge nurse uses the laissez-faire leadership style, the intention is to be a buddy or friend to team members. Being a friend is not the same as providing leadership. Attaining popularity with staff members is not a priority of an effective leader. Leading is a difficult task. When you lead, remember that your first responsibility is always to the clients whom you serve.

Democratic Style of Leadership

Between the two extreme methods of leadership just described is the **democratic** style. The focus of this assertive style is both task *and* human relations because the LPN/LVN charge nurse working in this style displays concern both for the work that needs to be done and for the team members who are performing the work. When using this leadership style, the LPN/LVN charge nurse encourages nursing assistants to communicate, offer input, make decisions, and problem-solve. The team is treated with sensitivity and respect. Nursing assistants are encouraged to offer suggestions to improve client care. Goals may be accomplished over a longer time period than with the autocratic style, but client outcomes are achieved with staff having positive feelings about both their supervisor and the experience. Examples of situations in which the democratic style of leadership is useful include the provision of daily nursing care, the unit meeting, and the review of client care plans. Matt Moatevatore's assertive style (in the Case Study) earned the respect of both his supervisors and the nursing assistants under his leadership.

Situational Leadership

As you read about the three styles of leadership, did you categorize yourself according to any one style? Perhaps you saw glimmers of yourself in each of the styles described. LPN/LVN charge nurses need to be aware of their personal tendencies in leadership style. Each leadership style can be ineffective when used consistently. Because situations are always changing in extended care, nursing assistants may need to be supervised at different times according to different leadership styles. **Situational leadership** is a style of leadership that encourages LPN/LVN charge nurses to be aware of individual situations and the needs of individual nursing assistants, and to be flexible in altering their leadership style to meet the demands of the circumstances. Use of a brisk autocratic style every workday may decrease motivation in team members and create a negative clinical climate. On the other hand, using a democratic style during a code situation, that is, seeking input and ideas from all team members involved, could breed disaster for the client. An inexperienced nursing assistant may need a more directive approach for client care than an experienced nursing assistant. Be aware of your personal style, and adapt it to match each clinical situation and the particular needs of team members.

PHYSICAL MANAGEMENT ACTIVITIES FOR THE LPN/LVN CHARGE NURSE

This book divides nursing care of the older adult into physical and psychosocial aspects. Management activities of the LPN/LVN charge nurse can be divided in the same manner. Two specific activities are discussed here as examples of physical management activities.

Assignment and Delegation

The terms assignment (**assigning**) and delegation (**delegating**) are defined here to clarify their use in the following discussion. The discussion emphasizes the role of the LPN/LVN charge nurse in assigning and delegating. The word "task" is used when assignment is discussed, and the word "duty" indicates a discussion of delegation. The term "charge nurse" is used only in the context of the LPN/LVN.

Assignment is the distribution of work during a particular shift. Effective assigning of clients and staff members is a skill that every LPN/LVN charge nurse needs to develop. Assignment occurs after report is received from the off-going shift. The need for assignment or reassignment can also occur at any time during the shift. The LPN/LVN charge nurse assigns to nursing assistants tasks that are in *their* job description. The assigned tasks involve work that nursing assistants are trained, hired, and paid to perform.

Delegation is transfer to nursing assistants of the authority to carry out a specific duty of the charge nurse; these nursing assistants must be capable of safely carrying out the duty in a selected nursing situation. The need to delegate can occur at any time during the shift. *Not every state in the United States allows LPN/LVNs to delegate duties in their charge nurse positions. Check a current copy of your state's nurse practice act to determine if you may delegate as an LPN/LVN charge nurse in your state.* Policies of the extended-care unit also need to be checked to determine if LPN/LVNs are allowed to delegate work in the facility. When work is

delegated, duties that are in the job description of the LPN/LVN charge nurse are offered to nursing assistants.

Major Similarities Between Assigning and Delegating

In extended care, the LPN/LVN as charge nurse manages and directs the activities of nursing assistants under the general supervision of a registered nurse (RN), who is ultimately responsible for the supervision of nursing assistants. However, the LPN/LVN charge nurse assists in the supervision of these health care workers and shares accountability with the RN supervisor for their actions. Nursing assistants are accountable for completing tasks or duties in a safe and timely manner.

There are four areas for which the LPN/LVN charge nurse is legally accountable when assigning tasks or delegating duties: (1) the task assigned or duty delegated; (2) the person to whom a task or duty is assigned or delegated; (3) communication; and (4) supervision and feedback.

Task Assigned or Duty Delegated. A legal consideration when tasks are assigned and duties are delegated by the LPN/LVN charge nurse is nursing judgment. When assigning or delegating, the LPN/LVN charge nurse must avoid real or potential danger to the client by assigning or delegating appropriate tasks or duties. Change-of-shift report gives the charge nurse the opportunity to appraise both the specific nursing needs of clients during the shift and the complexity of those needs. Specific tasks appropriate for assignment to nursing assistants based on their job description include routine bathing, feeding, turning, and ambulating; measuring vital signs and weight; providing assistance with elimination; and monitoring patient safety. The actual tasks assigned vary with the needs of clients on the unit, the level of training of nursing assistants, and the policies of the long-term care unit. Assignment of more complex tasks must be decided according to the stipulations of the state Nurse Practice Act, unit need, and the level of specialized training of nursing assistants.

A concise list of nursing duties that may be appropriately delegated or not delegated by an LPN/LVN charge nurse does not exist. The exact duties delegated to nursing assistants are determined according to each state's Board of Nursing policies and each individual client situation. The person doing the delegating is ultimately responsible for deciding when, to whom, and under what circumstances to delegate a particular duty. Duties that are part of your legal scope of practice as an LPN/LVN may never be delegated. Examples of duties not to delegate *might* include sterile technique procedures, crisis situations, and initial client education by an RN. Nursing duties must be delegated appropriately both for the good of the client and to ensure the protection of your professional license.

The Person to Whom a Task/Duty Is Assigned or Delegated. According to the law, you must know the job descriptions and skills lists of nursing assistants to whom you assign tasks or delegate duties. Know the strengths and weaknesses of nursing assistants whom you supervise. Have they completed training? Are they state certified? Have they completed orientation to your unit? Nursing assistants who are given the authority to perform a particular task or duty are accountable for their actions in safely performing that task or duty.

Communication. The objective in assigning a task or delegating a duty is to have it completed safely with client outcomes in view. Give clear, concise, objective directions to nursing assistants when you are assigning a task or delegating a duty. Be specific about the results you are expecting. Consider writing assignments in a concise, objective manner on a master assignment sheet. Make sure your directions are clear and complete. Explain what is expected at the nursing assistant's level of understanding. Clarify the message by asking nursing assistants to tell you what it is you expect them to do. Both "please" and "thank you" are in order as part of common courtesy and professional behavior.

Supervision and Feedback. When nursing assistants are assigned a task or accept a delegated duty, they accept the responsibility and accountability for safely and effectively completing that assignment. LPN/LVN charge nurses have the legal responsibility to periodically supervise the nursing assistant's ability and success in performing the task or duty and to check the outcome. Was the task or duty completed and performed

safely? Have patient outcomes been met? Observation and feedback concerning assigned tasks are essential.

Major Differences Between Assigning and Delegating

Although the suggestions so far in this chapter for assigning also apply to delegating, there are some important differences. Because assigning involves designating nursing care tasks to be done by nursing assistants within their job description, they cannot refuse the assignment. However, because nursing assistants assume responsibility for completing assigned tasks safely, they may refuse to complete assignments for which they are unqualified.

Delegating is a voluntary procedure that can be followed when one is allowed to delegate according to both the state nurse practice act and policies of extended care. The purpose of delegating is to provide time for the charge nurse to meet other responsibilities with the goal of improving client care. When delegating duties, the LPN/LVN charge nurse makes the decision to ask nursing assistants to do part of the charge nurse's job. Because the LPN/LVN is delegating duties that are part of the charge nurse job description, the nursing assistant must give approval to the delegated duty by voluntarily accepting it. In other words, the nursing assistant can refuse to accept the delegated duty.

Delegation: Concepts and Decision-Making Process (1995) was prepared by the National Council of State Boards of Nursing as a resource for licensed nurses in all types of health care settings. It provides a decision-making process to facilitate the provision of quality care by licensed nurses as they delegate nursing tasks in accord with their legal scope of practice and state Nurse Practice Act. See Internet Resources for access to the National Council's document. Also, Hill and Howlett (2001) provide a detailed explanation of assignment and delegation practices, written specifically for the LPN/LVN charge nurse.

Documentation

Use the guidelines for legal documentation that your instructors provide throughout your student education. Documentation in extended care follows the same general rules as documentation for other clinical sites. The client's record is a legal document and must contain details of the care received by the client, including a listing of all client problems and what was done in response to those problems. Be aware of the specific documentation policy of the extended-care facility and use it consistently.

Orientation to the extended-care facility includes information about federal and state laws that affect extended care. If the facility participates in accreditation, the requirements of accrediting agencies are also explained. In extended care, nursing documentation provides the basis for payment of resident fees or denial of payment. Documentation is especially important when participating agencies mandate resident outcomes. It is important to write all documentation in a specific and objective format. Avoid subjective comments and personal judgments in your documentation. Document what you see, hear, feel, smell, and so forth. How to supply objective documentation is sometimes a hard lesson for students to learn, especially if they see examples

of general and subjective entries on charts provided by licensed staff in the clinical area. It is tempting for students to chart "vital signs stable" because everyone on staff does the same. Use the client's actual numbers to convert this subjective entry into an **objective entry** (e.g., BP 126/78-82-24). Another example of a commonly used subjective entry is "Up. Tolerated well." Presented as an objective entry, it would be written as, "Up with help of one and cane. Walked to bathroom with steady gait." Box 15–4 provides suggestions for legally defensible documentation.

PSYCHOSOCIAL MANAGEMENT ACTIVITIES FOR THE LPN/LVN CHARGE NURSE

Communication

Each topic in this chapter provides examples of what an effective leader communicates. This chapter builds on basic communication skills taught in courses within the PN/VN nursing program. The

---

Box 15–4 Suggestions for Legally Defensible Documentation

- Consistently follow facility documentation policy.
- Periodically review prior documentation to help you improve current documentation. Imagine you are someone else (a lawyer?) reading your notes. Are your notes from yesterday easy to read? Do they say what you intended? Would you be able to understand the entries 5 years from now in a courtroom?
- Each entry must include the date and time of the event and your signature and legal title.
- Each entry must be objective and specific.
- Each entry must be legible (consider printing) with correct spelling and grammar. Unfair as it seems, sloppy, misspelled documentation combined with grammar mistakes could allow a lawyer to bring your ability to provide competent nursing care into question.
- Use permanent ink in the color specified by the facility. Erasable pens are not permitted.
- Draw a single, straight line to fill in any empty spaces before your signature. Avoid skipping lines.
- Draw a single line through incorrect entries and put the date and your name above the incorrect entry. Write "void" or "mistake in entry" before

your signature. Avoid "whiting out" or obliterating the entry. You have nothing to hide.
- All abnormal observations, including changes in client's condition, must be charted, along with whom you notified about the observation and what was done.
- Never document care you *intend* to give in the future. Document care as it is completed.
- Document with attention on flow sheets. Review the flowsheet's parameters for normal findings before you automatically place a checkmark.
- When documenting by computer, protect client privacy by avoiding entering information while visitors are passing by the computer screen.
- If you discover a record that has been tampered with, notify your nursing supervisor.
- Avoid placing personal criticism of prior shifts or other nurses in the record. Discuss your concerns directly with the persons involved.
- Document all reinforcement of client teaching that you have provided.
- Remember, if you did not document it, you did not do it, and a lawyer could conclude that you did not care.

focus of this section is assertive communication as a process by which the LPN/LVN charge nurse's messages are received and understood by nursing assistants, clients, physicians, families, visitors, and members of other departments within and outside of the facility.

Assertive Communication

Assertiveness is a communication style developed through practice. With **assertive communication**, LPN/LVN charge nurses communicate personal choices in their own best interests while being respectful of the feelings, choices, and opinions of others. Assertive communicators stand up for themselves without violating the rights of others.

Leadership styles are reflected in management behaviors, including style of communication. In the situation at the beginning of this chapter, Theresa's **aggressive communication** style got results, but use of military treatment as her predominant style eventually resulted in resentment among the nursing assistants. Jan resented that no one appreciated her efforts to make everyone happy. Jan's **passive**, conflict-avoiding **communication** style eventually resulted in stress and its consequent wear and tear. Matt was respected for his open, honest, and direct communication in explaining expectations and providing feedback. His **assertive communication** style promoted cooperation among the nursing assistants and encouraged them to participate in problem solving and in improving client care.

Verbal Communication

Matt chose assertive techniques that facilitate communication in all communication situations. These techniques show respect for the person and his feelings.

Open-ended questions, which encourage communication, are used instead of questions that can be answered with a single word, such as "Yes" or "No."

Example—Matt to new nursing assistant on staff: "What were the high and low points of your day?"

Validating allows the nurse to determine if needs are being met.

Example—Matt to physician who complained of Matt's need to keep running back to the nurses' station for supplies and charts during rounds: "I think the push cart has made it easier for me to access the charts and supplies you need during rounds. How is this system working for you?"

Reflecting encourages the speaker to continue expressing self.

Example—Matt in even tone to family member upset because his father was not walked today: "You are saying your dad did not walk in the hall today."

Acknowledging thoughts and feelings communicates acceptance of feelings and thoughts and encourages verbalizing.

Example—Matt to client with frown: "I see you are frowning. What's going on with you? Are you concerned about something?"

Some techniques block communication. Blocking does not enable one to recognize listeners as individuals or to respect their feelings. Reassurance minimizes feelings and communicates lack of interest in the individual.

Example—Jan to family member of a client needing a pacemaker: "Don't worry about a thing. Everything will be just fine."

Stereotyping communicates that the listener is not unique, and the nurse is not listening and is not interested.

Example—Theresa to a client who is anxious about an upcoming test: "Dry those tears! Every client tells me the test you are going to have is a piece of cake."

Leading statements ask for a particular response that the nurse wants to hear and intimidates the listener.

Example—Jan to a nursing assistant: "You're not planning to wear those shoes today, are you?"

Giving advice communicates that the speaker places importance on certain personal values and does not acknowledge the listener's right to her feelings.

Example—Theresa to physician she called to notify of change in condition of client: "If you traded in your car for a new one, then you could get here faster when I need you."

Listening. Listening is a powerful communication tool. Listening involves concentrating on understanding and interpreting the intended meaning of a speaker's verbal message. Focus on what the speaker is saying. Do not wander. It is not a coincidence that we were given two ears and one mouth.

Nonverbal Communication

Most communication is nonverbal. Receivers of verbal messages respond mostly to nonverbal communication. It is also not a coincidence that we were given two eyes and one mouth. Words may be assertive but the behavior of the speaker may give a different message. For example, a client may state he is "Fine" while shaking his head in a negative manner. Body language needs to be consistent with the words spoken. The speaker does not want a nonverbal message to cancel out or distract from the verbal message he is trying to communicate.

Professional Image. The verbal skills of a charge nurse can enhance or detract from professional image. A weak tone of voice, poor grammar, and/or a habit of using swear words can damage one's image and credibility. Appearance is included with nonverbal behavior and can make a strong statement to the people with whom you interact during a particular shift. It is impossible to avoid projecting an image through your dress and other nonverbal behavior. LPN/LVN charge nurses can strengthen their position by how they dress and groom themselves. Appropriate hairstyle, shoes, and accessories, as well as cleanliness, project a professional image consistent with your responsibilities. LPN/LVN charge nurses who plan their image enhance their role. If you ignore how you look and are perceived, you will have to work hard to overcome an image that is inconsistent with your responsibilities.

Table 15–1 provides suggestions of assertive verbal and nonverbal communication techniques for the LPN/LVN charge nurse.

Conflict Management

The stress, working conditions, and possibilities for communication errors that plague scores of individuals working within the extended-care unit create a ripe environment for conflict to be managed by the LPN/LVN charge nurse. Staff members can develop conflicts within themselves, especially when asked to work overtime while trying to meet family responsibilities. When two or more nursing assistants experience differences in values or goals while providing client care, the resulting tension can end in conflict. And two different groups, for example, the evening shift and the night shift, can become embroiled over what seems to be the pettiest of issues. Add to these situations the complaints of clients, the concerns of client families about quality of care issues, and the sometimes demeaning approach of physicians toward staff members, along with the need for health care staff members to collaborate with other departments both inside and outside of the extended-care facility, and it is easy to understand the importance for the LPN/LVN charge nurse of acquiring knowledge about how to manage conflicts.

Conflicts are *positive events* that can accompany change in the work environment or indicate the need for change and problem solving within the same environment. Conflicts are inevitable in the workplace and can be strong motivators for growth. When conflicts are left unresolved, team members can become frustrated, angry, and difficult to work with. Time with clients can be wasted and productivity hindered.

Strategies for Managing Conflicts

There are three basic strategies for managing conflicts: win-lose, lose-win, and win-win. Review the situation at the beginning of this chapter. Theresa Tanque would probably choose the aggressive **win-lose** strategy to manage conflicts. With this strategy, Theresa would use her power to force her ideas and opinions on those in conflict. The ideas and opinions of "the other side" would be ignored. Theresa would win and those at the other end of the conflict would lose. Jan Gelifisch might choose the passive **lose-win** strategy as her means of managing conflicts. According to this strategy, Jan would place the priority on accommodating those involved in the

Table 15–1
ASSERTIVE COMMUNICATION AND THE LPN/LVN CHARGE NURSE

Verbal

Oral Language

1. When talking to nursing assistants, deliver your message with clear, specific language. Spell out objectively what has to be done for clients. You might be working with nursing assistants who do not have English as a first language. Until you determine their proficiency with English, clarify that intended messages were received.
2. As an LPN/LVN charge nurse, you are a role model for nursing assistants. Discourage profanity, personal criticisms, gossip, and rumors.
3. Use "I" versus "You" messages. "I" messages indicate that you take the responsibility for the message (e.g., "I think you need to review how to apply a waist restraint"). "You" messages imply that you blame the person to whom you are speaking (e.g., "You really give poor nursing care"). Take responsibility for your messages. Propose solutions.

Written Language

1. Use language that all staff will understand.
2. Review your written messages to be sure that the intent of the message is clear.
3. Provide written client assignments that do not require the nursing assistant to make judgments.
4. Provide written reports of all meetings. If information is not restricted, a report from a meeting with management can dispel/prevent rumors about what "they" are doing now. The reports can be placed in a looseleaf binder in an area that is accessible to nursing assistants.

Telephone Communication

1. Gather your thoughts and think about the purpose for the call before you make a call.
2. With a smile in your voice, greet the person called by name and identify yourself. For routine calls, offer a brief inquiry as to his or her well-being if you know the person called (e.g., "Hello, Mrs. Jones. This is Matt Moatevatore from Sunnyside. How are things going?").
3. State the reason for the call (e.g., "I need to order a client care video and wanted to know if you had any specific needs?").
4. You initiated the conversation. Terminate it when your business is completed. The exception is when the person you called brings up a work-related question.
5. Avoid long conversations about non–work-related topics. This is what is considered allowing the telephone to cut into your time.
6. Arrange to have incoming calls answered quickly (e.g., by the second or third ring).
7. When you answer incoming calls, identify the facility and give your name and title (e.g., "Sunnyside, Matt Moatevatore, LVN Charge Nurse").
8. Keep a smile in your voice.
9. Speak clearly in a moderate tone of voice. Most people talk too loudly on the phone.
10. Callers are "customers." Treat the caller respectfully and cordially.
11. If it is necessary to put the person on hold, ask permission to do so.
12. If it was necessary to put the person on hold, try to get back to him or her within 30 seconds. If you are still delayed, ask for a number so you can call them back.
13. Provide information requested.

Listening Skills

1. Actively listen to the speaker. Avoid distraction and inattention. Avoid yawning, playing with hair, and scratching.
2. Stay focused on what the speaker is saying.
3. Avoid making a response while the speaker is speaking.
4. Avoid judging the message or the speaker.
5. Rephrase the message when the speaker is done to clarify that you understand the message.
6. Encourage comments. Your goal is to have the speaker say, "I feel as if that charge nurse really listened!"
7. Encourage constructive evaluation. Create an environment in which staff, clients, and family are encouraged to give their input—positive or negative.

Nonverbal

1. Make direct eye contact when speaking, but avoid staring at the listener.
2. Be sure your body language and message are consistent and professional. Face the person to whom you are speaking (e.g., avoid smiling when you are delivering a needed reprimand).
3. When delivering your message, convey that you are sure of yourself. Have an attentive posture. Keep hands at your sides, and use them appropriately to gesture while you speak. Avoid making fists or pointing a finger.
4. Speak in a firm, clear, audible voice. Avoid a whiny tone. Avoid ending sentences with a questioning inflection.

Adapted from Hill, S., & Howlett, H. (2001). *Success in practical/vocational nursing: From student to leader.* Philadelphia: W. B. Saunders.

conflict but at her own expense. Jan would lose and those involved in the conflict would win. Matt Moatevatore would probably choose the assertive **win-win** strategy. Win-win takes into consideration the conflict itself, the results of intervention, and the relationships of those involved in the conflict. This assertive strategy manages issues at the base of the conflict without compromising what is important to both sides. Win-win takes a collaborative approach.

Situational Conflict Management

Management of conflict is related to the principles of the three styles of leadership—autocratic, democratic, and laissez-faire—described earlier in

the chapter. The trap that the LPN/LVN charge nurse can fall into is the temptation to use the same strategy for all conflicts. Choose the most appropriate strategy for each situation. Be aware of your dominant style, and modify it for each event. Theresa's style is best used in emergency situations or when the conflict allows a majority vote to be taken, as in a staff meeting. When tempers are flaring, the lose-win strategy might be a good short-term tactic.

Conflicts can, at a minimum, be prevented from escalating. If the situation is not an emergency or the tempers of those involved are not flaring, the ideal approach would be a win-win strategy. Table 15–2 uses the nursing process to present elements of conflict resolution.

Table 15–2
THE NURSING PROCESS AND CONFLICT RESOLUTION

Assessment/Data Collection—Obtain all of the facts

1. When a conflict arises, avoid pursuing it on the spot. Arrange for involved parties to meet in an area that will provide privacy.
2. Separate the person from the problem. Attack the problem, and not the persons involved.
3. Each party has his or her own perception of, and strong emotions about, what happened. Unclear communication may result. Clarify subjective statements and generalizations. You need to get objective and specific facts. For example, clarify what is meant by "she always does that" and "they."
4. Actively listen to the person presenting the "facts."

Statement of the Problem—Identify the specific issue

1. After hearing all sides, state in your own words what you understand is the conflict. Use "I" messages when presenting your perspective.
2. Ask parties for feedback as to the accuracy of your understanding of the conflict.

Interventions (Planning)

1. Convey the attitude of working side by side to settle the conflict (e.g., sit side by side to work on the problem).
2. Involve all parties in identifying and discussing possible solutions to the conflict. The more alternatives the better. The goal is a solution that will be agreeable to everyone's interests.
3. Avoid bargaining over positions (what you want). Egos are identified with positions. The parties involved will focus on defending their position. In the end, the parties need to save face.
4. Focus on interests (why something is wanted). Behind a position is a motivating interest. Behind opposite positions often lie shared and compatible interests. **Compromise** involves giving up aspects of an issue that are important to one of the parties. This is not a good intervention. **Collaborate** for a win-win solution that focuses on shared or compatible interests.

Implementation—Implement the selected solution

On a sunny, cool day in the fall, two residents are sitting on the sun porch of Sunnyside extended-care facility. Resident A's position is that he wants a window open, and Resident B's position is that he wants the window closed. Matt Moatevatore asks Resident A why he wants a window open. He replies, "So I can get some fresh air." Matt asks Resident B why he wants the window closed. He replies, "So it won't be drafty." A solution built on *collaboration* would involve Matt wrapping Resident B in a blanket and moving his wheelchair to the North end of the sun porch. Matt would move Resident A to the South end of the sun porch and open a window near him. This is a "win-win" solution. A solution built on *compromise* would involve Matt returning both residents to their rooms, or returning one of the residents to his room and accommodating the other on the sun porch. This is an "I win–you lose" solution.

Evaluation—Evaluate the effectiveness of interventions toward meeting the intended outcome

In the above situation, Matt returns 30 minutes later and finds both residents fast asleep in their wheelchairs.

Adapted from Hill, S., & Howlett, H. (2001). *Success in practical/vocational nursing: From student to leader.* Philadelphia: W. B. Saunders.

Summary

- Extended care is a frequent site of employment for practical/vocational nurses, especially in their expanded role as LPN/LVN charge nurse. LPN/LVN charge nurses supervise, direct, and guide care given by nursing assistants.
- Each state's Nurse Practice Act describes the expanded role of the LPN/LVN and the conditions under which the charge nurse position may be assumed.
- Management involves *directing* nursing assistants to meet specific client outcomes by using resources effectively. Management tools, which include time management and organizational skills, allow the charge nurse to organize a shift "journey."
- Leadership refers to the style that the LPN/LVN charge nurse uses to *influence* nursing assistants in meeting client outcomes. The most important leadership tool, skill in assisting human relationships, allows nursing assistants not only to get to their destination, but also to enjoy the "trip."
- Leaders need good followers. Many of the desirable traits of successful leaders are also traits found in good followers.
- Three styles of leadership are autocratic, laissez-faire, and democratic.
- Situational leadership encourages flexibility in altering leadership style to meet the demands of particular circumstances.
- As part of their role, LPN/LVNs assign (distribute) tasks that are included in the job description of nursing assistants. The Nurse Practice Act of each state defines the LPN/LVN's legal scope in delegating duties to nursing assistants from the practical/vocational nurse's job description.
- Payment of client fees or denial of payment is based on the complete, accurate, and objective documentation of the LPN/LVN charge nurse.
- Assertive communication requires that LPN/LVNs communicate personal choices in their own best interests while being respectful of the feelings, choices, and opinions of others.
- Assertive communication consists of verbal and nonverbal messages, including the professional image that one projects.

- Using the nursing process and focusing on *why* parties involved in a conflict want something can help LPN/LVN charge nurses to manage conflicts.

STUDY QUESTIONS
Multiple-Choice Review

1. Select the strategy that allows the practical/vocational nurse to practice situational leadership.
   1. Tell subordinates what to do.
   2. Put subordinates first before the policies of the extended-care facility.
   3. Seek input from employees for emergency situations during the actual situation.
   4. Evaluate the situation in the work environment, and vary leadership style to meet the occasion.

2. Which strategy will help the practical/vocational nurse in managing a conflict?
   1. Develop a compromise solution.
   2. Limit the number of possible solutions to the conflict.
   3. Determine why parties in the conflict hold the positions that are in conflict.
   4. Investigate what the conflicting parties want to achieve as an outcome of the conflict.

3. Select the statement that applies to delegation.
   1. The nursing assistant cannot refuse a delegated task.
   2. Delegated duties are in the LPN/LVN job description.
   3. Delegated tasks are in the job description of nursing assistants.
   4. The practical/vocational nursing role is delegated to unlicensed personnel who have proved they are capable of assuming the role.

4. How does the assertive manager differ from the aggressive manager?
   1. Is respectful of others
   2. Tries to avoid conflict
   3. Intimidates team members
   4. Puts the happiness of the work group first

5. Choose the assertive communication strategy that allows the LPN/LVN to assess if client needs are being met.
   1. Reflecting
   —2. Validating
   3. Reassurance
   4. Leading statements

Critical Thinking

1. What are the stipulations of your state's Nurse Practice Act (NPA) with regard to assuming a charge nurse position and delegating as an LPN/LVN?

2. Where can you obtain information regarding your legal role as an LPN/LVN if an NPA does not address your expanded role, delegation, and so forth?

3. How do leadership and management overlap? How are they similar and different?

4. Discuss the differences between a leader and a follower.

Resources

Internet Resources

National Council of State Boards of Nursing
www.ncsbn.org
(use pull-down menu to obtain information on delegation)
National Federation of Licensed Practical Nurses, Inc.
www.nflpn.org

Organizations

American Nurses Association
600 Maryland Avenue, Suite 100W
Washington, DC 20024
(800) 274-4ANA

National League for Nursing
61 Broadway, 33rd Floor
New York, NY 10006
(212) 363-5555

Selected References

Boucher, M. (1998). Delegation alert. *American Journal of Nursing, 98*(2), 26, 28–32.

Cummings, J., & Nugent, L. (1997). Integrating management concepts into licensed practical nurse and associate degree in nursing student clinical experiences. *Nurse Educator, 22*(4), 41–43.

Delegation: Concepts and Decision-Making Process. Position statement of the National Council of State Boards of Nursing. Available at http://www.ncsbn.org Accessed 1/24/01.

Entry level competencies of graduates of educational programs in practical nursing. Available at www.cpnp@nln.org/ coun_cpnp_co.htm Accessed 1/24/01.

Fauber, G. (1999). Response (December 13, 1999) to issue of *Clinical Competence* of September 30, 1999. *1999 Online Journal of Issues in Nursing.*

Fiedler, F. (1967). *A theory of leadership effectiveness.* New York: McGraw-Hill.

Fisher, L., & Davidhizer, R. (1998). Every nurse is a leader. *Journal of Practical Nursing, 48*(2), 16–19.

Fisher, R., & Ury, W. (1991). *Getting to yes: Negotiating agreement without giving in.* New York: Penguin Books.

Hersey, P., & Blanchard, K. H. (1988). *Management of organizational behavior.* Englewood Cliffs, NJ: Prentice-Hall.

Hill, S., & Howlett, H. (2001). *Success in practical/vocational nursing: From student to leader* (4th ed). Philadelphia: W. B. Saunders.

Huber, D. (2000). *Leadership and nursing care management.* Philadelphia: W. B. Saunders.

Marrelli, T. (1997). *The nurse manager's survival guide: Practical answers to everyday problems.* St. Louis: Mosby Year-Book.

McGuffin, J. (1999). *The nurse's guide to successful management.* St. Louis: Mosby.

National Council of State Boards of Nursing (1995). *Delegation: Concepts and decision-making process.* Chicago: NCSBN.

National Council of State Boards of Nursing (2001). Linking the NCLEX-PN National Licensure Examination to Practice: 2000 Practice Analysis of Newly Licensed Practical/ Vocational Nurses in the U.S. Chicago: NCSBN, p. 16–17.

Osguthorpe, S. (April 1997). Managing a shift effectively: The role of the charge nurse. *Critical Care Nurse, 17*(2), 64, 66–70.

Porter-O'Grady, T. (1994). *The nurse manager's problem solver.* St. Louis: Mosby Year-Book.

Pugh, J., & Woodward-Smith, M. (1997). *Nurse manager: A practical guide to better employee relations.* Philadelphia: W. B. Saunders.

Wywialowski, E. (1997). *Managing client care.* St. Louis: Mosby Year-Book.

Yoder-Wise, P. (1999). *Leading and managing in nursing.* St. Louis: Mosby Year-Book.

Zerwekh, J., & Claborn, J. (2000). *Nursing today: Transition and trends.* Philadelphia: W. B. Saunders.

Appendices

Assessment Tools

MINI-MENTAL STATE EXAMINATION

Patient _____ Examiner _____ Date _____

Maximum Score	Score	
		Orientation
5	( )	What is the (year) (season) (date) (day) (month)?
5	( )	Where are we: (state) (county) (town) (hospital) (floor)
		Registration
3	( )	Name three objects: (Apple, Penny, Table) 1 second to say each. Then ask the patient all three after you have said them. Give 1 point for each correct answer. Then repeat them until he or she learns all three. Count trials and record.

Trials ___

		Attention and Calculation
5	( )	Serial 7's. 1 point for each correct. Stop after five answers. Alternatively spell "world" backwards.
		Recall
3	( )	Ask for the three objects repeated above. Give 1 point for each correct.
		Language
9	( )	Name a pencil and watch (2 points).

Repeat the following: "No ifs, ands, or buts." (1 point)
Follow a three-stage command:
  "Take a paper in your right hand, fold it in half,
    and put it on the floor." (3 points)
Read and obey the following:
  CLOSE YOUR EYES (1 point).
Write a sentence (1 point).
Copy design (overlapping pentagons) (1 point).

Overlapping pentagons

Total Score
ASSESS level of consciousness along a continuum_____

               Alert   Drowsy   Stupor   Coma

INSTRUCTIONS FOR ADMINISTRATION OF MINI-MENTAL STATE EXAMINATION

Orientation

(1) Ask for the date. Then ask specifically for parts omitted, e.g., "Can you also tell me what season it is?" One point for each correct.

(2) Ask in turn "Can you tell me the name of this hospital?" (town, country, etc.). One point for each correct.

Registration

Ask the patient if you may test his or her memory. Then say the names of three unrelated objects, clearly and slowly, about 1 second for each.

After you have said all three, ask him or her to repeat them. This first repetition determines his or her score (0–3), but keep saying them until he or she can repeat all three, up to six trials. If he or she does not eventually learn all three, recall cannot be meaningfully tested.

Attention and Calculation

Ask the patient to begin with 100 and count backwards by 7. Stop after five subtractions (93, 86, 79, 72, 65). Score the total number of correct answers.

If the patient cannot or will not perform this task, ask him or her to spell the word "world" backwards. The score is the number of letters in correct order, e.g., dlrow = 5, dlorw = 3.

Recall

Ask the patient if he or she can recall the three words you previously asked him or her to remember. Score 0–3.

Language

Naming: Show the patient a wristwatch and ask him or her what it is. Repeat for pencil. Score 0–2.

Repetition: Ask the patient to repeat the sentence after you. Allow only one trial. Score 0 or 1.

Three-stage command: Give the patient a piece of plain blank paper and repeat the command. Score 1 point for each part correctly executed.

Reading: On a blank piece of paper print the sentence "Close your eyes," in letters large enough for the patient to see clearly. Ask him or her to read it and do what it says. Score 1 point only if he or she actually closes his or her eyes.

Writing: Give the patient a blank piece of paper and ask him or her to write a sentence for you. Do not dictate a sentence, it is to be written spontaneously. It must contain a subject and verb and be sensible. Correct grammar and punctuation are not necessary.

Copying: On a clean piece of paper, draw intersecting pentagons, each side about 1 inch, and ask him or her to copy it exactly as it is. All 10 angles must be present, and 2 must intersect to score 1 point. Tremor and rotation are ignored.

Estimate the patient's level of sensorium along a continuum, from alert on the left to coma on the right.

From Folstein M. F., Folstein S. E., McHugh P. R. (1975). Mini-mental state. *Journal of Psychiatric Research, 12,* 189–198. Reprinted with permission. ©1975, 1998 Mini-Mental LLC.

MINIMUM DATA SET

Numeric Identifier_____

MINIMUM DATA SET (MDS) – VERSION 2.0
FOR NURSING HOME RESIDENT ASSESSMENT AND CARE SCREENING
BASIC ASSESSMENT TRACKING FORM

SECTION AA. IDENTIFICATION INFORMATION

1. RESIDENT NAME ✱ — (Exactly as appears on Medicare Card)
a. (First)   b. (Middle Initial)   c. (Last)   d. (Jr./Sr.)

2. GENDER ✱
1. Male   2. Female

3. BIRTHDATE ✱ — *(Complete all four digits)*
Month   Day   Year

4. RACE/ ETHNICITY
1. American Indian/Alaskan Native   4. Hispanic
2. Asian/Pacific Islander   5. White, not of
3. Black, not of Hispanic origin   Hispanic origin

5. SOCIAL ✱ SECURITY AND ✱ MEDICARE NUMBERS [C in 1st box if non Med. no.]
a. Social Security Number

b. Medicare number (or comparable railroad insurance number)

6. FACILITY PROVIDER NO. ✱
a. State No.   *(Facility Medicaid Provider number)*

(Facility Medicare Provider number)

b. Federal No.

7. MEDICAID NO. ["+" if pending, "N" if not a Medicaid ✱ recipient]
(Resident Medicaid number)

8. REASONS FOR ASSESSMENT
Use 8a if NOT Medicare covered, leave 8b blank. Use 8a & b if Medicare covered.

[Note–Other codes do not apply to this form]
a. Primary reason for assessment ☐
   1. Admission assessment (required by day 14)-may be ◆
   2. Annual assessment
   3. Significant change in status assessment-may be ◆
   4. Significant correction of prior full assessment-may be ◆
   5. Quarterly review assessment
   10. Significant correction of prior quarterly assessment
   0. NONE OF ABOVE

b. Codes for assessments required for Medicare PPS or the State
   1. Medicare 5 day assessment
   2. Medicare 30 day assessment
   3. Medicare 60 day assessment
   4. Medicare 90 day assessment
   5. Medicare readmission/return assessment
   6. Other state required assessment
   7. Medicare 14 day assessment
   8. Other Medicare required assessment

For MDS section AA8 use the following schedule for newly admitted and re-admitted residents expected to be covered by Medicare during the first 30 days.

Day 0 = Period prior to admission.
Day 1 = Resident admission day.
Day 1-8 = Reference date for the **Medicare** 5 day assessment (3 grace days available.
Day 11-19 = Reference date for the **Medicare** 14 day assessment (no grace days available if designated as initial admission assessment

✱ = Key items for computerized resident tracking
☐ = When box blank, must enter number or letter
a. = When letter in box, check if condition applies
Code "–" if information unavailable or unknown

◆ = Quality Indicator*
■ = Medicare covered care
☐ = Medicare noncovered care

QI LEGEND
❶ Incidence new fractures
❷ Prevalence of falls
❸ Prevalence of behavioral symptoms affecting others
❹ Prevalence of symptoms of depression
❺ Prevalence of depression w/o antidepressants
❻ 9+ medications

❼ Incidence of cognitive impairment
❽ Prevalence of bladder or bowel incontinence
❾ Prevalence of occasional bladder or bowel incontinence w/o plan
❿ Prevalence of indwelling catheter
⓫ Prevalence of fecal impaction*
⓬ Prevalence of UTI

⓭ Prevalence of weight loss
⓮ Prevalence of tube feeding
⓯ Prevalence of dehydration*
⓰ Prevalence of bedfast residents
⓱ Incidence of decline in late loss ADLs
⓲ Incidence of decline in ROM
⓳ Prevalence of antipsychotic use in absence of psychotic conditions

⓴ Prevalence of antianxiety/hypnotic use
㉑ Prevalence of hypnotic use > 2x/wk
㉒ Prevalence of daily restraints
㉓ Prevalence of little or no activity
㉔ Prevalence of stage 1-4 pressure ulcers*

*SENTINEL HEALTH EVENT

9. Signatures of Persons who Completed a Portion of the Accompanying Assessment or Tracking Form

I certify that the accompanying information accurately reflects resident assessment or tracking information for this resident and that I collected or coordinated collection of this information on the dates specified. To the best of my knowledge, this information was collected in accordance with applicable Medicare and Medicaid requirements. I understand that this information is used as a basis for ensuring that residents receive appropriate and quality care, and as a basis for payment from federal funds. I further understand that payment of such federal funds and continued participation in the government-funded health care programs is conditioned on the accuracy and truthfulness of this information, and that I may be personally subject to or may subject my organization to substantial criminal, civil, and/or administrative penalties for submitting false information. I also certify that I am authorized to submit this information by this facility on its behalf.

Signature and Title	Sections	Date
a.		
b.		
c.		
d.		
e.		
f.		
g.		
h.		
i.		
j.		
k.		
l.		

GENERAL INSTRUCTIONS

Complete this information for submission with all full and quarterly assessments (Admission, Annual, Significant Change, State or Medicare required assessments, or Quarterly Reviews, etc.).

MDS RUG III CASE MIX GROUPS

RU = Rehabilitation Ultra High   **CC**
RV = Rehabilitation Very High   **CB** = Clinically Complex
RH = Rehabilitation High   **CA**
RM = Rehabilitation Medium
RL = Rehabilitation Low
SE = Extensive Services
SS = Special Care

THESE GROUPS ARE CONSIDERED SKILLED CARE COVERED BY MEDICARE FOR ELIGIBLE RESIDENTS.

TRIGGER LEGEND
1 - Delirium
2 - Cognitive Loss/Dementia
3 - Visual Function
4 - Communication
5A - ADL-Rehabilitation
5B - ADL-Maintenance
6 - Urinary Incontinence and Indwelling Catheter
7 - Psychosocial Well-Being
8 - Mood State
9 - Behavioral Symptoms

10A - Activities (Revise)
10B - Activities (Review)
11 - Falls
12 - Nutritional Status
13 - Feeding Tubes
14 - Dehydration/Fluid Maintenance
15 - Dental Care
16 - Pressure Ulcers
17 - Psychotropic Drug Use
17* - For this to trigger, O4a, b, or c must = 1-7
18 - Physical Restraints

For additional information on MDS required schedule and documentation to justify skilled care, see page 8.

Form 1728EHH © 1997 Briggs Corporation, Des Moines, IA 50306 (800) 247-2343 PRINTED IN U.S.A.
R700 Copyright limited to addition of trigger, coding and QI recognition systems

Resident _____ Numeric Identifier_____

MINIMUM DATA SET (MDS) – *VERSION 2.0*
FOR NURSING HOME RESIDENT ASSESSMENT AND CARE SCREENING
BACKGROUND (FACE SHEET) INFORMATION AT ADMISSION

SECTION AB. DEMOGRAPHIC INFORMATION

1.	DATE OF ENTRY	Date the stay began. Note – Does not include readmission if record was closed at time of temporary discharge to hospital, etc. In such cases, use prior admission date. **Do NOT change this date on readmission** Month — Day — Year
2.	ADMITTED FROM (AT ENTRY)	1. Private home/apt. with no home health services 2. Private home/apt. with home health services 3. Board and care/assisted living/group home 4. Nursing home 5. Acute care hospital *(Not SNF unit of acute care hospital)* 6. Psychiatric hospital, MR/DD facility 7. Rehabilitation hospital 8. Other
3.	LIVED ALONE (PRIOR TO ENTRY)	0. No 1. Yes 2. In other facility
4.	ZIP CODE OF PRIOR PRIMARY RESIDENCE	
5.	RESIDENTIAL HISTORY 5 YEARS PRIOR TO ENTRY	*(Check all settings resident **lived in** during 5 years prior to date of entry given in item AB1 above.)* Prior stay at this nursing home — a. Stay in other nursing home — b. Other residential facility – board and care home, assisted living, group home — c. MH/psychiatric setting — d. MR/DD setting — e. *NONE OF ABOVE* — f.
6.	LIFETIME OCCUPATION(S) (Put "/" between two occupations)	
7.	EDUCATION (Highest level completed)	1. No schooling 5. Technical or trade school 2. 8th grade/less 6. Some college 3. 9-11 grades 7. Bachelor's degree 4. High school 8. Graduate degree
8.	LANGUAGE	*(Code for correct response)* **a.** Primary Language 0. English 1. Spanish 2. French 3. Other **b.** If other, specify
9.	MENTAL HEALTH HISTORY	Does resident's RECORD indicate any history of mental retardation, mental illness, or developmental disability problem? 0. No 1. Yes
10.	CONDITIONS RELATED TO MR/DD STATUS	*(Check all conditions that are related to MR/DD status that were manifested before age 22, and are likely to continue indefinitely)* Not applicable – no MR/DD (Skip to AB11) — a. MR/DD with organic condition Down's syndrome — b. Autism — c. Epilepsy — d. Other organic condition related to MR/DD — e. MR/DD with no organic condition — f.
11.	DATE BACKGROUND INFORMATION COMPLETED	*(This date must NOT be earlier than date of entry)* Month — Day — Year

SECTION AC. CUSTOMARY ROUTINE

1.	CUSTOMARY ROUTINE *(In year prior to DATE OF ENTRY to this nursing home, or year last in community if now being admitted from another nursing home)* **Review for possible care plan approaches**	*(Check all that apply. If all information UNKNOWN, check last box only.)*
		CYCLE OF DAILY EVENTS
		Stays up late at night (e.g., after 9 pm) — a.
		Naps regularly during day (at least 1 hour) — b.
		Goes out 1+ days a week — c.
		Stays busy with hobbies, reading, or fixed daily routine — d.
		Spends most of time alone or watching TV — e.
		Moves independently indoors (with appliances, if used) — f.
		Use of tobacco products at least daily — g.
		NONE OF ABOVE — h.
		EATING PATTERNS
		Distinct food preferences — i.
		Eats between meals all or most days — j.
		Use of alcoholic beverage(s) at least weekly — k.
		NONE OF ABOVE — l.
		ADL PATTERNS
		In bedclothes much of day — m.
		Wakens to toilet all or most nights — n.
		Has irregular bowel movement pattern — o.
		Showers for bathing — p.
		Bathing in PM — q.
		NONE OF ABOVE — r.
		INVOLVEMENT PATTERNS
		Daily contact with relatives/close friends — s.
		Usually attends church, temple, synagogue (etc.) — t.
		Finds strength in faith — u.
		Daily animal companion/presence — v.
		Involved in group activities — w.
		NONE OF ABOVE — x.
		UNKNOWN – Resident/family unable to provide information — y.

END

SECTION AD. FACE SHEET SIGNATURES

SIGNATURES OF PERSONS COMPLETING FACE SHEET:

a. Signature of RN Assessment Coordinator   Date

I certify that the accompanying information accurately reflects resident assessment or tracking information for this resident and that I collected or coordinated collection of this information on the dates specified. To the best of my knowledge, this information was collected in accordance with applicable Medicare and Medicaid requirements. I understand that this information is used as a basis for ensuring that residents receive appropriate and quality care, and as a basis for payment from federal funds. I further understand that payment of such federal funds and continued participation in the government-funded health care programs is conditioned on the accuracy and truthfulness of this information, and that I may be personally subject to or may subject my organization to substantial criminal, civil, and/or administrative penalties for submitting false information. I also certify that I am authorized to submit this information by this facility on its behalf.

Signature and Title	Sections	Date
b.		
c.		
d.		
e.		
f.		
g.		

▨ = When box blank, must enter number or letter

a. = When letter in box, check if condition applies

Code "–" if information unavailable or unknown

NOTE: Normally, the MDS Face Sheet is completed once, when an individual first enters the facility. However, the face sheet is also required if the person is readmitted to the facility after a discharge where return had not previously been expected. It is not completed following temporary discharges to hospitals or after therapeutic leaves/home visits.

Resident _____ Numeric Identifier _____

MINIMUM DATA SET (MDS) – *VERSION 2.0*
FOR NURSING HOME RESIDENT ASSESSMENT AND CARE SCREENING
FULL ASSESSMENT FORM
(Status in last 7 days, unless other time frame indicated)

SECTION A. IDENTIFICATION AND BACKGROUND INFORMATION

1. RESIDENT NAME (Exactly as appears on Medicare Card)

a. (First)　　b. (Middle Initial)　　c. (Last)　　d. (Jr./Sr.)

2. ROOM NUMBER

3. ASSESSMENT REFERENCE DATE
a. *Last day of MDS observation period*

Month — Day — Year

b. Original (0) or corrected copy of form (enter number of correction)

4a. DATE OF REENTRY Date of reentry from most recent temporary discharge to a hospital in last 90 days (or since last assessment or admission if less than 90 days)

Month — Day — Year

5. MARITAL STATUS
1. Never married　3. Widowed　5. Divorced
2. Married　4. Separated

6. MEDICAL RECORD NO.

7. CURRENT PAYMENT SOURCES FOR N.H. STAY
(Billing Office to indicate; check all that apply in last 30 days)

Medicaid per diem	a.	VA per diem	f.
Medicare per diem	b.	Self or family pays for full per diem	g.
Medicare ancillary part A	c.	Medicaid resident liability or Medicare co-payment	h.
Medicare ancillary part B	d.	Private insurance per diem (including co-payment)	i.
CHAMPUS per diem	e.	Other per diem	j.

8. REASONS FOR ASSESSMENT

[Note–If this is a discharge or reentry assessment, only a limited subset of MDS items need be completed]

See Section AA8 for explanation

a. Primary reason for assessment ⬚
1. Admission assessment (required by day 14)-may be ▉
2. Annual assessment
3. Significant change in status assessment-may be ▉
4. Significant correction of prior full assessment-may be ➤
5. Quarterly review assessment
6. Discharged–return not anticipated
7. Discharged–return anticipated
8. Discharged prior to completing initial assessment
9. Reentry
10. Significant correction of prior quarterly assessment
0. NONE OF ABOVE

b. *Codes for assessments required for Medicare PPS or the State* ▉
1. Medicare 5 day assessment
2. Medicare 30 day assessment
3. Medicare 60 day assessment
4. Medicare 90 day assessment
5. Medicare readmission/return assessment
6. Other state required assessment
7. Medicare 14 day assessment
8. Other Medicare required assessment

9. RESPONSIBILITY/ LEGAL GUARDIAN
(Check all that apply)

Legal guardian	a.	Durable power of attorney/ financial	d.
Other legal oversight	b.	Family member responsible	e.
Durable power of attorney/health care	c.	Patient responsible for self	f.
		NONE OF ABOVE	g.

10. ADVANCED DIRECTIVES
(For those items with supporting documentation in the medical record, check all that apply)

Living will	a.	Feeding restrictions	f.
Do not resuscitate	b.	Medication restrictions	g.
Do not hospitalize	c.	Other treatment restrictions	h.
Organ donation	d.	NONE OF ABOVE	i.
Autopsy request	e.		

SECTION B. COGNITIVE PATTERNS

1. COMATOSE (Persistent vegetative state/no discernible consciousness)

1 = ⬚CC　0. No ◆Q4.5　1. Yes (If yes, skip to Section G)

2. MEMORY (Recall of what was learned or known)

a1 = ⬚ IB / IA
a. Short-term memory OK–seems/appears to recall after 5 minutes
0. Memory OK　1. Memory problem 2

a1 = ◆Q7
b. Long-term memory OK–seems/appears to recall long past
0. Memory OK　1. Memory problem 2

---

3. MEMORY/ RECALL ABILITY (Check all that resident was **normally able to recall during** last 7 days)

Current season	a.	That he/she is in a nursing home	d.
Location of own room	b.	NONE OF ABOVE are recalled	e.
Staff names/faces	c.		

4. COGNITIVE SKILLS FOR DAILY DECISION-MAKING
(Made decisions regarding tasks of daily life)　1,2,3= ◆Q7
0. INDEPENDENT–decisions consistent/reasonable
1. MODIFIED INDEPENDENCE–some difficulty in new situations only 2
2. MODERATELY IMPAIRED–decisions poor; cues/ supervision required 2
3. SEVERELY IMPAIRED–never/rarely made decisions 2, 5B

2,3= ⬚ IB / IA

5. INDICATORS OF DELIRIUM– PERIODIC DISORDERED THINKING/ AWARENESS
(Code for behavior in the **last 7 days**.) [Note: Accurate assessment requires conversations with staff and family who have direct knowledge of resident's behavior over this time.]
0. Behavior not present
1. Behavior present, not of recent onset
2. Behavior present, over last 7 days appears different from resident's usual functioning (e.g., new onset or worsening)

a. EASILY DISTRACTED–(e.g., difficulty paying attention; gets sidetracked) 2 = **1, 17***

b. PERIODS OF ALTERED PERCEPTION OR AWARENESS OF SURROUNDINGS–(e.g., moves lips or talks to someone not present; believes he/she is somewhere else; confuses night and day) 2 = **1, 17***

c. EPISODES OF DISORGANIZED SPEECH–(e.g., speech is incoherent, nonsensical, irrelevant, or rambling from subject to subject; loses train of thought) 2 = **1, 17***

d. PERIODS OF RESTLESSNESS–(e.g., fidgeting or picking at skin, clothing, napkins, etc.; frequent position changes; repetitive physical movements or calling out) 2 = **1, 17***

e. PERIODS OF LETHARGY–(e.g., sluggishness; staring into space; difficult to arouse; little body movement) 2 = **1, 17***

f. MENTAL FUNCTION VARIES OVER THE COURSE OF THE DAY–(e.g., sometimes better, sometimes worse; behaviors sometimes present, sometimes not) 2 = **1, 17***

6. CHANGE IN COGNITIVE STATUS Resident's cognitive status, skills, or abilities have changed as compared to status of 90 days ago (or since assessment if less than 90 days)
0. No change　1. Improved　2. Deteriorated **1, 17***

SECTION C. COMMUNICATION/HEARING PATTERNS

1. HEARING (With hearing appliance, if used)
0. HEARS ADEQUATELY–normal talk, TV, phone
1. MINIMAL DIFFICULTY when not in quiet setting 4
2. HEARS IN SPECIAL SITUATIONS ONLY–speaker
3. has to adjust tonal quality and speak distinctly 4
4. HIGHLY IMPAIRED/absence of useful hearing 4

2. COMMUNICATION DEVICES/ TECHNIQUES
(Check all that apply during last 7 days)

Hearing aid, present and used	a.
Hearing aid, present and not used regularly	b.
Other receptive comm. techniques used (e.g., lip reading)	c.
NONE OF ABOVE	d.

3. MODES OF EXPRESSION (Check all used by resident to make needs known)

Speech	a.	Signs/gestures/sounds	d.
Writing messages to express or clarify needs	b.	Communication board	e.
American sign language or Braille	c.	Other	f.
		NONE OF ABOVE	g.

4. MAKING SELF UNDERSTOOD
(Expressing information content–however able)
0. UNDERSTOOD
1. USUALLY UNDERSTOOD–difficulty finding words or finishing thoughts 4
2. SOMETIMES UNDERSTOOD–ability is limited to making concrete requests 4
3. RARELY/NEVER UNDERSTOOD 4

2,3= ⬚ IB / IA

5. SPEECH CLARITY (Code for speech in the last 7 days)
0. CLEAR SPEECH–distinct, intelligible words
1. UNCLEAR SPEECH–slurred, mumbled words
2. NO SPEECH–absence of spoken words

6. ABILITY TO UNDERSTAND OTHERS
(Understanding verbal information content–however able)
0. UNDERSTANDS
1. USUALLY UNDERSTANDS–may miss some part/ intent of message 2, 4
2. SOMETIMES UNDERSTANDS–responds adequately to simple, direct communication 2, 4
3. RARELY/NEVER UNDERSTANDS 2, 4

7. CHANGE IN COMMUNICATION/ HEARING Resident's ability to express, understand, or hear information has changed as compared to status of 90 days ago (or since last assessment if less than 90 days)
0. No change　1. Improved　2. Deteriorated 17***

TRIGGER LEGEND
1 - Delirium
2 - Cognitive Loss/Dementia
4 - Communication
5B - ADL Maintenance
17* - Psychotropic Drugs
(For this to trigger, O4a, b, or c must = 1-7)

◆ = Quality Indicator*

▉ = When box blank, must enter number or letter.
a. = When letter in box, check if condition applies
▉ = Medicare covered care
⬚ = Medicare noncovered care

Code "–" if information unavailable or unknown

Resident _____   Numeric Identifier _____

SECTION D. VISION PATTERNS

1.	VISION	*(Ability to see in adequate light and with glasses if used)*
		0. ADEQUATE–sees fine detail, including regular print in newspapers/books
		1. IMPAIRED–sees large print, but not regular print in news-papers/books **3**
		2. MODERATELY IMPAIRED–limited vision; not able to see newspaper headlines, but can identify objects **3**
		3. HIGHLY IMPAIRED–object identification in question, but eyes appear to follow objects **3**
		4. SEVERELY IMPAIRED–no vision or sees only light, colors, or shapes; eyes do not appear to follow objects

2.	VISUAL LIMITATIONS/ DIFFICULTIES	Side vision problems–decreased peripheral vision (e.g., leaves food on one side of tray, difficulty traveling, bumps into people and objects, misjudges placement of chair when seating self) **3**	a.
		Experiences any of following: sees halos or rings around lights; sees flashes of light; sees "curtains" over eyes	b.
		NONE OF ABOVE	c.

3.	VISUAL APPLIANCES	Glasses; contact lenses; magnifying glass	
		0. No 1. Yes	

SECTION E. MOOD AND BEHAVIOR PATTERNS

1.	INDICATORS OF DEPRES-SION, ANXIETY, SAD MOOD	*(Code for indicators observed in last 30 days, irrespective of the assumed cause)*
		0. Indicator not exhibited in last 30 days
		1. Indicator of this type exhibited up to five days a week
		2. Indicator of this type exhibited daily or almost daily (6, 7 days a week)

Any 2 coded 1 or 2 = **BB**

VERBAL EXPRESSIONS OF DISTRESS
a. Resident made negative statements–e.g., "Nothing matters; Would rather be dead; What's the use; Regrets having lived so long; Let me die" 1 or 2 = **8** **Q4,5**
b. Repetitive questions– e.g., "Where do I go; What do I do?" 1 or 2 = **8**
c. Repetitive verbal-izations– e.g., calling out for help ("God help me") **1** or 2 = **8**
d. Persistent anger with self or others–e.g., easily annoyed, anger at placement in nursing home; anger at care received 1 or 2 = **8**
e. Self deprecation–e.g., "I am nothing; I am of no use to anyone" 1 or 2 = **8**
f. Expressions of what appear to be unreal-istic fears–e.g., fear of being abandoned, left alone, being with others 1 or 2 = **8**
g. Recurrent statements that something terrible is about to happen– e.g., believes he or she is about to die, have a heart attack **Q4,5**

h. Repetitive health com-plaints–e.g., persistently seeks medical attention, obsessive concern with body functions 1 or 2 = **8**
i. Repetitive anxious com-plaints/concerns (non-health related) e.g., per-sistently seeks attention/ reassurance regarding schedules, meals, laundry/ clothing, relationship 1 or 2 = **8**

SLEEP-CYCLE ISSUES
j. Unpleasant mood in morning 1 or 2 = **8** **Q4,5**
k. Insomnia/change in usual sleep pattern 1 or 2 = **8**

SAD, APATHETIC, ANXIOUS APPEARANCE
l. Sad, pained, worried facial expressions– e.g., furrowed brows 1 or 2 = **8**
m. Crying, tearfulness 1 or 2 = **8**
n. Repetitive physical move-ments–e.g., pacing, hand wringing, restlessness, fidgeting, picking 1 or 2 = **8, 17*** **Q4,5**

LOSS OF INTEREST
o. Withdrawal from activities of interest–e.g., no interest in longstanding activities or being with family/friends 1 or 2 = **7, 8** **Q4,5**
p. Reduced social interaction 1 or 2 = **8** **Q4,5**

2.	MOOD PERSIS-TENCE	One or more indicators of depressed, sad or anxious mood were not easily altered by attempts to "cheer up", console, or reassure the resident over last 7 days 1,2 = **Q4,5**
		0. No mood 1. Indicators present, 2. Indicators present, indicators easily altered **8** not easily altered **8**

3.	CHANGE IN MOOD	Resident's mood status has changed as compared to status of 90 days ago (or since last assessment if less than 90 days)
		0. No change 1. Improved 2. Deteriorated **1, 17***

4.	BEHAVIORAL SYMPTOMS	*(A) Behavioral symptom frequency in last 7 days*
		0. Behavior not exhibited in last 7 days
		1. Behavior of this type occurred 1 to 3 days in last 7 days
		2. Behavior of this type occurred 4 to 6 days, but less than daily
		3. Behavior of this type occurred daily
		(B) Behavioral symptom alterability in last 7 days
		0. Behavior not present OR behavior was easily altered
		1. Behavior was not easily altered

a,b,c, 4+ coded = **BB**

E4b,c,d Box A = 1,2,3 = **Q3**

d,e = **BA**

E4e Box A = 1,2,3 = **Q4,5**

			(A)	(B)
a.	WANDERING (moved with no rational purpose, seemingly oblivious to needs or safety) A = 1, 2, or 3 = **9, 11**			
b.	VERBALLY ABUSIVE BEHAVIORAL SYMPTOMS (others were threatened, screamed at, cursed at) A = 1, 2, or 3 = **9**			
c.	PHYSICALLY ABUSIVE BEHAVIORAL SYMPTOMS (others were hit, shoved, scratched, sexually abused) A = 1, 2, or 3 = **9**			
d.	SOCIALLY INAPPROPRIATE/DISRUPTIVE BEHAVIORAL SYMPTOMS (made disruptive sounds, noisiness, screaming, self-abusive acts, sexual behavior or disrobing in public, smeared/threw food/feces, hoarding, rummaged through others' belongings) A = 1, 2, or 3 = **9**			
e.	RESISTS CARE (resisted taking medications/injections, ADL assistance, or eating) A = 1, 2, or 3 = **9**			

* ADL INDEX used to calculate all RUG III catagories except default

---

5.	CHANGE IN BEHAVIORAL SYMPTOMS	Resident's behavior status has changed as compared to **status of 90 days ago** (or since last assessment if less than 90 days)
		0. No change 1. Improved **9** 2. Deteriorated **1, 17***

SECTION F. PSYCHOSOCIAL WELL-BEING

1.	SENSE OF INITIATIVE/ INVOLVE-MENT	At ease interacting with others	a.
		At ease doing planned or structured activities	b.
		At ease doing self-initiated activities	c.
		Establishes own goals **7**	d.
		Pursues involvement in life of facility (e.g., makes/keeps friends; involved in group activities; responds positively to new activities; assists at religious services)	e.
		Accepts invitations into most group activities	f.
		NONE OF ABOVE	g.

2.	UNSETTLED RELATION-SHIPS	Covert/open conflict with or repeated criticism of staff **7**	a.
		Unhappy with roommate **7**	b.
		Unhappy with residents other than roommate **7**	c.
		Openly expresses conflict/anger with family/friends **7**	d.
		Absence of personal contact with family/friends	e.
		Recent loss of close family member/friend	f.
		Does not adjust easily to change in routines	g.
		NONE OF ABOVE	h.

3.	PAST ROLES	Strong identification with past roles and life status **7**	a.
		Expresses sadness/anger/empty feeling over lost roles/status **7**	b.
		Resident perceives that daily routine (customary routine, activities) is very different from prior pattern in the community **7**	c.
		NONE OF ABOVE	d.

SECTION G. PHYSICAL FUNCTIONING AND STRUCTURAL PROBLEMS

1.	(A) ADL SELF-PERFORMANCE–(Code for resident's PERFORMANCE OVER ALL SHIFTS during last 7 days–Not including setup)
	0. INDEPENDENT–No help or oversight–OR–Help/oversight provided only 1 or 2 times during last 7 days
	1. SUPERVISION–Oversight, encouragement or cueing provided 3 or more times during last 7 days–OR–Supervision (3 or more times) plus physical assistance provided only 1 or 2 times during last 7 days
	2. LIMITED ASSISTANCE–Resident highly involved in activity; received physical help in guided maneuvering of limbs or other nonweight bearing assistance 3 or more times–OR–More help provided only 1 or 2 times during last 7 days
	3. EXTENSIVE ASSISTANCE–While resident performed part of activity, over last 7-day period, help of following type(s) provided 3 or more times: –Weight-bearing support –Full staff performance during part (but not all) of last 7 days
	4. TOTAL DEPENDENCE–Full staff performance of activity during entire 7 days
	8. ACTIVITY DID NOT OCCUR during entire 7 days

(B) ADL SUPPORT PROVIDED–(Code for MOST SUPPORT PROVIDED OVER ALL SHIFTS during last 7 days; code regardless of resident's self-performance classification)		(A)	(B)
0. No setup or physical help from staff 3. Two+ persons physical assist		SELF-PERF	SUPPORT
1. Setup help only 8. ADL activity itself did not			
2. One person physical assist occur during entire 7 days			

a. *	BED MOBILITY **ADL INDEX**	How resident moves to and from lying position, turns side to side, and positions body while in bed **Q17** A = 1 = **5A**; A = 2, 3, or 4 = **5A, 16**; A = 8 = **16**		
b. *	TRANSFER **ADL INDEX**	How resident moves between surfaces–to/from: bed, chair, wheelchair, standing position (EXCLUDE to/from bath/toilet) **Q17** A = 1, 2, 3, or 4 = **5A**		
c.	WALK IN ROOM	How resident walks between locations in his/her room A = 1, 2, 3, or 4 = **5A**		
d.	WALK IN CORRIDOR	How resident walks in corridor on unit A = 1, 2, 3, or 4 = **5A**		
e.	LOCOMO-TION ON UNIT	How resident moves between locations in his/her room and adjacent corridor on same floor. If in wheelchair, self-sufficiency once in chair A = 1, 2, 3, or 4 = **5A**		
f.	LOCOMO-TION OFF UNIT	How resident moves to and returns from off unit locations (e.g., areas set aside for dining, activities, or treatments). If facility has only one floor, how resident moves to and from distant areas on the floor. If in wheelchair, self-sufficiency once in chair A = 1, 2, 3, or 4 = **5A**		
g.	DRESSING	How resident puts on, fastens, and takes off all items of street clothing, including donning/removing prosthesis A = 1, 2, 3, or 4 = **5A**		
h. *	EATING **ADL INDEX**	How resident eats and drinks (regardless of skill). Includes intake of nourishment by other means (e.g., tube feeding, total parenteral nutrition) **Q17** A = 1, 2, 3, or 4 = **5A**		
i. *	TOILET USE **ADL INDEX**	How resident uses the toilet room (or commode, bedpan, urinal); transfers on/off toilet, cleanses, changes pad, manages ostomy or catheter, adjusts clothes **Q17** A = 1, 2, 3, or 4 = **5A**		
j.	PERSONAL HYGIENE	How resident maintains personal hygiene, including combing hair, brushing teeth, shaving, applying makeup, washing/ drying face, hands, and perineum (EXCLUDE baths and showers) A = 1, 2, 3, or 4 = **5A**		

Form 1728EHH   © 1997 Briggs Corporation, Des Moines, IA 50306   (800) 247-2343   PRINTED IN U.S.A.
Copyright limited to addition of trigger, coding and QI recognition systems

Resident _____

Numeric Identifier _____

2.	BATHING	How resident takes full-body bath/shower, sponge bath, and transfers in/out of tub/shower (EXCLUDE washing of back and hair). *Code for most dependent in self-performance and support.* A = 1, 2, 3 or 4 =**5A** (A) BATHING SELF-PERFORMANCE codes appear below. 0. Independent–No help provided 1. Supervision–Oversight help only 2. Physical help limited to transfer only 3. Physical help in part of bathing activity 4. Total dependence 8. Activity itself did not occur during entire 7 days *(Bathing support codes are as defined in Item 1, code B above)*	(A) (B)

3.	TEST FOR BALANCE (See training manual)	*(Code for ability during test in the last 7 days)* 0. Maintained position as required in test 1. Unsteady, but able to rebalance self without physical support 2. Partial physical support during test; or stands (sits) but does not follow directions for test 3. Not able to attempt test without physical help
		a. Balance while standing
		b. Balance while sitting–position, trunk control 1, 2, or 3 = **17***

4.	FUNCTIONAL LIMITATION IN RANGE OF MOTION (see training manual) † Loss a–f >0 but sum of a–f is <12 = ◆ Q18	*(Code for limitations during last 7 days that interfered with daily functions or placed resident at risk of injury)* **(A)** *RANGE OF MOTION* **(B)** *VOLUNTARY MOVEMENT* 0. No limitation 0. No loss 1. Limitation on one side 1. Partial loss 2. Limitation on both sides 2. Full loss	(A) (B)
		a. Neck	
		b. Arm–Including shoulder or elbow	
		c. Hand–Including wrist or fingers	
		d. Leg–Including hip or knee	
		e. Foot–Including ankle or toes	
		f. Other limitation or loss	

5.	MODES OF LOCOMOTION	*(Check all that apply during last 7 days)*
		Cane/walker/crutch	a.	Wheelchair primary mode of locomotion	d.
		Wheeled self	b.		
		Other person wheeled	c.	NONE OF ABOVE	e.

6.	MODES OF TRANSFER a = ◆ Q16 Transfer included in ADL Index	*(Check all that apply during last 7 days)*
		Bedfast all or most of time **16**	a.	Lifted mechanically	d.
		Bed rails used for bed mobility or transfer	b.	Transfer aid (e.g., slide board, trapeze, cane, walker, brace)	e.
		Lifted manually	c.	NONE OF ABOVE	f.

7.	TASK SEGMEN-TATION	Some or all of ADL activities were broken into subtasks during **last 7 days** so that resident could perform them 0. No 1. Yes

8.	ADL FUNCTIONAL REHABILITA-TION POTENTIAL	Resident believes he/she is capable of increased independence in at least some ADLs **5A**	a.
		Direct care staff believe resident is capable of increased independence in at least some ADLs **5A**	b.
		Resident able to perform tasks/activity but is very slow	c.
		Difference in ADL Self-Performance or ADL Support, comparing mornings to evenings	d.
		NONE OF ABOVE	

9.	CHANGE IN ADL FUNCTION	Resident's ADL self-performance status has changed as compared to status of **90 days ago** (or since last assessment if less than 90 days) 0. No change 1. Improved 2. Deteriorated

SECTION H. CONTINENCE IN LAST 14 DAYS

1.	CONTINENCE SELF-CONTROL CATEGORIES *(Code for resident's PERFORMANCE OVER ALL SHIFTS)* 0. *CONTINENT*–Complete control *(includes use of indwelling urinary catheter or ostomy device that does not leak urine or stool)* 1. *USUALLY CONTINENT*–BLADDER, incontinent episodes once a week or less; BOWEL, less than weekly 2. *OCCASIONALLY INCONTINENT*–BLADDER, 2 or more times a week but not daily; BOWEL, once a week 3. *FREQUENTLY INCONTINENT*–BLADDER, tended to be incontinent daily, but some control present (e.g., on day shift); BOWEL, 2-3 times a week 4. *INCONTINENT*–Had inadequate control. BLADDER, multiple daily episodes; BOWEL, all (or almost all) of the time

a.	BOWEL CONTI-NENCE	Control of bowel movement, with appliance or bowel continence programs, if employed 1, 2, 3 or 4 = **16** 3,4 = ◆ Q8 2,3 = ◆ Q9
b.	BLADDER CONTI-NENCE	Control of urinary bladder function (if dribbles, volume insufficient to soak through underpants), with appliances (e.g., foley) or continence programs, if employed 2, 3 or 4 = **6** 3,4 = ◆ Q8 2,3 = ◆ Q9

2.	BOWEL ELIMIN-ATION PATTERN	Bowel elimination pattern regular–at least one movement every three days	a.	Diarrhea	c.
				Fecal impaction **17*** ◆ Q11	d.
		Constipation **17***	b.	NONE OF ABOVE	e.

3.	APPLIANCES AND PROGRAMS a,b not √ d = ◆ Q8 ★	Any scheduled toileting plan	a.	Did not use toilet room/ commode/urinal	f.
		Bladder retraining program	b.	Pads/briefs used **6**	g.
		External (condom) catheter **6**	c.	Enemas/irrigation	h.
		Indwelling catheter **6** ◆ Q10	d.	Ostomy present	i.
		Intermittent catheter **6**	e.	NONE OF ABOVE	j.

4.	CHANGE IN URINARY CONTI-NENCE	Resident's urinary continence has changed as compared to status of **90 days ago** (or since last assessment if less than 90 days) 0. No change 1. Improved 2. Deteriorated

★ H3 a & b included in Nursing Rehab calculation

SECTION I. DISEASE DIAGNOSES

Check only **those diseases that have a relationship** to current ADL status, cognitive status, mood and behavior status, medical treatments, nursing monitoring, or risk of death. (Do not list inactive diagnoses)

1.	DISEASES *Insulin →* 14 days & 2 order changes = **CC**	*(If none apply, CHECK the NONE OF ABOVE box)*				
		ENDOCRINE/METABOLIC/ NUTRITIONAL		Hemiplegia/Hemiparesis **CC**	v.
		Diabetes mellitus	a.	Multiple sclerosis **SS**	w.
		Hyperthyroidism	b.	Paraplegia	x.
		Hypothyroidism	c.	Parkinson's disease	y.
		HEART/CIRCULATION		Quadriplegia **SS**	z.
		Arteriosclerotic heart disease (ASHD)	d.	Seizure disorder	aa.
		Cardiac dysrhythmias	e.	Transient ischemic attack (TIA)	bb.
		Congestive heart failure	f.	Traumatic brain injury	cc.
		Deep vein thrombosis	g.	**PSYCHIATRIC/MOOD**	
		Hypertension	h.	Anxiety disorder	dd.
		Hypotension **17***	i.	Depression **17*** affects CC, C8, CA codes	ee.
		Peripheral vascular disease **16**	j.	Manic depression (bipolar disease)	ff.
		Other cardiovascular disease	k.	Schizophrenia	gg.
		MUSCULOSKELETAL		**PULMONARY**	
		Arthritis	l.	Asthma	hh.
		Hip fracture	m.	Emphysema/COPD	ii.
		Missing limb (e.g., amputation)	n.	**SENSORY**	
		Osteoporosis	o.	Cataracts **3**	jj.
		Pathological bone fracture	p.	Diabetic retinopathy	kk.
		NEUROLOGICAL		Glaucoma **3**	ll.
		Alzheimer's disease	q.	Macular degeneration	mm.
		Aphasia **SS**	r.	**OTHER**	
		Cerebral palsy **SS**	s.	Allergies	nn.
		Cerebrovascular accident (stroke)	t.	Anemia	oo.
		Dementia other than Alzheimer's disease	u.	Cancer	pp.
				Renal failure	qq.
				NONE OF ABOVE	rr.

2.	INFECTIONS W/Fever →	*(If none apply, CHECK the NONE OF ABOVE box)*				
		Antibiotic resistant infection (e.g., Methicillin resistant staph)	a.	Septicemia **CC**	g.
		Clostridium difficile (c. diff.)	b.	Sexually transmitted diseases	h.
		Conjunctivitis	c.	Tuberculosis	i.
		HIV infection	d.	Urinary tract infection in last 30 days **14** ◆ Q12	j.
		Pneumonia **CC**	e.	Viral hepatitis	k.
		Respiratory infection	f.	Wound infection	l.
				NONE OF ABOVE	m.

3.	OTHER CURRENT OR MORE DETAILED DIAGNOSES AND ICD-9 CODES	Dehydration 276.5 = **14** ◆ Q15 Fever & dehydration = **SS**
		a. _____ •
		b. _____ •
		c. _____ •
		d. _____ •
		e. _____ •

SECTION J. HEALTH CONDITIONS

1.	PROBLEM CONDITIONS W/Fever → **SS** W/Fever → **SS**	*(Check all problems present in last 7 days unless other time frame is indicated)*				
		INDICATORS OF FLUID STATUS		Dizziness/Vertigo **11, 17***	f.
		Weight gain or loss of 3 or more pounds within a 7 day period **14**	a.	Edema	g.
		Inability to lie flat due to shortness of breath	b.	Fever **14** w/dehyd. **SS**	h.
				Hallucinations **17*** **BA**	i.
		Dehydrated; output exceeds input **14** ◆ Q15 **CC**	c.	Internal bleeding **14** **CC**	j.
				Recurrent lung aspirations in **last 90 days 17***	k.
		Insufficient fluid; did **NOT** consume all/almost all liquids provided during **last 3 days 14**	d.	Shortness of breath	l.
				Syncope (fainting) **17***	m.
		OTHER		Unsteady gait **17***	n.
		Delusions **BA**	e.	Vomiting w/wt. loss & fever **17***	o.
				NONE OF ABOVE **SS**	p.

Form 1728EHH   © 1997 Briggs Corporation, Des Moines, IA 50306   (800) 247-2343   PRINTED IN U.S.A.
 Copyright limited to addition of trigger, coding and QI recognition systems

Resident _____   Numeric Identifier _____

2.	PAIN SYMPTOMS	(Code the *highest level of pain* present in **the last 7 days**)
		a. FREQUENCY with which resident complains or shows evidence of pain **0.** No pain *(skip to J4)* **1.** Pain less than daily **2.** Pain daily	**b. INTENSITY** of pain **1.** Mild pain **2.** Moderate pain **3.** Times when pain is horrible or excruciating

3.	PAIN SITE	(If pain present, **check all sites** that apply in **last 7 days**)			
		Back pain	a.	Incisional pain	f.
		Bone pain	b.	Joint pain (other than hip)	g.
		Chest pain while doing usual activities	c.	Soft tissue pain (e.g., lesion, muscle)	h.
		Headache	d.	Stomach pain	i.
		Hip pain	e.	Other	j.

4.	ACCIDENTS a = ◀ Q2 ▶ c,d = ◀ Q1 ▶	(Check all that apply)		Hip fracture in **last 180 days 17***	c.
		Fell in past 30 days **11, 17***	a.	Other fracture in last 180 days	d.
		Fell in past 31-180 days **11, 17***	b.	*NONE OF ABOVE*	e.

5.	STABILITY OF CONDITIONS	Conditions make resident's cognitive, ADL, mood or behavior patterns unstable–(fluctuating, precarious, or deteriorating)	a.
		Resident experiencing an acute episode or a flare-up of a recurrent or chronic problem	b.
		End-stage disease, 6 or fewer months to live	c.
		NONE OF ABOVE	d.

SECTION K. ORAL/NUTRITIONAL STATUS

1.	ORAL PROBLEMS	Chewing problem	a.
		Swallowing problem **17***	b.
		Mouth pain **15**	c.
		NONE OF ABOVE	d.

2.	HEIGHT AND WEIGHT	Record (a.) **height in inches** and (b.) **weight in pounds**. Base weight on most recent measure in **last 30 days**; measure weight consistently in accord with standard facility practice–e.g., in a.m. after voiding, before meal, with shoes off, and in nightclothes.		
		a. HT (in.)		**b. WT (lb.)**

3.	WEIGHT CHANGE	**a. Weight loss**–5% or more in **last 30 days**; or 10% or more in **last 180 days** **0.** No **1.** Yes **12** SS Q4 Q5 Q13	a.
		b. Weight gain–5% or more in **last 30 days**; or 10% or more in **last 180 days** **0.** No **1.** Yes	b.

4.	NUTRI-TIONAL PROBLEMS	Complains about the taste of many foods **12**	a.	Leaves 25% or more of food uneaten at most meals **12**	c.
		Regular or repetitive complaints of hunger	b.	*NONE OF ABOVE*	d.

5.	NUTRI-TIONAL APPROACH-ES *Tube Fed & Fever or Aphasia =* SS	(Check all that apply in last 7 days)			
		Parenteral/IV **12, 14** SE	a.	Dietary supplement between meals	f.
		Feeding tube **13, 14** CC Q14	b.	Plate guard, stabilized built-up utensil, etc.	g.
		Mechanically altered diet **12**	c.	On a planned weight change program	h.
		Syringe (oral feeding) **12**	d.	*NONE OF ABOVE*	i.
		Therapeutic diet **12**	e.		

6.	PARENTERAL OR ENTERAL INTAKE *If a,b=2,3,4* = SS OR CC	(Skip to Section L if neither 5a nor 5b is checked)
		a. Code the proportion of **total calories** the resident received through parenteral or tube feedings in the **last 7 days** **0.** None **3.** 51% to 75% **1.** 1% to 25% **4.** 76% to 100% **2.** 26% to 50%
		b. Code the average **fluid intake** per day by IV or tube in **last 7 days** **0.** None **3.** 1001 to 1500 cc/day **1.** 1 to 500 cc/day **4.** 1501 to 2000 cc/day **2.** 501 to 0 **5.** 2001 or more cc/day

SECTION L. ORAL/DENTAL STATUS

1.	ORAL STATUS AND DISEASE PREVEN-TION	Debris (soft, easily movable substances) present in mouth prior to going to bed at night **15**	a.
		Has dentures or removable bridge	b.
		Some/all natural teeth lost–does not have or does not use dentures (or partial plates) **15**	c.
		Broken, loose, or carious teeth **15**	d.
		Inflamed gums (gingiva); swollen or bleeding gums; oral abscesses; ulcers or rashes **15**	e.
		Daily cleaning of teeth/dentures or daily mouth care–by resident or staff Not ✓ = **15**	f.
		NONE OF ABOVE	g.

TRIGGER LEGEND
10A - Activities (Revise)
10B - Activities (Review)
11 - Falls
12 - Nutritional Status
13 - Feeding Tubes
14 - Dehydration/Fluid Maintenance
15 - Dental Care
16 - Pressure Ulcers
17* - Psychotropic Drugs
(*For this to trigger, O4a, b, or c must = 1-7)

SECTION M. SKIN CONDITION

1.	ULCERS (Due to any cause) 2+ sites any stage or any stage 3 or 4 = SS	(Record the number of ulcers at each ulcer stage–regardless of cause. If none present at a stage, record "0" (zero). Code all that apply during **last 7 days**. Code 9 = 9 or more.) [Requires full body exam.]	Number at Stage
		a. Stage 1. A persistent area of skin redness (without a break in the skin) that does not disappear when pressure is relieved.	
		b. Stage 2. A partial thickness loss of skin layers that presents clinically as an abrasion, blister, or shallow crater.	
		c. Stage 3. A full thickness of skin is lost, exposing the subcutaneous tissues–presents as a deep crater with or without undermining adjacent tissue.	
		d. Stage 4. A full thickness of skin and subcutaneous tissue is lost, exposing muscle or bone.	

2.	TYPE OF ULCER a = SS a > o = Q24	(For each type of ulcer, **code for the highest stage in the last 7 days** using scale in item M1–i.e., 0=none; stages 1, 2, 3, 4)	
		a. Pressure ulcer–any lesion caused by pressure resulting in damage of underlying tissue 1 = **16**; 2, 3, or 4 = **12, 16**	
		b. Stasis ulcer–open lesion caused by poor circulation in the lower extremities	

3.	HISTORY OF RESOLVED ULCERS	Resident had an ulcer that was resolved or cured in **LAST 90 DAYS** **0.** No **1.** Yes **16**	

4.	OTHER SKIN PROBLEMS OR LESIONS PRESENT	(Check all that apply during last 7 days)	
		Abrasions, bruises	a.
		Burns (second or third degree) CC	b.
		Open lesions other than ulcers, rashes, cuts (e.g., cancer lesions) SS	c.
		Rashes–e.g., intertrigo, eczema, drug rash, heat rash, herpes zoster	d.
		Skin desensitized to pain or pressure **16**	e.
		Skin tears or cuts (other than surgery)	f.
		Surgical wounds SS	g.
		NONE OF ABOVE	h.

5.	SKIN TREAT-MENTS a thru h = SS	(Check all that apply during last 7 days)	
		Pressure relieving device(s) for chair	a.
		Pressure relieving device(s) for bed	b.
		Turning/repositioning program	c.
		Nutrition or hydration intervention to manage skin problems	d.
		Ulcer care	e.
		Surgical wound care	f.
		Application of dressings (with or without topical medications) other than to feet	g.
		Application of ointments/medications (other than to feet)	h.
		Other preventative or protective skin care (other than to feet)	i.
		NONE OF ABOVE	j.

6.	FOOT PROBLEMS AND CARE	(Check all that apply during last 7 days)	
		Resident has one or more foot problems–e.g., corns, calluses, bunions, hammer toes, overlapping toes, pain, structural problems	a.
		Infection of the foot–e.g., cellulitis, purulent drainage CC	b.
		Open lesions on the foot CC	c.
		Nails/calluses trimmed during **last 90 days**	d.
		Received preventative or protective foot care (e.g., used special shoes, inserts, pads, toe separators)	e.
		Application of dressings (with or without topical medications) CC	f.
		NONE OF ABOVE	g.

SECTION N. ACTIVITY PURSUIT PATTERNS

1.	TIME AWAKE 10B only if BOTH N1a = ✓ and N2 = 0	(Check appropriate time periods over last 7 days) Resident awake all or most of time (i.e., naps no more than one hour per time period) in the: d = CC = Q4.5			
		Morning Q4.5 10B	a.	Evening Q4.5	c.
		Afternoon Q4.5	b.		

	(IF RESIDENT IS COMATOSE, SKIP TO SECTION O)

2.	AVERAGE TIME INVOLVED IN ACTIVITIES	(When awake and not receiving treatments or ADL care) **0.** Most–more than 2/3 of time **10B** **1.** Some–from 1/3 to 2/3 of time **2.** Little–less than 1/3 of time **10A** Q23 **3.** None **10A** Q23	

3.	PREFERRED ACTIVITY SETTINGS	(Check all settings in which activities are **preferred**)			
		Own room	a.		
		Day/activity room	b.	Outside facility	d.
		Inside NH/off unit	c.	*NONE OF ABOVE*	e.

4.	GENERAL ACTIVITY PREFER-ENCES (Adapted to resident's current abilities)	(Check all PREFERENCES whether or not activity is currently available to resident)			
		Cards/other games	a.	Trips/shopping	g.
		Crafts/arts	b.	Walking/wheeling outdoors	h.
		Exercise/sports	c.	Watching TV	i.
		Music	d.	Gardening or plants	j.
		Reading/writing	e.	Talking or conversing	k.
		Spiritual/religious activities	f.	Helping others	l.
				NONE OF ABOVE	m.

Resident _____   Numeric Identifier _____

| 5. | PREFERS CHANGE IN DAILY ROUTINE | Code for resident preferences in daily routines
0. No change **1.** Slight change **2.** Major change
a. Type of activities in which resident is currently involved 1 or 2 = **10A**
b. Extent of resident involvement in activities 1 or 2 = **10A** | |

SECTION O. MEDICATIONS

1.	NUMBER OF MEDICATIONS	*(Record the number of different medications used in the last 7 days; enter "0" if none used)* 9+ = ◆Q6	
2.	NEW MEDICATIONS	*(Resident currently receiving medications that were initiated during the last 90 days)* **0.** No **1.** Yes	
3.	INJECTIONS	*(Record the number of DAYS injections of any type received during the last 7 days; enter "0" if none used)* ▪CA	
4.	DAYS RECEIVED THE FOLLOWING MEDICATION c = Affects CC, CB, CA	*(Record the number of DAYS during last 7 days; enter "0" if not used. Note–enter "1" for long-acting meds used less than weekly)* **(NOTE:** For 17 to actually be triggered, O4a, b, or c MUST = 1–7 AND at least one additional item marked **17*** must be indicated. See sections B, C, E, G, H, I, J, and K.) **a.** Antipsychotic ≥1= ◆Q19 1-7 = **17** **b.** Antianxiety ≥1= ◆Q20 1-7 = **11, 17** **c.** Antidepressant 0 = ◆Q5 1-7 = **11, 17** **d.** Hypnotic ≥1= ◆Q20 2+= ◆Q21 **e.** Diuretic 1-7 = **14**	

SECTION P. SPECIAL TREATMENTS AND PROCEDURES

| 1. | SPECIAL TREATMENTS, PROCEDURES, AND PROGRAMS | **a. SPECIAL CARE**–Check treatments or programs received during the **last 14 days** | |

TREATMENTS

		PROGRAMS	
Chemotherapy ▪CB	a.	Alcohol/drug treatment program	m.
Dialysis ▪CB	b.	Alzheimer's/dementia special care unit	n.
IV medication ▪SE	c.	Hospice care	o.
Intake/output	d.	Pediatric unit	p.
Monitoring acute medical condition	e.	Respite care	q.
Ostomy care	f.	Training in skills required to return to the community (e.g., taking medications, house work, shopping, transportation, ADLs)	r.
Oxygen therapy ▪CC	g.		
Radiation ▪SS	h.		
Suctioning ▪SE	i.		
Tracheostomy care ▪SE	j.		
Transfusions ▪CC	k.	*NONE OF ABOVE*	s.
Ventilator or respirator ▪SE	l.		

b. THERAPIES–Record the number of days and total minutes each of the following therapies was administered (for at least 15 minutes a day) in the **last 7 calendar days** (Enter 0 if none or less than 15 min. daily) [Note–count only post admission therapies]

	DAYS	MIN
(A) = # of days administered for **15 minutes or more**	(A)	(B)
(B) = total # of minutes provided in last 7 days		
a. Speech-language pathology and audiology services		
b. Occupational therapy		
c. Physical therapy		
d. Respiratory therapy ▪SS		
e. Psychological therapy (by any licensed mental health professional)		

2.	INTERVENTION PROGRAMS FOR MOOD, BEHAVIOR, COGNITIVE LOSS	(Check all interventions or strategies used in **last 7 days**–no matter where received)	
		Special behavior symptom evaluation program	a.
		Evaluation by a licensed mental health specialist in **last 90 days**	b.
		Group therapy	c.
		Resident-specific deliberate changes in the environment to address mood/behavior patterns–e.g., providing bureau in which to rummage	d.
		Reorientation–e.g., cueing	e.
		NONE OF ABOVE	f.

| 3. | NURSING REHABILITATION/ RESTORATIVE CARE

Any 2, 6x wk = Nursing Rehab. =
**
▪RL = 2 Nsg. rehab & therapy 3 days/45 min. | *Record the NUMBER OF DAYS each of the following rehabilitation or restorative techniques or practices was provided to the resident for more than or equal to 15 minutes per day in the last 7 days (Enter 0 if none or less than 15 min. daily.)* | |

a. Range of motion (passive)		**f.** Walking	
b. Range of motion (active)		**g.** Dressing or grooming	
c. Splint or brace assistance		**h.** Eating or swallowing	
TRAINING AND SKILL PRACTICE IN:		**i.** Amputation/ prosthesis care	
d. Bed mobility		**j.** Communication	
e. Transfer		**k.** Other	

4.	DEVICES AND RESTRAINTS If c,d,e = 2 = ◆Q22	*(Use the following codes for last 7 days:)* **0.** Not used **1.** Used less than daily **2.** Used daily Bed rails **a.** –Full bed rails on all open sides of bed **b.** –Other types of side rails used (e.g., half rail, one side) **c.** Trunk restraint 1 = **11, 18**; 2 = **11, 16, 18** **d.** Limb restraint 1 or 2 = **18** **e.** Chair prevents rising 1 or 2 = **18**	
5.	HOSPITAL STAY(S)	Record number of times resident was admitted to hospital with an overnight stay in **last 90 days** (or since last assessment if less than 90 days). *(Enter 0 if no hospital admissions)*	
6.	EMERGENCY ROOM (ER) VISIT(S)	Record number of times resident visited ER without an overnight stay in **last 90 days** (or since last assessment if less than 90 days). *(Enter 0 if no ER visits)*	
7.	PHYSICIAN VISITS	In the **LAST 14 DAYS** (or since admission if less than 14 days in facility) how many days has the physician (or authorized assistant or practitioner) examined the resident? *(Enter 0 if none)* ▪CB ▪CA	
8.	PHYSICIAN ORDERS	In the **LAST 14 DAYS** (or since admission if less than 14 days in facility) how many days has the physician (or authorized assistant or practitioner) changed the resident's orders? *Do not include order renewals without change. (Enter 0 if none)* ▪CB ▪CA	
9.	ABNORMAL LAB VALUES	Has the resident had any abnormal lab values during the **last 90 days** (or since admission)? **0.** No **1.** Yes	

SECTION Q. DISCHARGE POTENTIAL AND OVERALL STATUS

| 1. | DISCHARGE POTENTIAL | **a.** Resident expresses/indicates preference to return to the community
0. No **1.** Yes
b. Resident has a support person who is positive toward discharge
0. No **1.** Yes
c. Stay projected to be of a short duration–discharge projected **within 90 days** (do not include expected discharge due to death)
0. No **2.** Within 31-90 days
1. Within 30 days **3.** Discharge status uncertain | |
| 2. | OVERALL CHANGE IN CARE NEEDS | Resident's overall self sufficiency has changed significantly as compared to status of **90 days ago** (or since last assessment if less than 90 days)
0. No change
1. Improved–receives fewer supports, needs less restrictive level of care
2. Deteriorated–receives more support | |

SECTION R. ASSESSMENT INFORMATION

1.	PARTICIPATION IN ASSESSMENT	**a.** Resident: **0.** No **1.** Yes	
		b. Family: **0.** No **1.** Yes **2.** No family	
		c. Significant other: **0.** No **1.** Yes **2.** None	

2. SIGNATURE OF PERSON COORDINATING THE ASSESSMENT:

a. Signature of RN Assessment Coordinator (sign on above line)

b. Date RN Assessment Coordinator signed as complete

completion date for full and quarterly assessments

Month	—	Day	—	Year

Must NOT be dated before A3a (Assessment reference date)

** may affect IB, IA, BB, BA, PE, PD, PC, PB, PA

◆ = Quality Indicator

Form 1728EHH   © 1997 Briggs Corporation, Des Moines, IA 50306   (800) 247-2343   PRINTED IN U.S.A.
Copyright limited to addition of trigger, coding and QI recognition systems

Resident _____

Numeric Identifier _____

SECTION T. THERAPY SUPPLEMENT FOR MEDICARE PPS		
1. **SPECIAL TREAT-MENTS AND PROCE-DURES**	**a. RECREATION THERAPY**–*Enter number of days and total minutes of recreation therapy administered* (**for at least 15 minutes a day**) *in the* **last 7 days** *(Enter 0 if none)*	

Section T is used to recognize ordered and scheduled PT, OT, ST therapy services a resident will likely receive through the fifteenth day from admission.

	DAYS (A)	MIN (B)
(A) = # of days administered for 15 minutes or more		
(B) = total # of minutes provided in last 7 days		

Skip unless this is a Medicare 5 day or Medicare readmission/return assessment.

b. ORDERED THERAPIES–*Has physician ordered any of following therapies to begin in FIRST 14 days of stay–physical therapy, occupational therapy, or speech pathology service?*

0. No   **1.** Yes

If not ordered, skip to item 2

c. Through day 15, provide an estimate of the number of days when at least 1 therapy service can be expected to have been delivered.

d. Through day 15, provide an estimate of the number of therapy minutes (across the therapies) than can be expected to be delivered.

2. **WALKING WHEN MOST SELF SUFFICIENT**	*Complete item 2 if ADL self–performance score for* **TRANSFER (G.1.b.A)** *is 0, 1, 2, or 3 AND at least one of the following are present:*

- Resident received physical therapy involving gait training (**P.1.b.c**)
- Physical therapy was ordered for the resident involving gait training (**T.1.b**)
- Resident received nursing rehabilitation for walking (**P.3.f**)
- Physical therapy involving walking has been discontinued within the past 180 days

Skip to item 3 if resident did not walk in last 7 days
FOR FOLLOWING FIVE ITEMS, BASE CODING ON THE EPISODE WHEN THE RESIDENT WALKED THE FARTHEST WITHOUT SITTING DOWN. INCLUDE WALKING DURING RE-HABILITATION SESSIONS.)

a. **Furthest distance walked** without sitting down during this episode.

  0. 150+ feet   **3.** 10-25 feet
  1. 51-149 feet   **4.** Less than 10 feet
  2. 26-50 feet

b. **Time walked** without sitting down during this episode.

  0. 1-2 minutes   **3.** 11-15 minutes
  1. 3-4 minutes   **4.** 16-30 minutes
  2. 5-10 minutes **5.** 31+ minutes

c. **Self-Performance in walking** during this episode.

  0. *INDEPENDENT*–No help or oversight
  1. *SUPERVISION*–Oversight, encouragement or cueing provided
  2. *LIMITED ASSISTANCE*–Resident highly involved in walking; received physical help in guided maneuvering of limbs or other nonweight bearing assistance
  3. *EXTENSIVE ASSISTANCE*–Resident received weight bearing assistance while walking

d. **Walking support provided** associated with this episode. (code regardless of resident's self–performance classification).

  0. No setup or physical help from staff
  1. Setup help only
  2. One person physical assist
  3. Two+ persons physical assist

e. **Parallel bars** used by resident in association with this episode.

  0. No   **1.** Yes

3. **CASE MIX GROUP**	Medicare					State					

RU = 720 minutes minimum, 2 disciplines total, 1 discipline 5x/week, 2nd 3x/week

RV = 500 minutes minimum, 1 discipline 5x/week

RH = 325 minutes minimum, 1 discipline 5x/week

RM = 150 minutes minimum, 3 days a week across 3 disciplines.

RL = Therapy 3 days a week/45 min. minimum + Nsg. rehab 6 days a week/2 activities.

In Sections P of the MDS, record the number of days and minutes of PT, OT, ST received by the resident during the observation period that ends on the Assessment Reference Date (A3a).

How time the therapist spends evaluating the resident is counted, depends on whether it is an <u>INITIAL</u> evaluation or an evaluation performed after the course of therapy has begun. The time it takes to perform an initial evaluation and developing the treatment goals and plan of care for the resident CANNOT BE COUNTED AS MINUTES OF THERAPY received by the resident (P1a, b, c). However, reevaluations that are performed once a therapy regimen is under way may be counted as minutes of therapy received. Documentation time may not be counted in P1a, b, c.

RAPS MUST BE COMPLETED WITH THE 5 OR 14 DAY ASSESSMENT, WHICHEVER IS DESIGNATED AS INITIAL ADMISSION ASSESSMENT

Day 21-34 = Last day for assessment reference date for **Medicare** 30 day assessment (RAPs not required unless significant change in status occurred).

Day 50-64 = Last day for assessment reference date for **Medicare** 60 day assessment (RAPs not required unless significant change in status occurred).

Day 80-94 = Last day for assessment reference date for **Medicare** 90 day assessment (RAPs not required unless significant change in status occurred).

Day 100 = Last possible day of **Medicare** coverage.

RETURN TO THE STATE REQUIRED OR CLINICAL MDS ASSESSMENT SCHEDULE.

DOCUMENTATION REQUIRED TO JUSTIFY SKILLED CARE

| IB |
| IA | = Impaired Cognition **(NOT AUTOMATIC MEDICARE SKILLED LEVEL OF CARE)**

| BB |
| BA | = BEHAVIOR ONLY **(NOT AUTOMATIC MEDICARE SKILLED LEVEL OF CARE)**

| PE |
| PD |
| PC | = Physical Function Reduced **(NOT AUTOMATIC MEDICARE SKILLED LEVEL OF CARE)**
| PB |
| PA |

Form 1728EHH   © 1997 Briggs Corporation, Des Moines, IA 50306   (800) 247-2343   PRINTED IN U.S.A.
Copyright limited to addition of trigger, coding and QI recognition systems

Required for Comprehensive Assessments
SECTION V. RESIDENT ASSESSMENT PROTOCOL SUMMARY   Numeric Identifier_____

Resident's Name:	Medical Record No.:

1. Check if RAP is triggered.

2. For each triggered RAP, use the RAP guidelines to identify areas needing further assessment. Document relevant assessment information regarding the resident's status.

   • Describe:
   – Nature of the condition (may include presence or lack of objective data and subjective complaints).
   – Complications and risk factors that affect your decision to proceed to care planning.
   – Factors that must be considered in developing individualized care plan interventions.
   – Need for referrals/further evaluation by appropriate health professionals.

   • Documentation should support your decision-making regarding whether to proceed with a care plan for a triggered RAP and the type(s) of care plan interventions that are appropriate for a particular resident.

   • Documentation may appear anywhere in the clinical record (e.g., progress notes, consults, flowsheets, etc.).

3. Indicate under the Location of RAP Assessment Documentation column where information related to the RAP assessment can be found.

4. For each triggered RAP, indicate whether a new care plan, care plan revision, or continuation of current care plan is necessary to address the problem(s) identified in your assessment. The Care Planning Decision column must be completed within 7 days of completing the RAI (MDS and RAPs).

A. RAP Problem Area	(a) Check if Triggered	Location and Date of RAP Assessment Documentation	(b) Care Planning Decision–check if addressed in care plan
1. DELIRIUM			
2. COGNITIVE LOSS			
3. VISUAL FUNCTION			
4. COMMUNICATION			
5. ADL FUNCTIONAL/ REHABILITATION POTENTIAL			
6. URINARY INCONTINENCE AND INDWELLING CATHETER			
7. PSYCHOSOCIAL WELL-BEING			
8. MOOD STATE			
9. BEHAVIORAL SYMPTOMS			
10. ACTIVITIES			
11. FALLS			
12. NUTRITIONAL STATUS			
13. FEEDING TUBES			
14. DEHYDRATION/FLUID MAINTENANCE			
15. ORAL/DENTAL CARE			
16. PRESSURE ULCERS			
17. PSYCHOTROPIC DRUG USE			
18. PHYSICAL RESTRAINTS			

B. _____
   1. Signature of RN Coordinator for RAP Assessment Process

2. ☐☐ – ☐☐ – ☐☐☐☐
   Month   Day   Year

_____
   3. Signature of Person Completing Care Planning Decision

4. ☐☐ – ☐☐ – ☐☐☐☐
   Month   Day   Year

STROKE RISK SCREENING

Site and address of assessment: _____ Date ___/___/___

PART I. DEMOGRAPHICS

Name (last) _____ (first) _____ (middle initial) _____

Gender: __ Male __ Female   Highest Level of Education: __ High School or Less __ College __ Graduate School

Address: _____ City _____ State _____ ZIP _____ County _____

Telephone: (home) (_____) _____-_____ (work) (_____) _____-_____

Do you have a primary healthcare provider? . . . . ____ Yes ____ No

Have you seen a healthcare provider in the past year? . . . . ____ Yes ____ No

Do you have any type of medical insurance? . . . . ____ Yes ____ No

PART II. HISTORY OF KNOWN AND ESTABLISHED RISK FACTORS FOR STROKE

1. Have you ever been told that you have high blood pressure? . . . . ____ Yes ____ No

2. Do you take medication for high blood pressure? . . . . ____ Yes ____ No

3. Do you have a history of abnormal heart rate or rhythm called atrial fibrillation? . . . . . . ____ Yes ____ No

4. Have you ever been checked for, or been told that you have,
   narrowing of the arteries to the brain? . . . . ____ Yes ____ No

5. Have you had a heart attack, heart bypass surgery, angioplasty,
   or another disease of the heart? . . . . ____ Yes ____ No

6. Have you had a previous stroke, mini-stroke, or TIA? . . . . ____ Yes ____ No

7. Do you have diabetes mellitus (DM) or are you on insulin or medication
   for high blood sugar? . . . . ____ Yes ____ No

8. Have you ever smoked cigarettes? . . . . ____ Yes ____ No

9. Do you currently smoke cigarettes? . . . . ____ Yes ____ No

PART III. HISTORY OF SIGNIFICANT BUT SLIGHTLY LOWER RISK FACTORS FOR STROKE

10. Has a family member had a stroke or heart attack when he or his was
    less than 45 years of age? . . . . ____ Yes ____ No
11. Do you consume more than two ounces of alcohol per day on a daily basis? . . . . ____ Yes ____ No
12. Do you have a cholesterol level greater than 200? . . . . ____ Yes ____ No

PART IV. HISTORY OF UNCOMMON BUT IMPORTANT RISK FACTORS FOR STROKE

13. Do you smoke cigarettes and take birth control pills? . . . . ____ Yes ____ No
14. Do you have sickle cell anemia? . . . . ____ Yes ____ No
15. Do you use one or more of the following drugs: cocaine, crack, heroin, amphetamines? . . . . . . ____ Yes ____ No

PART V. ASSESSMENT

Blood pressure (BP) recorded sitting: _____ (systolic)/ _____ (diastolic) _____ Right arm or _____ Left arm

Radial pulse rate for 60 seconds ___ (beats/minute)   Irregular pulse rate? . . . . ____ Yes ____ No

PART VI. AGE AND ETHNICITY

Date of Birth (DOB): _____/_____/_____   Age in years: _____

Ethnicity/Race:____ African American ____ Caucasian ____ Hispanic White ____ Hispanic Non-White
_____ Asian/Pacific Islander ____ American Indian or Alaskan Native ____ Other and Unknown

PART VII. IDENTIFICATION OF RISK FOR STROKE AND RECOMMENDATION

1. ____ *Low Risk for Stroke:*
   Under the age of 55, responded "NO" to questions 1–15 (self-reported risk factors), and was not identified as having an irregular pulse or a systolic BP ≥140 or a diastolic BP ≥90 on assessment
   Recommendation: Take this completed assessment to your healthcare provider at your next appointment.

2. ____ *Moderate Risk for Stroke:*
   Age ≥55 with no self-reported risk factors and no risk factors identified on assessment
   OR
   Up to age 64 with: one self-reported risk factor, or an irregular pulse, or a systolic BP ≥140 or a diastolic BP ≥90
   Recommendation: Notify your healthcare provider within a week with the results of your screening and request an appointment for evaluation and care to prevent a stroke.

3. ____ *High Risk for Stroke:*
   Age ≥65 with: one self-reported risk factor, or an irregular pulse, or a systolic BP ≥140 or a diastolic BP ≥90
   OR
   Any age with two or more risk factors (includes self-reported risk factors and those identified on assessment)
   Recommendation: Notify your healthcare provider *today* with the results of your screening and request an appointment for evaluation and care to prevent a stroke.

4. ____ *Presents with warning signs of stroke, or TIA (mini-stroke)*
   Recommendation: Call "911" immediately!
   Individual signs here that he/she received this recommendation.
   (Signature) _____

PART VIII. THE WARNING SIGNS OF STROKE

▶ WEAKNESS, NUMBNESS, OR PARALYSIS OF THE ARMS OR LEGS

▶ SUDDEN BLURRED VISION OR BLINDNESS IN ONE EYE

▶ DIFFICULTY SPEAKING OR SLURRING OF SPEECH

▶ SEVERE HEADACHE WITH SUDDEN ONSET THAT OCCURS WITHOUT APPARENT REASON

▶ LOSS OF BALANCE OR FALLING WITHOUT ANY APPARENT REASON

Individual was taught the warning signs of stroke, how to access emergency care by calling "911" for transportation to a hospital for emergent care for stroke, and the need to seek treatment *immediately:* __ Yes

Signature of healthcare provider completing assessment: _____ Title _____

The Stroke Risk Screening was developed by the Division on Research of the Delaware Nurses Association and Ellen Barker, RN, MSN, CNRN, Neuroscience Nursing Consultants, Wilmington, Delaware. Marian P. LaMonte, MD, MSN, Assistant Professor of Neurology and Director of the Maryland Brain Attack Center, University of Maryland Medical Center, Baltimore, Maryland served as Nurse/Neurologist advisor. There is no copyright. This screening tool may be photocopied and distributed without the permission of the authors or publisher.

BRADEN SCALE
FOR PREDICTING PRESSURE SORE RISK

Patient's Name _____   Evaluator's Name _____   Date of Assessment

SENSORY PERCEPTION ability to respond meaningfully to pressure-related discomfort	**1. Completely limited:** Unresponsive (does not moan, flinch, or gasp) to painful stimuli, due to diminished level of consciousness or sedation OR limited ability to feel pain over most of body surface.	**2. Very Limited:** Responds only to painful stimuli. Cannot communicate discomfort except by moaning or restlessness OR has a sensory impairment which limits the ability to feel pain or discomfort over 1/2 of body.	**3. Slightly Limited:** Responds to verbal commands, but cannot always communicate discomfort or need to be turned OR has some sensory impairment which limits ability to feel pain or discomfort in 1 or 2 extremities.	**4. No Impairment:** Responds to verbal commands. Has no sensory deficit which would limit ability to feel or voice pain or discomfort.
MOISTURE degree to which skin is exposed to moisture	**1. Constantly Moist:** Skin in kept moist almost constantly by perspiration, urine, etc. Dampness is detected every time patient is moved or turned.	**2. Very Moist:** Skin is often, but not always moist. Linen must be changed at least once a shift.	**3. Occasionally Moist:** Skin is occasionally moist, requiring an extra linen change approximately once a day.	**4. Rarely Moist:** Skin is usually dry, linen only requires changing at routine intervals.
ACTIVITY degree of physical activity	**1. Bedfast:** Confined to bed	**2. Chairfast:** Ability to walk severely limited or non-existent. Cannot bear own weight and/or must be assisted into chair or wheelchair.	**3. Walks Occasionally:** Walks occasionally during day, but for very short distances, with or without assistance. Spends majority of each shift in bed or chair.	**4. Walks Frequently:** Walks outside the room at least twice a day and inside room at least once every 2 hours during waking hours.
MOBILITY ability to change and control body position	**1. Completely Immobile:** Does not make even slight changes in body or extremity position without assistance.	**2. Very Limited:** Makes occasional slight changes in body or extremity position but unable to make frequent or significant changes independently.	**3. Slightly Limited:** Makes frequent though slight changes in body or extremity position independently.	**4. No Limitations:** Makes major and frequent changes in position without assistance.
NUTRITION *usual* food intake pattern	**1. Very Poor:** Never eats a complete meal. Rarely eats more than 1/3 of any food offered. Eats 2 servings or less of protein (meat or dairy products) per day. Takes fluids poorly. Does not take a liquid dietary supplement OR is NPO and/or maintained on clear liquids or IV's for more than 5 days.	**2. Probably Inadequate:** Rarely eats a complete meal and generally eats only about 1/2 of any food offered. Protein intake includes only 3 servings of meat or dairy products per day. Occasionally will take a dietary supplement OR receives less than optimum amount of liquid diet or tube feeding.	**3. Adequate:** Eats over half of most meals. Eats a total of 4 servings of protein (meat, dairy products) each day. Occasionally will refuse a meal, but will usually take a supplement if offered OR is on a tube feeding or TPN regimen which probably meets most of nutritional needs.	**4. Excellent:** Eats most of every meal. Never refuses a meal. Usually eats a total of 4 or more servings of meat and dairy products. Occasionally eats between meals. Does not require supplementation.
FRICTION AND SHEAR	**1. Problem:** Requires moderate to maximum assistance in moving. Complete lifting without sliding against sheets is impossible. Frequently slides down in bed or chair, requiring frequent repositioning with maximum assistance. Spasticity, contractures or agitation leads to almost constant friction.	**2. Potential Problem:** Moves feebly or requires minimum assistance. During a move skin probably slides to some extent against sheets, chair, restraints, or other devices. Maintains relatively good position in chair or bed most of the time but occasionally slides down.	**3. No Apparent Problem:** Moves in bed and in chair independently and has sufficient muscle strength to lift up completely during move. Maintains good position in bed or chair at all times.	

At risk = 15–18; Moderate risk = 13–14; High risk = 10–12; Severe Risk = 9.   Total Score

NPO = nothing by mouth; IV = intravenously; TPN = total parenteral nutrition.

The warning signs of poor nutritional health are often overlooked. Use this checklist to find out if you or someone you know is at nutritional risk.

DETERMINE YOUR NUTRITIONAL HEALTH

Read the statements below. Circle the number in the yes column for those that apply to you or someone you know. For each yes answer, score the number in the box. Total your nutritional score.

	YES
I have an illness or condition that made me change the kind and/or amount of food I eat.	2
I eat fewer than 2 meals per day.	3
I eat few fruits or vegetables, or milk products.	2
I have 3 or more drinks of beer, liquor or wine almost every day.	2
I have tooth or mouth problems that make it hard for me to eat.	2
I don't always have enough money to buy the food I need.	4
I eat alone most of the time.	1
I take 3 or more different prescribed or over-the-counter drugs a day.	1
Without wanting to, I have lost or gained 10 pounds in the last 6 months.	2
I am not always physically able to shop, cook and/or feed myself.	2
TOTAL	

Total Your Nutritional Score. If it's —

0-2 **Good!** Recheck your nutritional score in 6 months.

3-5 **You are at moderate nutritional risk.** See what can be done to improve your eating habits and lifestyle. Your office on aging, senior nutrition program, senior citizens center or health department can help. Recheck your nutritional score in 3 months.

6 or more **You are at high nutritional risk.** Bring this checklist the next time you see your doctor, dietitian or other qualified health or social service professional. Talk with them about any problems you may have. Ask for help to improve your nutritional health.

These materials developed and distributed by the Nutrition Screening Initiative, a project of:

 AMERICAN ACADEMY OF FAMILY PHYSICIANS

 THE AMERICAN DIETETIC ASSOCIATION

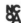 NATIONAL COUNCIL ON THE AGING, INC.

* Remember that warning signs suggest risk, but do not represent diagnosis of any condition.

From Nutrition Screening Initiative: Implementing Nutrition Screening and Intervention Strategies. Washington, DC, Nutrition Screening Initiative, 1993. (Reprinted with permission by the Nutrition Screening Initiative, a project of the American Academy of Family Physicians, the American Dietetic Association and the National Council on Aging, Inc., and funded in part by a grant from Ross Products Divisions, Abbott Laboratories.)

Sample Advance Directives

FLORIDA LIVING WILL

Declaration made this _____ day of _____, _____,
                          (day)   *(month)*   *(year)*

I, _____, willfully and voluntarily make known
my desire that my dying not be artificially prolonged under the circumstances set
forth below, and I do hereby declare that:

If at any time I am incapacitated and
  __ I have a terminal condition, or
  __ I have an end-stage condition, or
  __ I am in a persistent vegetative state

and if my attending or treating physician and another consulting physician have
determined that there is no reasonable medical probability of my recovery from
such condition, I direct that life-prolonging procedures be withheld or withdrawn
when the application of such procedures would serve only to prolong artificially
the process of dying, and that I be permitted to die naturally with only the administration of medication or the performance of any medical procedure deemed necessary to provide me with comfort care or to alleviate pain.

It is my intention that this declaration be honored by my family and physician as
the final expression of my legal right to refuse medical or surgical treatment and to
accept the consequences for such refusal.

In the event that I have been determined to be unable to provide express and
informed consent regarding the withholding, withdrawal, or continuation of life-
prolonging procedures, I wish to designate, as my surrogate to carry out the provisions of this declaration:

Name: _____
Address: _____
_____ Zip Code: _____
Phone: _____

I wish to designate the following person as my alternate surrogate, to carry out the provisions of this declaration should my surrogate be unwilling or unable to act on my behalf:

Name: _____

Address: _____

_____ Zip Code: _____

Phone: _____

Additional instructions (optional):

I understand the full import of this declaration, and I am emotionally and mentally competent to make this declaration.

Signed: _____

Witness 1:
  Signed: _____
  Address: _____

Witness 2:
  Signed: _____
  Address: _____

_____

Courtesy of *Partnership for Caring, Inc.*, 1035 30th Street, NW Washington, DC 20007 800-989-9455 10/99

FLORIDA DESIGNATION OF HEALTH CARE SURROGATE

Name: _____

              (Last)   *(First)*   *(Middle Initial)*

In the event that I have been determined to be incapacitated to provide informed consent for medical treatment and surgical and diagnostic procedures, I wish to designate as my surrogate for health care decisions:

Name: _____
Address: _____
_____ Zip Code: _____
Phone: _____

If my surrogate is unwilling or unable to perform his or her duties, I wish to designate as my alternate surrogate:

Name: _____
Address: _____
_____ Zip Code: _____
Phone: _____

I fully understand that this designation will permit my designee to make health care decisions and to provide, withhold, or withdraw consent on my behalf; to apply for public benefits to defray the cost of health care; and to authorize my admission to or transfer from a health care facility.

Additional instructions (optional):

I further affirm that this designation is not being made as a condition of treatment or admission to a health care facility. I will notify and send a copy of this document to the following persons other than my surrogate, so they may know who my surrogate is:

Name: _____
Address: _____
Name: _____
Address: _____

Signed: _____
Date: _____

Witness 1:
  Signed: _____
  Address: _____

Witness 2:
  Signed: _____
  Address: _____

Courtesy of *Partnership for Caring, Inc.*, 1035 30th Street, NW Washington, DC 20007 800-989-9455 10/99

Laboratory Value Alterations with Aging

Test	Unchanged/Same as Younger Reference	Decrease With Older Subjects	Increase With Older Subjects
CBC			
RBC	Unchanged	or Slight decrease	
Hgb	Unchanged	or Slight decrease	
Hct	Unchanged	or Slight decrease	
RBC indices	Unchanged		
WBC count	Unchanged		
Differential			
Basophils	Unchanged		
Eosinophils	Unchanged		
Myelocytes	Unchanged		
Bands	Unchanged		
Monocytes	Unchanged		
Lymphocytes	Unchanged	or Slight decrease	
Platelets	Unchanged		
ESR			Slight increase
B_{12}		Decrease	
Folate/folic acid		Decrease	
TIBC/transferrin	Unchanged		
Serum Fe	Unchanged		
Blood chemistry			
Electrolytes			
Na	Unchanged	or Slight decrease	
K	Unchanged		or Slight increase
Cl	Unchanged		
Ca	Unchanged	or Slight decrease	
P	Unchanged		
Mg		Decrease	
Glucose			
FBS	Unchanged	or Slight increase	
PPBS			Increase
OGTT			Increase
HgA_{1c}			Increase
End products of metabolism			
BUN	Unchanged		or Slight increase
Creatinine	Unchanged		or Slight increase
Creatinine clearance		Decrease	
Bilirubin	Unchanged		
Uric acid			Slight increase
Liver function tests			
ALAT (SGPT)	Unchanged		
AST (SGOT)	Unchanged		
LDH	Unchanged		or Slight increase
Alkaline phosphatase			Gradual increase

Test	Unchanged/Same as Younger Reference	Decrease With Older Subjects	Increase With Older Subjects
Total protein	Unchanged	or Slight decrease	
Albumin		Decrease	
Globulin	Unchanged		
Lipoproteins			
Total cholesterol			Gradual increase
LDL			Increase
HDL	Unchanged	or Slight decrease in women	or Slight increase in men
Triglycerides			Increase
Thyroid function tests			
T_4	Unchanged	or Slight decrease	
T_3		Decrease	
TSH			Slight increase

Reproduced with permission from the article "Interpretation of Laboratory Values in Older Adults" by K.D. Mellillo, from the July, 1993 issue of *The Nurse Practitioner,* © Springhouse Corporation.

CBC = complete blood count; RBC = red blood cell; WBC = white blood cell; Hgb = hemoglobin; Hct = hematocrit; ESR = erythrocyte sedimentation rate; TIBC = total iron-binding capacity; FBS = fasting blood sugar; PPBS = postprandial blood sugar; OGTT = oral glucose tolerance test; HgA_{1c} = hemoglobin A_{1c}; BUN = blood urea nitrogen; ALAT (SGPT) = alanine aminotransferase (serum glutamic-pyruvic transaminase); AST (SGOT) = aspartate aminotransferase (serum glutamic-oxaloacetic transaminase); LDH = lactate dehydrogenase; LDL = low-density lipoprotein; HDL = high-density lipoprotein; T_4 = thyroxine; T_3 = tri-iodothyronine; TSH = thyroid-stimulating hormone.

Glossary

Abduction: Movement of a limb away from the body.

Absorption: Passage of substances across and into tissues (e.g., digested food molecules into intestinal cells or liquids into kidneys).

Abuse: To physically or verbally attack or injure.

Accessory muscles: Additional or reinforcing muscles, such as muscles of the neck, back, and abdomen, that may play a more prominent role in respiration during a breathing disorder or during exercise.

Activity theory: Theory that supports the continuation of activities and hobbies, as well as substitution when necessary, in order to sustain interest in, and quality of, life.

Activities of daily living (ADLs): Activities usually performed in the course of a normal day in a person's life, such as eating, toileting, dressing, bathing, and brushing the teeth.

Acute care: A pattern of health care in which a patient is treated for a brief but severe episode of illness, following an accident or other trauma, or during recovery from surgery.

Acute pain: Short severe course of pain, as may follow surgery or trauma or may accompany myocardial infarction or other conditions and diseases.

Adduction: Movement of a limb toward the center of the body.

Advance directive: A written declaration made in advance by a person regarding treatment preferences if he or she should become unable to communicate his or her wishes. Examples are *durable power of attorney for health care* and a *living will.*

Adverse drug reaction: A harmful, unintended reaction to a drug administered at a normal dosage.

Afferent arteriole: Central artery, such as the renal artery.

Age-associated memory impairment: Changes in short-term memory that occur with age.

Ageism: An attitude that discriminates, separates, stigmatizes, or otherwise places older adults at a disadvantage on the basis of chronological age.

Aggressive communication: Communication that is characterized by forceful behavior, action, or attitude that is expressed physically, verbally, or symbolically; it is manifested by either constructive or destructive acts directed toward oneself or against others.

Alcohol-dependent: Having a psychological reliance (dependency) on alcohol.

Alcoholic: A person who has developed a dependency on alcohol through abuse of the substance.

Alveoli: Small outpouchings of walls of alveolar space through which gas exchange between alveolar air and pulmonary capillary blood takes place.

Angina: Descriptive feature of various diseases characterized by a feeling of choking, suffocation, or crushing pressure and pain.

Anterior-posterior diameter: Distance from the front toward the back, as in the anterior-posterior diameter of the thoracic cavity.

Anxiety: Nursing diagnosis defined as a vague, uneasy feeling, the source of which is often nonspecific or unknown to the individual.

Aphakia: Condition in which part or all of the crystalline lens of the eye is absent, usually because it has been surgically removed, as in the treatment of cataracts.

Aphasia: Abnormal neurologic condition in which language function is defective or absent because of injury to certain areas of the cerebral cortex.

Arcus senilis: An opaque ring, gray or white in color, that surrounds the periphery of the cornea, caused by deposits of fat granules in the cornea with hyaline degeneration and occurring primarily in older adults.

Aspiration: Inspiration of foreign material into the airway.

Assertive communication: Communication that is characterized by behavior directed toward claiming one's rights without denying those of others.

Assigning: Distributing work during a particular nursing shift.

Assisted living: Facility that provides the older adult who is relatively independent with supervision, help, and some health care services provided in a homelike environment.

Atelectasis: Abnormal condition characterized by collapse of the alveoli in the lungs, thus preventing respiratory exchange of gas. Symptoms include diminished breath sounds, fever, and increased discomfort with breathing.

Atherosclerosis: Common arterial disorder characterized by yellow plaques of cholesterol, lipids (fats), and cellular debris in the inner layers of the walls of arteries.

Atrophy: Wasting or decrease in size of a part of the body, such as a limb, because of disease or other influences.

Atypical presentation: Irregular signs and symptoms of a disorder, or lack of the usual signs and symptoms (e.g., myocardial infarction without chest pain).

Autocratic: Referring to a style of communication or leadership by which one person rules with unlimited authority.

Autonomic nervous system: Part of the nervous system that regulates involuntary function, including activity of the heart muscle, smooth muscles, and glands.

Autonomy: Self-determination that is free from both controlling influences of others and personal limitations.

Belief: State of mind in which trust or confidence is placed in a particular person or thing.

Beneficence: Ethical principle of doing good.

Benign senile tremor: Fine, quick movements, especially of the hands, along with rhythmic head nodding and increased trembling during purposeful movement, occurring in older adults.

Bladder training: System of therapy for incontinence in which the person, while maintaining a normal intake of fluid, practices withholding urine for intervals that begin at 1 hour and increase over a period of 10 days. The person also learns to recognize and react to the urge to urinate.

Body mass index: Formula for determining obesity, calculated by dividing a person's weight in kilograms by the square of the person's height in meters.

Busyness: Keeping stressful feelings and thoughts temporarily in check by staying busy, a commonly used defense mechanism.

Capillary refill time: Time it takes blood to return to a portion of the capillary system after being interrupted briefly. When cardiac output is reduced, capillary refill is slow.

Cardiac output: Volume of blood expelled by the ventricles of the heart; it is equal to the amount of blood ejected at each beat (the stroke output) multiplied by the heart rate per minute (number of beats in the period of time used in the computation).

Centenarian: Person who is 100 years of age or older.

Central vision: Vision that results from images falling on the macula of the retina.

Cerumen: Yellowish or brownish waxy secretion produced by the apocrine sweat glands in the external ear canal; also called earwax.

Chemical restraint: Psychotropic medications given to subdue agitated or confused clients.

Cholinesterase inhibitors: Classifications of drugs that slow the breakdown of acetylcholine at the synapse, thus improving the transmission of nerve impulses.

Chronic illness: Any disorder that persists over a long period and affects physical, emotional, intellectual, social, or spiritual functioning.

Chronic pain: Pain that continues or recurs over a prolonged period and is caused by various diseases or abnormal conditions, such as rheumatoid arthritis.

Cilia: Hairlike processes that extend from a cell surface.

Circulation: Movement of a substance through a circular course so that it returns to its starting point, such as the circulation of blood through the circuitous network of arteries and veins.

Clinical pathway: Description of interventions likely to result in favorable outcomes for a particular diagnosis that uses prospectively defined resources to minimize cost. Also called *critical pathway*.

Cochlea: A cone-shaped, bony structure of the inner ear, perforated by numerous openings for passage of the cochlear part of the vestibulocochlear nerve.

Collaborate: Work jointly with others or together; work cooperatively.

Compromise: To come to agreement by mutual concession; a settlement reached in a particular manner.

Conductive hearing loss: A form of hearing loss in which sound is inadequately conducted through the external or middle ear to the inner ear. Sensitivity of sound is diminished, but clarity is not changed as long as the sound is loud enough.

Confidentiality: Nondisclosure of certain information except to another authorized person.

Confusion: Mental state characterized by disorientation regarding time, place, person, or situation, causing bewilderment, lack of orderly thought, and inability to choose or act decisively and perform activities of daily living.

Continuing stressor: Anything that causes wear and tear on the body's physical or mental resources on an ongoing basis.

Continuity theory: The concept that an individual's personality does not change as the person ages, with the result that his or her behavior becomes more predictable.

Contractility: A property of muscle tissue, particularly cardiac muscle, that allows it to contract.

Cortical bone: The compact bone in the bone shaft that surrounds the marrow cavity.

Creatinine clearance: A diagnostic test for kidney function that measures the rate at which creatinine is cleared from the blood by the kidney.

Crepitation: A dry, crackling sound or sensation, such as that produced by the grating of the ends of a fractured bone.

Cultural diversity: Mixture of people from different cultures, races, religions, and backgrounds.

Culturally sensitive care: Concept recognizing that every culture has developed a unique way of understanding health and responding to illness. Stresses that the dominant culture's ways are not the "right" ways, and advocates increased appreciation, awareness, and inclusion of different perspectives in the care of clients.

Culture: The shared values, beliefs, and practices of a particular group of people, which are transmitted from one generation to the next and are identified as patterns that guide the thinking and action of the group members.

Cyanosis: Bluish discoloration of the skin and mucous membranes caused by an excess of deoxygenated hemoglobin in the blood.

Débridement: Removal of dirt, foreign objects, damaged tissue, and cellular debris from a wound or a burn to prevent infection and to promote healing.

Delegating: Transferring responsibility or authority to someone.

Delirium: Acute mental disorder characterized by confusion, disorientation, restlessness, incoherence, fear, anxiety, excitement, and often hallucinations, usually of visual origin.

Democratic: Socially equal; available to all.

Denial: An unconscious defense mechanism in which emotional conflict and anxiety are avoided by refusal to acknowledge those thoughts, feelings, desires, impulses, or facts that are consciously intolerable.

Diagnosis-related group: A group of clients classified for the purpose of measuring a medical facility's delivery of care in order to determine appropriate Medicare payments, usually for inpatient care.

Diplopia: Double vision caused by defective function of the extraocular muscles or a disorder of the nerves in the muscles.

Disengagement theory: Psychosocial concept that normally aging individuals and society mutually withdraw from normal interaction. It assumes that older adults are a homogenous group whose members prefer the company of others of their own age.

Disorientation: A state of mental confusion characterized by inadequate or incorrect perceptions of place, time, or identity.

Dispense: To prepare and issue drugs or drug mixtures from a pharmaceutical outlet or department.

Displacement: An unconscious defense mechanism for avoiding emotional conflict and anxiety by transferring emotions, ideas, or wishes from one object to a substitute that is less anxiety-producing.

Distribution: The location of medication in various organs and tissues after administration.

Diuresis: Increased formation and secretion of urine, occurring in conditions such as diabetes mellitus and acute renal failure.

Do not resuscitate: Orders written by a physician when the client has indicated a desire to be allowed to die if breathing ceases or the heart stops.

Dorsiflexion: Backward flexion or bending, as of the hand or foot.

Drug toxicity: The degree to which a drug is poisonous.

Durable power of attorney: A document that designates an agent or proxy to make personal decisions if the person is no longer able to make them.

Duty: A moral or legal obligation.

Dysarthria: Difficult, poorly articulated speech, resulting from interference in control over the muscles of speech, usually caused by damage to a central or peripheral motor nerve.

Dyspnea: A stressful sensation of uncomfortable breathing that may be caused by certain heart or lung conditions, strenuous exercise, or anxiety.

Dyssomnia: Category of sleep disorders consisting of disturbances in the quality, amount, or timing of sleep.

Dysthymic disorder: A disorder of mood in which the essential feature is a chronic disturbance of mood of at least 2 years' duration. Involves either depressed mood or loss of interest or pleasure in all or almost all usual activities or pastimes, but is not sufficiently severe to be classified as a major depressive episode.

Dysuria: Painful urination.

Eastern medicine: Traditional Chinese medicine, used to prevent and treat illness.

Ecchymosis: Bluish discoloration of an area of skin or mucous membrane caused by the passage of blood into the subcutaneous tissues as a result of trauma to the underlying blood vessels.

Edentulous: Toothless.

Embolism: An abnormal circulatory condition in which a foreign body, such as air or fat, travels through the bloodstream and becomes lodged in a blood vessel.

Emotional: Characterized by an intense mental state accompanied by physiologic changes; having strong feelings.

Enteral nutrition: Nutrients provided through the gastrointestinal tract when the client cannot ingest, chew, or swallow food but can digest and absorb nutrients; also known as tube feeding.

Erythema: Redness or inflammation of the skin or mucous membranes.

Ethical dilemma: Problem or conflict that results when people hold different values, such as regarding provision of life support.

Ethnic group: A population of individuals organized on the basis of an assumed common cultural origin.

Ethnicity: Ethnic quality or affiliation.

Exacerbation: An increase in the seriousness of a disease or disorder as marked by greater intensity in the signs or symptoms of the client being treated.

Expanded role of the LPN/LVN: Changing duties and responsibilities of the LPN/LVN. In extended care, for example, the charge nurse may supervise, direct, and guide the care given by nursing assistants on assigned units and wings.

Exploiting age or illness: Gaining advantage, attention, or favor based on age or illness.

Excretion: The process of eliminating, shedding, or getting rid of a drug from the body, usually through the kidneys.

Extrapulmonary: Outside of the lungs.

Extravasation: Passage or escape into the tissues, usually of blood, serum, or lymph.

Failure to thrive: Severe malnutrition.

Fidelity: The ethical principle of being loyal.

Flexion: Movement by certain joints that decreases the angle between two adjoining bones (e.g., bending the elbow).

Food Guide Pyramid: A guide developed by the U.S. Department of Agriculture showing the six food groups necessary for good nutrition and the recommended daily intake of each group.

Forced expiratory volume (FEV): The volume of air that can be forcibly expelled during a fixed period following full inspiration.

Formal authority: Power assigned to another in accordance with accepted rules and regulations.

Functional assessment: Health history that includes observation of the older adult's ability to perform activities of daily living and instrumental activities of daily living; this assessment is used to help the health care professional determine which activities the older adult is capable of performing and which should be done with assistance.

Gangrene: Necrosis or death of tissue, usually as the result of loss of blood supply (ischemia) or bacterial invasion and subsequent putrefaction.

Gerontological nursing: Nursing care of older adults.

Gerotranscendence: A psychosocial theory of aging in which life crisis speeds up, or accelerates, the process of personality development in a positive, constructive way.

Glomerular filtration rate: Kidney function test in which results can be determined from the amount of ultrafiltrate formed by plasma flowing through the glomeruli of the kidney.

Habit training: Scheduled voiding by the client, along with voiding between scheduled times if the desire to void occurs.

Half-life: A measure of drug metabolism, defined as the time it takes for the body to inactivate half of the medication.

Halitosis: Offensive breath resulting from poor oral hygiene, dental or oral infection, ingestion of certain foods, or some systemic diseases.

Health promotion: Activities that develop an individual's resources to maintain and enhance well-being and protect against illness.

Hemiarthroplasty: Surgical procedure done to repair an injured or diseased hip joint; hip replacement surgery.

Herbal therapy: Alternative or complementary medicine that uses herbs to treat diseases or disorders.

Home care: Health service provided in the client's home, either by a member of the client's family or by a home health nurse.

Homeostasis: Tendency of biological systems to maintain stability in the internal environment while continually adjusting to changes necessary for survival.

Homocysteine: Amino acid, high levels of which are associated with an increased risk of collagen cardiovascular disorders, particularly thromboembolic stroke.

Hospice: Program that provides a continuum of home and client care for the terminally ill and their families.

Hyperglycemia: Excess glucose (sugar) in the blood.

Hyperkalemia: Excess potassium in the blood.

Hypernatremia: Excess sodium (salt) in the blood, or a loss of body water.

Hyperopia: Farsightedness, or the inability of the eye to focus on near objects.

Hypertension: Blood pressure elevated above the normal range.

Hyperthermia: Higher than normal body temperature.

Hypertrophy: Increase in the size of an organ caused by an increase in the size of the cells, rather than the number of cells. The heart and kidney are particularly prone to hypertrophy.

Hypochlorhydria: Deficiency of hydrochloric acid in the stomach.

Hypodermoclysis: Injection of an isotonic or hypotonic solution into subcutaneous tissue to supply a continuous and large amount of fluid, electrolytes, and nutrients when a client is unable to take fluids intravenously, orally, or rectally.

Hypokalemia: Abnormally low level of potassium in the blood.

Hyponatremia: Abnormally low level of sodium in the blood.

Hypothermia: Subnormal body temperature.

Hypoxemia: Deficiency of oxygen in the blood.

Hypoxia: Inadequate oxygen at the cellular level.

Idealization: Making something or someone perfect in one's eyes.

Illness-wellness continuum: A simple linear model in which illness and wellness are at opposite ends.

Illusion: A false interpretation of an external sensory stimulus, usually through sight or hearing.

Infarction: A localized area of necrosis in a tissue, vessel, organ, or part resulting from tissue oxygen deprivation.

Informal authority: Power conferred on a leader by others.

Inhalation: Breathing in or drawing in of breath.

Integrity vs. despair: Stage or task of the older adult, according to Erikson.

Intellectually: Through the power and ability of the mind to know and understand, as contrasted with feeling.

Interdisciplinary team: Health care professionals, such as those in medicine, nursing, and physical therapy, working together as a team to meet the needs of the client.

Intermittent claudication: Cramplike pains in the calves caused by poor circulation of the blood to the leg muscles, manifested only at certain times, usually after an extended period of walking, and relieved by rest.

Interstitial: Pertaining to the space between cells, as interstitial fluid. Also called *intercellular.*

Intima: The innermost layer of a structure, such as the lining membrane of an artery or vein.

Intrapulmonary: Pertaining to the interior of the lungs.

Ischemia: Deficiency of blood in a body part, usually due to functional constriction or actual obstruction of a blood vessel.

Justice: The ethical principle of fairness.

Kyphosis: Excessive curve in the thoracic spine.

Laissez-faire: Opposite extreme of the autocratic style of leadership, this type of leadership avoids conflict and favors peace at any price.

Leadership: The capacity to lead; guidance, direction.

Leadership style: The manner in which a leader creates an environment that encourages people working under the leader to be productive and to work toward achieving common goals.

Level of consciousness: Degree of cognitive function involving arousal mechanisms in the brain.

Living will: An advance directive by a terminally ill client, which specifies that the person does not want to be connected to life support equipment.

Long-term care: Provision of medical, social, and personal care services on a continuing basis to clients with chronic physical or mental disorders.

Long-term memory: Ability to recall sensations, events, ideas, and other information for long periods without apparent effort.

Lose-win: A passive strategy for managing conflict in which one places priority on accommodating those involved in the conflict, but at one's own expense.

Loyalty: Within the ethical principle of fidelity, the keeping of promises.

Macular: Related to a gray scar on the cornea of the eye that is visible without magnification.

Management: In the case of the LPN/LVN charge nurse, directing the nursing assistants under the manager's supervision to achieve specific client outcomes by providing safe, timely, and cost-effective nursing care.

Maximum heart rate: The upper limit, in beats per minute, that the heart is able to pump.

Medical directives: A general term for documents that provide direction on the type of care a client desires (advance directives).

Medicare: Federally funded U.S. national health insurance program for people age 65 and older.

Metabolism: Cellular chemical reactions in the body.

Multitasking: Performing multiple tasks simultaneously.

Muscle wasting: Decrease in muscle mass that occurs as a result of a decreased number of muscle fibers and general atrophy of organs and tissues due to the aging process.

Myocardium: Contractile heart muscle.

Myopia: Nearsightedness, or the inability to see objects far away.

Necrosis: Local death of tissue from disease or injury.

Negative pressure: Pressure less than the atmosphere, such as within the lungs, which keeps them inflated.

Neglect: As pertains to care of the older adult, a lack of the services necessary to maintain the physical and mental health of older adults who live alone or who are unable to provide self-care.

Neovascularization: New blood vessel formation.

Nephrotoxic: Toxic or destructive to a kidney.

Neurofibrillary tangles: Intracellular clumps of neurofibrils made of insoluble protein that develop in the brain of a person with Alzheimer's disease.

Noncompliance: An informed decision on the part of the client not to adhere to a therapeutic suggestion.

Nonmaleficence: Ethical principle to do no harm.

Nonpharmacologic pain treatment: Measures other than medication for reducing pain, such as heat/warmth, cold, distraction, relaxation techniques, massage, imagery, acupuncture, and hypnosis.

Nonproductive cough: Sudden, noisy cough that may be caused by irritation or inflammation and does not remove sputum from the respiratory tract.

Nosocomial infection: An infection originating in the hospital; hospital acquired.

Objective entry: In charting and documenting client care, the use of objective data, that is, information obtained by observation of the client during assessment, not subjective data provided by the client himself or herself.

Obstructive lung disease: Also called COPD (chronic obstructive pulmonary disease). A progressive and irreversible condition characterized by limited breathing capacity of the lungs.

Oldest old: Adults aged 85 and above.

Orientation: Awareness of one's physical environment with regard to time, place, and the identity of other people.

Orthostatic hypotension: Abnormally low blood pressure that occurs when a person stands up; also called postural hypotension.

Otosclerosis: Hereditary condition of unknown cause in which irregular ossification (bone creation) occurs in the ossicles of the middle ear, causing hearing loss.

PaCO$_2$: Abbreviation for partial pressure of carbon dioxide in arterial blood.

Palliative care: Therapy designed to relieve or reduce the intensity of uncomfortable symptoms but not to produce a cure, for example, the use of narcotics to relieve pain in people with cancer.

Pallidotomy: Surgical production of lesions on the globus pallidus (a part of the brain) for the treatment of extrapyramidal disorders (neurologic disorders that cause involuntary movement, changes in muscle tone, and abnormal posture).

Pallor: Paleness of the skin.

PaO$_2$: Abbreviation for partial pressure of alveolar oxygen (oxygen through the lungs).

Parenteral nutrition: Administration of nutrients (usually saline solution with glucose, amino acids, electrolytes, vitamins, and medications) by a route other than the alimentary canal, such as subcutaneously, intravenously, intramuscularly, or intradermally.

Paresis: Motor weakness or partial paralysis.

Passive communication: Communication style whereby conflict is avoided at all costs.

Patient-controlled analgesia: Analgesia doses controlled by the client.

Pelvic exercises: Kegel exercises; isometric exercises in which a person performs a series of voluntary contractions of the muscles of her pelvic floor to improve retention of urine.

Pelvic floor electrical stimulation: Treatment for urinary incontinence whereby mild electrical pulses stimulate muscle contractions.

Pharmacodynamics: The study of a drug's effect on cellular physiology and biochemistry, as well as its mechanism of action.

Pharmacokinetics: The study of how drugs enter the body, are metabolized, reach their site of action, and are excreted.

Pharmacologic pain treatment: Narcotic and nonnarcotic medications for reducing or eliminating pain.

Physical restraint: Device, such as a vest or waist, wrist, or ankle tie, used to restrict movement.

Plantar flexion: Reflex bending of the toes and foot.

Plaque: Microscopic mass seen in small amounts in the brains of normal elderly people, and in larger amounts in those with Alzheimer's disease.

Polydipsia: Excessive thirst.

Polyphagia: Excessive, uncontrolled eating.

Polypharmacy: Use of a number of different drugs by a client who may have one or several health problems.

Polysomnography: Polygraphic recording during sleep of multiple physiologic changes to assess possible biological causes of sleep disorders.

Polyuria: The excretion of an abnormally large quantity of urine.

Presbycusis: Inability to hear high-pitched sounds or spoken words; occurs in old age.

Presbyopia: Age-related decreased ability to focus on near objects.

Preventive health care: A pattern of nursing and medical care that focuses on disease prevention and health maintenance, including early diagnosis of disease, identification of risk factors for disease, and client education.

Primary prevention: Early health promotion efforts designed to foster well-being, such as promoting effective family communication.

Prodromal: Early symptoms or beginning stage, as of an illness.

Productive cough: Sudden noisy cough that effectively removes sputum or mucus from the respiratory tract and helps clear the airways, permitting oxygen to reach the lungs.

Projection: The unconscious attributing of one's own wishes, emotional feelings, or motivation to another person.

Prospective payment: A system of reimbursement whereby payment is made based on client diagnosis.

Protein binding: The affinity of a drug to bind with protein in the bloodstream.

Pulse oximetry: A noninvasive, safe method of assessing oxygenation by passing a beam of light through tissue, then having the amount of light absorbed by oxygen-saturated hemoglobin measured through a sensor attached to the fingertip, toe, or ear lobe.

Quality of life: A measure of the optimum energy or force that gives a person the power to cope successfully with the challenges encountered in the real world.

Recommended Dietary Allowances: Recommended amounts of various nutrients for diet planning.

Regression: A retreat or backward movement in conditions, signs, or symptoms; a return to an earlier, more primitive form of behavior.

Rehabilitative techniques: Techniques employed in attempting to restore a person's ability to live and work as normally as possible following a disabling injury or illness.

Religion: System of faith or belief in a higher power.

Restrictive lung disease: Respiratory disorder characterized by restricted expansion of the lungs or chest wall, resulting in diminished lung volumes and capacities.

Role reversal: Switching roles with another person (e.g., grown children caring for aged parent).

Rubor: Redness, especially with inflammation.

Safety habits: Habits designed to prevent accidental injury.

Sarcopenia: Loss of skeletal muscle that occurs with aging.

Secondary prevention: Efforts directed toward early detection and treatment of a disorder, before adverse effects have been felt.

Selective memory: Recalling only positive or negative aspects of a situation.

Selective sensory intake: Responding only to what you can deal with.

Sensorineural hearing loss: Form of hearing loss in which sound is conducted normally through the external and middle ear, but a defect in the inner ear or auditory nerve results in hearing loss.

Sepsis: Severe, overwhelming infection.

Septicemia: Systemic infection in which the pathogens (e.g., bacteria) are present in the bloodstream, having spread from an infection in any part of the body.

Shearing forces: Forces or pressure exerted against the surface or layers of the skin as tissues slide in opposite but parallel planes, causing pressure ulcers.

Short-term memory: Memory of recent events, generally the first to be affected in Alzheimer's disease.

Sinoatrial (SA) node: A small area of conducting tissue that starts the heartbeat. Located in the upper wall of the right atrium.

Situational leadership: A style of leadership that encourages the leader to be aware of the situation, to be flexible, and to alter his or her leadership style to meet the demands of the circumstances.

Skilled nursing facility: An institution that meets the criteria for accreditation established by the sections of the Social Security Act that determine the basis for Medicaid and Medicare reimbursement for skilled nursing care, including rehabilitation and various medical and nursing procedures.

Sleep log: A journal that is kept to document quality, quantity, and other aspects of sleep.

Socially: Pertaining to one's behavior in society or in groups.

Somatization: Process by which a mental event is expressed in a body disorder or physical symptom, such as a peptic ulcer.

Spiritually: Pertaining to one's spiritual beliefs.

Stroke volume: Amount of blood ejected by the ventricle during contraction of the heart.

Subacute care: Level of health care between acute (hospital-based) and chronic (long-term settings); also, treatment of a disease that is of moderate severity or duration.

Subintentional suicide: Long-standing self-destructive behavior.

Superior vena cava: The large vein that carries unoxygenated blood from the head, shoulders, and upper extremities to the right atrium.

Tachycardia: Heart rate greater than 100 beats per minute.

Tachypnea: Increased or rapid breathing.

Thalamotomy: Surgical production of lesions within the nuclei of the thalamus, generally performed to treat disease of the basal ganglia.

Thready: As in thready pulse, a pulse that is weak, somewhat difficult to palpate, and often fairly rapid, in which the artery does not feel full and the rate may be difficult to assess.

Thrombolytic agents: Drugs that dissolve blood clots (thrombi).

Thrombosis: Formation of a blood clot (thrombus).

Tinnitus: Noise in the ears, such as ringing, buzzing, or roaring.

Total hip arthroplasty: Surgical procedure to correct a hip joint damaged by degenerative disease, often arthritis; total hip replacement.

Trabecular bone: The spongy, honey-combed inner part of a bone.

Traditional healers: In some cultures, medicine men or women who practice traditional spiritual-based treatments for illness.

Transcultural nursing: Nursing care that recognizes cultural diversity and is sensitive to the needs of the client and family.

Transurethral resection of the prostate: Surgical procedure through the urethra, in this case a prostatectomy.

Tryptophan: Amino acid essential for nitrogen balance in adults and found in dietary protein, such as green, leafy vegetables, grains, and seeds.

24-Hour recall method: Method of nutritional assessment whereby an individual traces back 24 hours and documents all nutrients consumed during that period.

Typical presentation: The usual signs and symptoms of a disorder, such as burning on urination with a urinary tract infection.

Urgency: A feeling of the need to void urine immediately.

Urinary incontinence: Involuntary passing of urine, with failure of voluntary control over the bladder and uretheral sphincters.

Urinary retention: State in which an individual experiences incomplete emptying of the bladder.

Urinary tract infection: An infection in the urinary tract.

Values: Morals; strong beliefs.

Veracity: Truthfulness.

Well-being: Achievement of a good and satisfactory existence as defined by the individual.

Wellness: A dynamic state of health in which an individual progresses toward a higher level of functioning, achieving an optimum balance between internal and external environments.

Western medicine: System of medical care practiced primarily in Europe and the United States and having its foundation in the scientific, biomedical model of disease.

White noise: A sound in which the intensity is the same at all frequencies within a designated band; background noise.

Win-lose: Aggressive conflict management strategy in which one's ideas and opinions are forced on another.

Win-win: Assertive conflict management strategy that takes into consideration the conflict itself, the result of the intervention, and the relationships of those involved in the conflict.

Xerosis: Condition in which the skin lacks moisture, characterized by a pattern of fine lines, scaling, and itching; dry skin.

Xerostomia: Dryness of the mouth caused by lack of normal salivary secretion.

Young old: Older adults up to and including age 75 years.

Zoonotic: Describing a disease that is transmissible from animals to humans under natural conditions.

Index

Note: Page numbers followed by the letter f refer to figures; those followed by the letter b refer to boxed material, and those followed by t to tables.

A

Abdomen, assessment of, 71
Abduction pillow, 81
Absorption, of medications, 36–37
Abuse, 253
  alcohol. *See* Alcohol abuse.
  assessment of, 255
  intervention in cases of, 255–256
  neglect as, 254–255
  prevention of, 256, 257t
  reporting, legal requirement for, 255
  signs and symptoms of, 256t
  types of, 253–254
Activities of daily living (ADL), 31
  assistance with, resources for, 56b
  in functional assessment, 43, 56–57
  instrumental, 43
  motivations for performing, 57
Activity
  assessment of, 76–77, 77t
  promoting, 68–83
Activity theory, 224
Acute care, 4, 30–32
ADL. *See* Activities of daily living (ADL).
Advance directives, 262–263
  sample of, 302–305
Adverse drug reactions, 38, 39. *See also* Medication(s); Medication safety tip(s).
  resulting from polypharmacy, 38
  risk factors for, 39b
Afferent arteriole, 111
African Americans, health and aging views of, 19
Age-associated memory impairment (AAMI), 62
Ageism, 8
Age-related changes
  cultural views of health and, 17–18
    African American, 19
    American Indian, 18–19

Age-related changes *(Continued)*
    Asian American, 20–21
    European American, 21–22
    Hispanic American, 19–20
    Jewish American, 22
  in brain and nervous system, 198–200
  in cardiovascular system, 137
  in endocrine system, 111–113, 114t
  in gastrointestinal tract, 90–92, 92t
  in genitourinary tract, 111–113, 112b
  in laboratory test values, 306–307
  in learning, 199b
  in musculoskeletal system, 68–69
  in reproductive system, 111–113, 112b
  in respiratory system, 158–160, 159t
  in sensory organs, 181–183
  in skin, 69
  in sleep cycle, 69–70, 71f
  misconceptions about, 8–10
  psychosocial, 222–223
  theories of, 10–11
Aggressive communication style, 278
Aging. *See* Age-related changes.
Aging population
  caring for, 8
  demographics of, 8, 9f, 9t
  misconceptions about, 8–10
Alcohol abuse, 229–230
  categories of, 230–231
  physical disorders associated with, 231–232
  psychosocial disorders associated with, 231–232
  reasons for, 230–231
  signs and symptoms of, 230
  susceptibility to, 231
Alzheimer's disease, 208–210
  brain anomalies in, 209
  causes of, 208–209
  communicating with clients with, 212b
  sample outcomes for, 212t

Alzheimer's disease *(Continued)*
  signs and symptoms of, 209
  stages of, 209t
  treatment of, 209–210, 210t
American Indians, health and aging views of, 18–19
American Nurses Association (ANA), 6
Analgesia, patient-controlled, 81
Angina, 140
  toleration of, 147
Anxiety, 227–228
Aphasia, in stroke, 204t
Arcus senilis, 183
Arms, assessment of, 71–72
Arteriole, afferent, 111
Asian Americans, health and aging views of, 20–21
Assertive communication style, 278
Assessment, of older adult
  cardiovascular system in, 137–139
  diagnosis after, 76–77
  endocrine system in, 113–114
  functional, 43
  gastrointestinal tract in, 92
  genitourinary tract in, 113–114
  hydration status in, 92–93
  intervention implementation after, 78–85. *See also* Interventions, implementing.
  musculoskeletal system in, 70–72
  nervous system in, 200–202
  nutritional status in, 93–95
  physical examination in, 42–43
  plan of care collaboration in, 77–78
  presentation of illness in, 43–44
  reproductive system in, 113–114
  respiratory system in, 160–162
  section vs. resident protocol in, 296
  sensory and perceptual function in, 183–184
  sleep in, 72–73
  tools for, 286–299
  vital sign ranges in, 42t